# THE MANY FACES OF SHAME

*Edited by*

Donald L. Nathanson, M.D.

THE GUILFORD PRESS
*New York* *London*

*Dedicated to*

*my wife*
*Rosalind Helene Nathanson*

*and my daughter*
*Julie Ann Nathanson*



Printed in the United States of America

*Last digit is print number* 9 8 7 6 5 4 3

Library of Congress Cataloging-in-Publication Data

The Many faces of shame.

Partially based on a symposium held in Los Angeles, 1984 for the 137th Annual Meeting of the American Psychiatric Association.
Includes bibliographies and index.
1. Shame—Congresses. 2. Psychology, Pathological—Congresses. I. Nathanson, Donald L. II. American Psychiatric Association. Meeting (137th : 1984 : Los Angeles, Calif.) [DNLM: 1. Guilt. 2. Psychoanalytic Theory. BF 575.S45 M295]
RC455.4.S53M36 1987 616.85′2 86–31937
ISBN 0–89862–705–2

# Contributors

Joseph H. Berke, MD. Director, Arbours Association, London, England.

Warren Kinston, MD. Institute of Organisation and Social Studies, Brunel University, Uxbridge, Middlesex, England.

Melvin R. Lansky, MD. Adjunct Professor of Psychiatry, UCLA Medical School; Staff Psychiatrist and Chief, Family Treatment Program, Brentwood V.A. Medical Center; Faculty, Los Angeles Psychoanalytic Institute, Los Angeles, California.

Helen Block Lewis, PhD. Late Professor Emerita (Adjunct) of Psychology, Yale University; Former Editor, Psychoanalytic Psychology.

Andrew P. Morrison, MD. Assistant Clinical Professor of Psychiatry, Harvard Medical School, Massachusetts Mental Health Center.

Donald L. Nathanson, MD. Senior Attending Psychiatrist, The Institute of Pennsylvania Hospital. Clinical Associate Professor, Mental Health Sciences, Hahnemann University, Philadelphia, Pennsylvania.

Carl D. Schneider, PhD. Senior Pastoral Psychotherapist and Director, Divorce Mediation Service, Pastoral Psychotherapy Institute, Parkside Human Services Corporation, a member of the Lutheran General Health Care System, Park Ridge, Illinois.

Robert J. Stoller, MD. Professor of Psychiatry, UCLA School of Medicine, Los Angeles, California.

Silvan S. Tomkins, PhD. Department of Social Systems Sciences, University of Pennsylvania, Philadelphia, Pennsylvania.

Otto Allen Will, Jr., MD. Private Practice, Richmond, California.

Emmett Wilson, Jr., MD, PhD. Private Practice, Princeton, New Jersey.

Léon Wurmser, MD. Clinical Professor of Psychiatry, University of West Virginia; Lecturer on Psychiatry, Harvard Medical School.

# Preface

> There is a Zen teaching story about a man whose farm was on the cliff overlooking a seacoast town. From his fields he saw, in the distance, the unmistakable specter of a tsunami, a tidal wave. Realizing the village would be engulfed before he could run to warn anyone, the farmer set fire to his home. All who ran to help him were saved.

For some years I have taken the study of emotion, of affect psychology, as my prime interest. The pleasant sense of security offered by years of immersion in such work was shattered when I realized that I did not know anything about the affect *shame*. Elsewhere in this book I have described some of the details of that awakening, and of its effect on me. Suddenly I became aware that this ignorance had caused me to misunderstand a great many of my patients, whose conflicts had remained obscure, and who had profited little from my work as their therapist.

Recognition of, and acceptance of my ignorance was followed by intense study, which created as many problems as it solved. Each of the articles and books I read contributed something, each required that I change some aspect of my therapeutic technique, each forced me to think about previously unexplored realms of my own psyche. Shame seems to be an emotion little discussed in our clinical work: In the 20 years I have stayed awake at case conferences, attended lectures, professional meetings, and symposia, I have never heard a single case in which embarassment, ridicule, humiliation, mortification, or any other of the shame family of emotions was discussed. The curiosity that impelled my original search turned into a passion as I began to comprehend that the ubiquity of shame-laden situations was matched by what appeared to be a culture-wide avoidance of pertinent discussion. During the past decade or so, many articles and books about shame have appeared in the literature of Western culture. The nearly simultaneous appearance of these writings and the astonishing regularity with which they have been ignored signified to me the sort of ferment (attended by cultural denial) that usually precedes a major shift in cultural understanding.

Every therapist is used to this experience of ignorance and inadequacy. The doing of psychotherapy is intrinsically humbling, for no one can know enough to understand everybody. Most people outside this branch of the helping professions are unaware of the amount of time spent by psychotherapists in the pursuit of answers to such puzzles presented by those who come to us for help. It began to dawn on me that my own ignorance was only a symptom of a larger ignorance, that my profession was largely blind to shame, despite the many competent studies available. A new dimension of the problem appeared, for if therapists are themselves treated and trained by therapists who fail to understand the importance of shame, then the cultural tendency to overlook shame is compounded or amplified by a system of therapy that itself ignores shame. The problem was far larger than that of my own momentary feeling of inadequacy and the embarrassment consequent to it.

The study of shame draws one into other areas. Surely equal in significance to the general ignorance about shame is the understanding that shame does not fit well into any of the existing popular theories of psychological functioning. One might even say that shame represents a hole in contemporary theory. But how important is theory to the therapist? The answer to that question is more difficult than one might guess, for theory only becomes important when therapy does not work. I was fascinated to observe that most of those who have made major contributions to our understanding of shame had been drawn to it by the sober analysis of therapeutic failure. The new theories about shame illuminate all of psychological and psychoanalytic theory.

Try as I might, I was unable to understand shame from the excellent writings already available. So many authors described shame from such highly individual points of view that sometimes it seemed as if they were describing different emotions. I made the assumption that my own confusion might be a logical response to a deeper level of confusion in our field, and began to correspond with all of those whom I could identify as working in areas directly or peripherally related to my growing interest in the nature of shame. Each came to my assistance with alacrity. As in the Zen epigram quoted above, I used my own ignorance to call attention to a situation which I felt dangerous to us all. As word of this project spread, others, previously unknown to me, asked if they might participate.

To each author I posed a series of questions in an attempt to develop two themes. My first goal was to produce a fair and complete summary of all the theories about shame, major and minor, currently under discussion in the literature. Beneath this surface request lay my hope that by assembling this new work, by laying it out in some new pattern, a new understanding might emerge. Each chapter is the result of a lengthy dialogue between editor and author, and is testimony to the willingness of many busy professionals to write, not as dictated by their inner voices, but in response to my requests for increasing amounts of information and clarification. Rather than write a lengthy introduction to the entire volume I have elected to insert a brief commentary before each author's text, hoping thereby to draw into a cohesive whole this rather broad-based group of contributions.

As editor, studying each chapter in its many versions, trying to find a way to link these disparate views of shame into a coherent whole, I began to see the chapters in a visual metaphor. Initially appearing as a group of separate islands, in some cases completely cut off from each other by waters too wide to bridge, they began to group in my mind as an archipelago, a series of geographical formations connected beneath the surface. All that remained was to drop below the surface of the water and establish a new topography. The opening chapter represents this attempt to go below the surface of shame as we know it in the many adult presentations so well described in the remainder of the book, and to build a new developmental theory. That this theory requires us to go well beyond the traditional boundaries set by drive theory (and the rigid limitations of libido theory in particular) will come as no surprise to those who have been reading the work of contemporary thinkers in psychoanalysis, psychiatry, and psychology. While drive theory is not "dead," it is being slowly eroded by this increasing attention to the affects. As many of the authors represented herein state with special emphasis, shame does not fit into conventional psychoanalytic theory. Since we can't make shame disappear, we simply have to make new theories. My own synthesis of the extensive work done by many researchers in related fields may serve as a guide to others who will later refine it into a more sure and certain scheme. Here it is offered as one possible explanation, one map of the seabed which may underlie the archipelago.

One might expect that so richly varied a group of authors might fail to achieve concord on more than one issue. Each of us is aware that the English language treats the masculine gender as representative of all humanity, and the feminine gender as "special," for we have no gender-neutral pronoun which describes the human. As editor I must take responsibility for the inclusion of the neologism "s/he" or such phrases as "himself or herself" wherever possible, in my attempt to replace the masculine tone of psychoanalytic writing with something closer to our experience as people. Some authors have objected that this stylistic preference makes for an awkward prose, and have asked for relief from such a rule. I suspect that the change to gender neutrality will come slowly, but will achieve more validity if evolutionary rather than revolutionary. It is my hope that the reader will feel I have struck a fair balance between the old way and the new.

Many friends and colleagues surrounded and supported me during this venture. Drs. Vernon C. Kelly, Neal Satten, and Eric Stake joined with me in a study group that concentrated initially on the specific affect *shame*, but now has expanded in focus to include the entire field of affect psychology. Dr. Léon Wurmser was kind enough to help me organize a symposium ("Shame: New Clinical and Theoretical Aspects") for a national meeting of the American Psychiatric Association, and has continued to help me in every conceivable way. I cannot adequately express my gratitude to him for this valuable support. In addition to the suggestions offered by the many colleagues who responded to early versions of my opening chapter, I was grateful for the opportunity to present this work at an intense and thought-provoking meeting of the American Psychoanalytic Association. The questions raised there allowed the chapter to assume its final form. New friends appeared in the context of my growing interest in psychoanalytic theory and the special branch called *affect theory*. These included Drs. Michael Franz Basch, Francis J. Broucek, E. Virginia Demos, and especially Silvan Tomkins, who made available unending amounts of time both at his home and by telephone to help me over the rough spots of theory.

With great good humor, Helen Block Lewis referred to all of us who study shame as "shameniks." She earned the right to coin maternal sobriquets by writing the landmark 1971 volume *Shame and Guilt in Neurosis*, which many credit as the start of our current reexamination of the superego, and by her stewardship of a legion of scholars. Despite the pressure of the enormous number of responsibilities assumed during her version of "retirement," she agreed to contribute a chapter to this book, but on condition that I write a chapter for her next book as a fair trade. Uncharacteristically fatigued after giving a speech last November, Helen sought medical attention only to find out some weeks later that she harbored an otherwise asymptomatic disseminated terminal malignancy. Quietly she went about the final arrangements for her last book and for her journal, passing into death on 18 January 1987. Her respect for the new approach which permeates *The Many Faces of Shame* was of great importance to me; my respect for Helen and my gratitude to her shows throughout this book, and in my contribution to her last book, *The Role of Shame in Symptom Formation*.

The decision to mount a major symposium, and to assemble a book, all of which sound like quite simple tasks for the ordinary academician, were formidable indeed for a full-time clinician with no secretarial support. None of this would have been possible save for the enlightened assistance of Alan Ellenbogen, president of Word Systems, Incorporated (WSI), our region's preeminent purveyor of word-processing equipment, who took a personal interest in my project. At a time when few of my colleagues had even heard of word processing, he outfitted me with a state-of-the-art NBI office system at his cost, and provided 2 years of maintenance. Such a relationship between the business and scholarly communities is rare indeed, and most welcome. Similarly, the Ciba-Geigy Corporation, through the kind intervention of my long-time friend Dr. George Ehrlich, and Dr. Mark Roffman, contributed funds to cover certain secretarial and communications expenses incurred in the production of the symposium. I am very appreciative of this assistance.

Not enough is said in writing about the importance of great clinicians who do not write. For many years, I had the opportunity to work in analysis, later in therapy and supervision with Dr. Reuben Robert Pottash. His kindness and understanding were matched by a powerful intellect that cut across boundaries to allow the synthesis of previously disparate fields of knowledge. For nearly a generation his rumbling voice was the dominant force shaping the lives and training of psychiatrists and psychologists in the Philadelphia area. Books and articles by those who worked with him are now beginning to emerge; none of them really related to his life work, yet all made possible by his remarkable skill. Kohut said that mother provides the first opportunity for empathic mirroring; when she fails we can be saved by an empathic father. To the extent that both are imperfect, we rely on our therapists to help us rebuild and reconstitute a self. Bob Pottash was that and more for many of us, and we are all the better for his work.

Whenever I felt lost in the world of publishing companies I was assisted by the remarkably capable literary agent John Ware, who established my connection with Guilford and handled all negotiations. My editor, Sharon Panulla, took on this project with such grace and enthusiasm that in her company I finally came to believe that the book would actually get to press. That a sheaf of manuscripts might turn into a coherent and elegant book was the work of Rennie Childress; his skill as production editor shows throughout.

Most of all I have been sustained by my wife Rosalind and my daughter Julie. Julie, who was 9 when I started to study shame, became a real expert on the theory of embarrassment, and reported regularly on her observations at school. I suspect that her cronies have had the benefit of a most unusual education. Roz fed the study group when it arrived hungry, supported all of us at the symposium in Los Angeles, welcomed all the scholars who visited us from other parts of the country, and most of all helped me carve out the space within which I could write; this, while running her own business and handling a myriad of volunteer activities for my hospital. These many months of writing intruded greatly into our shared space, and she sacrificed much to allow the accomplishment of what she knew was so important to me.

It is my belief that we are witnessing the beginnings of the "affect era" in the helping professions. This book may be viewed as a series of conversations between the editor and 11 experts on the affect shame. If the material is found trivial, the editor will be happy to assume the blame, for, like the Japanese farmer, he has set fire to his reputation. It is our hope that the reader may find herein much to add to a therapeutic armamentarium. Finally, it is the hope of the editor that the study of shame may draw to the attention of the reader this new wave of interest in the nature of affect.

# Contents

# 1

# A Timetable for Shame*

DONALD L. NATHANSON

*This contribution represents an attempt to develop a new understanding of shame that reconciles the data from neurophysiology, psychopharmacology, and infant observation with classical psychoanalytic thinking. In an era when all emotion could be explained on the basis of the hydraulics and mechanics of drive theory, it was acceptable to ignore the importance of shame, or to demean it as little worthy of investigation. The contributions which comprise the present volume, which describe* The Many Faces of Shame, *demonstrate the centrality of shame as a primary source of human discomfort and make it and the related emotions all but impossible to overlook. Just as our methods of therapy must be changed significantly by this new attention to such matters as shyness, modesty, embarrassment, ridicule, and humiliation, so must our theoretical structures be altered to accommodate data from laboratories undreamed of in the early days of psychoanalytic theory.*

*Freud used hypnosis, later the techniques of psychoanalytic investigation, to minimize the reticence which prevented the adult from disclosure, discussion, or even awareness of certain noxious memories and the emotions associated with them. Although this initiated the modern*

*Portions of this chapter were presented at the American Psychoanalytic Association meeting of 20 December 1986.

Donald L. Nathanson. Senior Attending Psychiatrist, The Institute of Pennsylvania Hospital. Clinical Associate Professor, Mental Health Sciences, Hahnemann University.

*scientific study of the inner life of man, one unfortunate byproduct of such investigation was a tendency to understand the normal infant and child in terms of the disturbed adult. The normal infant, and the normal relationship between infant and care-giver, were either ignored or viewed in the language of psychopathology. The major early psychoanalytic investigators of childhood (A. Freud, 1966; Spitz, 1965) studied children in drastically altered conditions of nurturance, like hospitals and foundling homes. Thus, much that we take for granted in our understanding of normal development derives from the study of the abnormal. The modern investigator of neonatal and child development studies happy, healthy children as they interact with normal parents, both in their natural home, and in laboratories designed to make the participants feel at home.*

*There is a sizable body of information about early life, and about the emotions, that rarely enters into psychoanalytic theory. This statement takes on particular importance when one begins to study shame. The classical developmental construct, based on the idea that an invisible force called libido leaks from oral and anal portals until organized into its proper sexual channels during the oedipal phase, encourages attention to anxiety and guilt. The actual presence of shame much earlier in development than can be explained on the basis of libido theory (as will be demonstrated in this chapter) forces our attention to other theoretical systems.*

*Where once Landauer (1938) could state with authority that the emotions were inherited hysterical attacks, that "an affective attack is a storm of instinct in which every zone pursues the aim determined for it by its structure" (p. 408) and that "affects represent reactions to stimuli from the external world" (p. 388), we have begun to recognize that the affects comprise a biological system quite separate from the drives, one which may be the major motivational force in human development. Much of this new attitude derives from the work of Tomkins (1962, 1963), and it is Tomkins's understanding that is central to my own.*

*In this chapter, Tomkins's concept of the affect* interest *is introduced and linked to attachment theory and affective communication; his theoretical position regarding the innate affect shame as a mechanism for the reduction of the affects interest, excitement, and enjoyment is discussed. Using this concept as a base, I suggest that one can explain the enormous variation in the adult manifestations of shame by likening the mature emotion shame to a molecule, constructed over time, made of specific component atoms which achieve different significance for each person. Components such as innate affects, affect modulators, drives, cognitions, and personal experience as held in memory are co-assembled to produce each major attribute of the mature emotion, including the phenomena of hiding and blushing, the relationship of shame to the self, the tendency of shame to cause a sense of isolation, as well as its relationship to excretory function, gender identity, the genital organs, and the significance attached to genital prowess. A construct for the development of the mature emotion* guilt *from an incomplete form of the shame "molecule" is suggested. Finally, the phenomenology of manic–depressive illness is re-evaluated in terms of the affect interest and this new approach to shame. Where speculation is unaccompanied by objective data, suggestions for future research are offered. The psychological portion of this research must be based on the direct observation of developing children rather than on the inherently distorted anecdotal reports elicited from adult patients; opportunities for neurophysiological investigation are also presented.*

*It is not my intent to declare this timetable as an immutable schedule "defining" shame for every individual in every situation. Rather, I present it as an introduction to this current volume, a new way of understanding the remarkable number of approaches and attitudes which allow shame to take on so many faces for so many observers. It will be successful in direct proportion to the number of questions it raises, and to the amount of new thinking so encouraged.*

That shame is a universal experience is both a boon and a hindrance to our understanding of it. While it is true that each of us "knows" what it feels like to be embarrassed or to be humiliated, we do not know with any certainty what another person means to express when using these words. To our list of words implying the acute lowering of self esteem, we may add shyness, bashfulness, and modesty, as well as the experiences of being put down, slighted, and thought of as contemptible. Disgrace, dishonor, degradation, and debasement involve closely related states. Wurmser (1981) approaches this problem in a direct and clear manner, suggesting that we consider as cognates the many words by which the shame experience is described. Thus, we speak of the "shame family of emotions," rather than any specific member.

Certainly most people would understand that mortification implies being mortally shamed, and see humiliation as the result of an aggressive shaming attack. Nevertheless, our work as therapists suggests that a situation, or an experience, which one person might describe as mildly embarrassing is treated as abject shame by another. Even the observing clinician is first and foremost an individual with a personal lexicon of emotions. So variably are shame words used by the population at large, so different is the perception of these emotion states that it is not possible to use these names with any confidence that another person knows precisely what we mean when we talk about shame. Such a belief infuses this chapter, in which I shall attempt to demonstrate some reasons for the inherent variability of the shame experience.

There is greater concord about other aspects of shame. Most writers (Lynd, 1958; Wurmser, 1981) agree that shame follows a moment of *exposure*, and that this uncovering reveals aspects of the self of a peculiarly sensitive, intimate, and vulnerable nature. Wurmser (1981) summarizes the *content* of this complex emotion: "What one is ashamed for or about clusters around several issues: (1) I am weak, I am failing in competition; (2) I am dirty, messy, the content of my self is looked at with disdain and disgust; (3) I am defective, I have shortcomings in physical and mental makeup; (4) I have lost control over my body functions and my feelings; (5) I am sexually excited about suffering, degradation, and distress; (6) watching and self-exposing are dangerous activities and may be punished" (pp. 27–28). Kaufman (1985) points out that the interpersonal trigger to shame is a sundering of the "interpersonal bridge," alluding to that quality of the shame experience in which we feel shorn from our fellow humans; moments in which we wish a hole would open up and swallow us. Betrayal, treachery, and abandonment can activate shame.

Shame, like guilt, is an unpleasant emotion experienced as if it were directed by one agency of the self against another. Whereas guilt refers to punishment for wrongdoing, for violation of some sort of rule or internal law, shame is about some quality of the self. Guilt implies action, while shame implies that some quality of the self has been brought into question (Alexander, 1938; Lewis, 1971; Wurmser, 1981). Experience teaches us that wrongdoing may be punished by guilt; while unwarranted opinions about the self, when exposed, will be punished by shame. With experience comes the ability to predict the effects of our actions—therefore guilt limits action, while shame limits narcissism. It is not possible to discuss narcissism without a full understanding of shame, for no quality of the self can be perceived as narcissistic unless called to attention by shame, and "pathological narcissism" must imply disavowal or denial of shame.

Shame is a vital aspect of the psychopathology of our times, of what has been called an "age of narcissism." Whereas, in Freud's late Victorian era, anxiety was declared the proper focus of attention for the symptom neurosis, shame now seems central to the characterologic illnesses which are more commonly seen as we approach the end of the twentieth century. Shame is a response to exposure—by forcing attention to the self it protects us from narcissism, as when we are made to accept that the viewing other does not share our opinion of ourselves. One may wonder about the fairly recent swing from privacy and modesty toward public nakedness and display; away from the seclusion of curtained windows toward glass walls that reveal interior rooms; from social acceptance of the privacy of personal grief and pain to the canonization of the intruding investigative reporter. Perhaps it is the devaluation of the affect shame that has allowed our culture to slip into its current "narcissistic" preoccupation with exposure. Shame is the matrix within which narcissism is embedded.

There is so much talk of narcissism today. Wurmser (1981) calls it a "rubber concept" (p. 48), a word that has been stretched to include so many meanings that it has, for many of us, lost validity. The young boy Narcissus, hardly noticing that he was the object of amorous pursuit by the nymph Echo, was arrested by the beauty of his own reflection in the pool of water toward which he had bent to drink. Spellbound by the image of the handsome stranger in the water he remained there forgetting to eat or drink, and wasted to death. In that same spot, there sprang up the narcissus flower; Echo stood by this symbol of her departed love until nothing of her remained save her voice "which to this day can be heard senselessly repeating the words of others" (I. D'Aulaire & E. D'Aulaire, 1962, p. 92). Since Greek mythology leaves no doubt that narcissism implies psychopathology, one must enquire how the concept has acquired other meanings.

In his attempt to derive a developmental psychology from the analysis of adults, Freud (1914) came to the erroneous conclusion that narcissism was not an acquired illness but rather the persistence into adult life of the "normal" self-involvement of the infant. Only upon renouncing the pleasures of this narcissistic phase did the infant begin to accept the existence of others and develop true relatedness. Stern (1985) describes such reasoning as having forced psychoanalysis "to position pathomorphically chosen clinical issues seen in adults in a central developmental role" (p. 20). Still working backward toward infancy from the analysis of the adult, Kohut (1971) described a group of patients who were refractory to the usual methods of treatment. These patients experienced grave difficulty in forming intimate relationships; like infants, they responded to apparently minimal stimuli with unmodulated displays of affect; in addition, their sense of self seemed distorted. Such observations pointed the way to a psychology of the self for which Kohut coined the unfortunate term "narcissistic development"; reading Kohut and his followers one is asked to accept the oxymoron "normal narcissism." We need a language of the self, but one based on the healthy and normal, not the pathologic.

The two major attitudes toward shame (i.e., whether one views the early development of the self from the pathomorphic standpoint of "normal infantile narcissism" or from the cribside position of infant observation) have vast and divergent implications for the timetable of shame. If narcissism is limited by shame, and if infants are "normally" narcissistic, then shame "cannot" appear before there is failure to renounce narcissism. If theory states that the child does not possess a self, does not differentiate a self-concept out of the primordial slush of primary process thinking until s/he has begun the contest of toilet training, then investigators will not see shame before the anal phase. Speculating from the analysis of adults, Piers and Singer (1953) link shame to urination, while Erikson (1950) sees shame as derivative of anal phase struggles involving autonomy and the search for self-control. There may be considerable shame about failure to control bodily functions, but much data exists to demonstrate that this is not the root of shame.

If self is a function of the separation/individuation process, then shame "cannot" appear until the 18-month stage. The earlier in development we push the development of the self, the earlier we are allowed to see shame. And this has great importance for our work as therapists, for it is axiomatic that whatever is earliest must affect us for the greatest period of time, and cast its influence during the most significant formative periods. We might pay more attention to shame if we saw it as operational from infancy.

Neither looking for shame, nor sensitive to its appearance, Spitz (1965) saw the reaction to strangers of the 6- to 8-month-old in terms of Freud; he called it anxiety rather than shame.

> If a stranger approaches him, this will release an unmistakable, characteristic and typical behavior in the child; he shows varying intensities of apprehension or anxiety and rejects the stranger. . . . He may lower his eyes "shyly," he may cover them with his hands, lift his dress to cover the face, throw himself prone on his cot and hide his face in the blankets, he may weep or scream. The common denominator is a refusal of contact, a turning away, with a shading, more or less, of anxiety. . . . I have called this pattern the *eight-month-anxiety* and consider it the earliest manifestation of *anxiety proper*. (p. 150; emphasis in original)

Unless one is burdened by a theory that says shame cannot appear for another year or so, it is difficult to conceptualize shyness, lowered eyes, and the (pathognomic for shame) action of hiding the face as anything but shame. The 8-month-old child may exhibit distress or fear when first placed in contact with a new adult, but only after repeated episodes of the pattern described by Spitz have sensitized the infant to expect a specific type of noxious experience with a stranger. The infant decides to curtail communication because not everybody is mother, the primary mirror and communicant for his or her affective transmission. If we analyze the data without bias, Spitz seems to be describing a primitive form of anticipatory shame, incorrectly labelled "anxiety." Possible reasons for this will be discussed below, but for the moment I wish only to call attention to the presence of observable behaviors suggesting the presence of shame in the 6- to 8-month old.

Broucek (1982) concurs: "So-called 'stranger anxiety' in the first year of life is probably as much shame-shyness as anxiety"

(p. 370), while Anthony (1984a) referred to shame as a "separate developmental track for anxiety." And finally, Lichtenberg (1983) suggests that "the most developmentally normal response to the not-mother person (often no 'stranger') is one of wary exploratory interest" (p. 102).

The very word shame is derived from an Indo-European root (*skam* or *skem*) which means "to hide," and from which also derive our words *skin*, and *hide*, the latter in both of its meanings: the hide which covers us naturally, and that within which we seek cover. We learn to hide first for the sake of shame, and later for protection from physical danger.

Today it appears that we must disregard much or most of Freud's schema of infancy and early childhood development. During the past two decades the intense study of infancy and of the relationship between infant and caregiver has forced us to reexamine much that was once held sacred. Most important of the early attempts to reconsider child development through the actual observation of parents and children was that of Mahler, Pine, & Bergman (1975) who saw the infant oscillating between some form of total self-involvement (a theoretical extension of Freud's idea of early infantile narcissism to its furthest possible limit: "normal" infantile autism) and fusion with the inner state of the mother. Yet even if we accept for the moment that included in development is a phase during which the infant learns slowly how to pull away from this hypothesized state of fusion on the way to a secure identity, this very awareness of the intensity and power of the links between infant and mother makes it difficult to conceptualize as narcissistic an organism so thoroughly involved with its care-giver.

In a recent lecture, James Anthony (1984b) paused as his audience studied a slide of a smiling, enraptured mother—her chin resting on the mattress of her 2-week-old's crib, each utterly engrossed in the other's face—and commented "We now feel that if this situation obtains during the first few weeks of extra-uterine life the child will grow up without serious emotional difficulty." Such an opinion is incompatible with the view that the infant is born into a world of "blooming, buzzing confusion" (James, 1890) with an undifferentiated mind capable only of narcissistic activity and protected from external impression by an inherent barrier to stimuli.

Stern (1977, 1985) argues that the infant is interactive from birth. During the 3- to 5-month period, for example, the infant can be observed to take control of the social activities surrounding the initiation and termination of mutual gaze: "When watching the gazing patterns of mother and infant during this life period, one is watching two people with almost equal facility and control over the same social behavior" (1985, p. 21). Robson (1967) suggests that mutual gaze acts as a releaser of attachment. Tomkins (1962) points out that shared interocular contact is the most intimate of human experiences. With such shifts in our understanding of the infant must come alterations in our view of shame. During mutual gaze we feel attached. In the moment of shame, we feel shorn not just from the other but from all possible others.

In the adult, shame certainly has a great deal to do with our links to the object world (Lewis 1971, 1981; Wurmser, 1981), and for this reason some have asked whether its operation as a monitor of interpersonal relatedness might be the inherent function of shame. The considerable early literature on attachment theory (Ainsworth, 1979; Bowlby, 1969; Harlow, Harlow, & Hansen, 1963; Sroufe, 1979) has, according to Lichtenberg (1983), been well substantiated by solid research:

> This theory of how attachment occurs is at considerable variance with the theory that states that, subsequent to biological caretaking, the infant only gradually awakens psychologically to the existence of mother as an oral-need-satisfying "part-object." In the view of contemporary infant research, attachment is a continuous process, from the first few minutes of postnatal experience. It extends throughout life, taking different forms at different times. (p. 158)

Lewis (1981) states directly that the human is social from birth, that both shame and guilt are affects that serve to repair lost affectionate bonds, and that they are *inherently* social affects. Further, she suggests that the blush evolved to inform the viewing other that we wish to be accepted back into human society. This, from one of the most dedicated and productive scholars of shame, is no small alteration of current theory. It bears on a question of central interest to therapist and theologian alike: Is the human born "individual" and trained to be social, or is the human born into a community and inherently social? In the former view narcissism is the foundation from which the infant builds the structure of a personality, and to which the adult returns in times of stress; while in the latter, social behavior is viewed as the foundation of the personality, and narcissism constitutes a defense against failures in the social realm.

In both theoretical systems shame affects the individual with equal power. Where they differ, of course, is in the meaning attributed to shame. In the former view, shame cannot appear until the child has built enough personality structure to have left the narcissistic foundation to which shame forces a return. In the latter view, shame (and guilt) operate from birth to inform the growing organism of its transgressions against the social system, to threaten it with isolation, and to provide, through penance for guilt and self-correction for shame, a system for return from exile. In neither system is shame viewed apart from its relationship to the self as illuminated by interpersonal interaction.

Both systems take for granted that shame and guilt are experienced by the developing child pretty much as we know them to be in the adult, despite our observation that the adult experience of shame is quite variable. Lewis (1981) assumes this equivalence when she postulates the *inherent* function of shame as a modulator of social interaction. Yet there is another way of understanding shame, one which views the adult manifestations of both shame and guilt as the result of the slow, steady accumulation of experience added to an innate physiological mechanism, a mechanism to which the social or interactional is merely an accretion, rather than its essence.

## A DEVELOPMENTAL THEORY FOR SHAME

During the past 25 years psychoanalytic theory has undergone revolutionary change. Just as the youngest science was trying to build for itself a solid base, the foundation for a secure establishment, it was threatened by an avalanche of new data about human cognition and emotion. The success of psychoanalytic therapy had not stopped the neurophysiologist, psychopharmacologist, communication scientist, or psychologist from asking questions or from devising experiments that shed light on the human condition. The resultant data must be integrated into the great body of psychoanalytic thinking, lest the natural gulf between sober thinkers of different backgrounds become the barrier between entrenched, warring camps.

The careful study of any affect can form the basis for such an integration. Using the data available to him in the early part of this century, Freud did this for anxiety. The psychoanalytic detective of today must leave the comfort of the analytic cloister and roam the teeming agora of science. In the pages which follow I will demonstrate a little of what can be done using shame as a focus of attention.

## *AFFECT THEORY AND THE WORK OF TOMKINS*

Anyone who studies the affects must eventually come in contact with the pioneering work of Silvan Tomkins (1962, 1963, 1981) who developed a concept of the affects as comprising a biological system with a clear-cut function entirely apart from that of the drives, and showed their importance as a major motivating force. To Basch (1976, 1983a) must be given the credit for providing the first link between psychoanalysis and Tomkins's affect theory. Today it would be as great an omission for someone to ignore Tomkins when writing seriously about biological or developmental aspects of the emotional life of the human species as to avoid reference to Freud when discussing the unconscious. Tomkins's challenge to conventional suppositions about emotion remains untested. However, until direct neurophysiologic evidence is found to counter his synthesis of the data currently available to us, Tomkins's work remains the most complete system on the affects yet devised.

Rather than attempt a "brief" exploration of Tomkins's affect system, it may be useful merely to introduce his terminology. Simply stated, Tomkins celebrated the birth of his son by taking a few months' vacation to remain at home with his wife and child. Like all of us who have observed a newborn, he was fascinated by the display of "emotion" on the face of his infant son, but noted that what looked like emotion was being displayed on the face of an organism with none of the history, none of the life experience we have always considered necessary for the development of emotion. "Certainly the infant who emits his birth cry upon exit from the birth canal has not 'appraised' the new environment as a vale of tears before he cries" (Tomkins 1982, p. 362). Nonetheless, the crying infant looks quite like a crying adult—this cry of distress must have been *available* to the infant courtesy of some preexistent mechanism triggered by some stimulus acceptable to that mechanism.

Tomkins sees nine of these mechanisms, a group of primarily facial responses that he calls "innate affects," as operating from birth. In general, the innate affects are given a two-word group name that describes both the nature of the affect and the range over which it may be elaborated, with the first word indicating the mildest form of the affect and the second indicating the most extreme.

The first seven of these innate affects share one common characteristic—each is triggered by a specific pattern of neural activity (which will be discussed below) and is elaborated as a specific pattern of facial display. The positive affects are as follows; first, *interest-excitement*, with the eyebrows down and the stare fixed or tracking an object; second, *enjoyment-joy*, the smiling response. *Surprise-startle*, with the eyebrows raised and eyes blinking, functions as a neutral affect that allows the organism to halt its previous activity and pay attention to new data. (Since this new data is capable of activating either further surprise or any other affect, surprise is usually confused with the affect that follows it.) The negative innate affects, also present from birth and visible on the face of the newborn, are: first, *distress-anguish*, the crying response; second, *anger-rage*, with a frown, clenched jaw, and red face; third, *fear-terror*, with the eyes held open or frozen in a fixed stare, or (alternatively) looking to the side, away from the source of this fear; and fourth, *shame-humiliation*, with the eyes and head lowered. These seven affects may be added to any drive to give it intensity or power by what Tomkins calls analogic amplification, but none of them has any intrinsic relationship to any drive.

The two remaining innate affects are drive-related in that they stem from mechanisms that Tomkins calls "drive auxiliaries," mechanisms that interact with, modulate, or control the specific drive *hunger*. The olfactory system provides a group of chemosensory receptors that allow possible foodstuffs to be detected and evaluated at a distance by their emitted odor. When these receptors sense that a distant object is noxious we are protected by a mechanism Tomkins calls *dissmell*, which is elaborated in adult life as an affect and seen in such responses as turning one's nose up at something or calling an offensive person a "stinker." The power of this particular affect can be judged by recollecting the violence with which Southern whites claimed that black people "smelled bad" and by a cursory evaluation of our society's expenditure on commercial products that alter or mask emitted personal odors.

Taste is the final sentinel of the gastrointestinal system: It allows us to spit out something noxious and turn off the hunger drive. When we reject with *disgust* a person or relationship previously found pleasing, a mechanism initially functioning as a drive auxiliary—protecting us from unselective hunger—now functions as an affect and turns off the relationship. Angry rejection of an object for reasons related to dissmell or disgust may describe the complex communication called *contempt*.

Each of these innate affects has its own subcortical "address," or location in the brain, that contains the affect "program." Each is triggered by discrete activators of affect. Tomkins's theory is brain-centered, not mind-centered; thus he postulates that the seven affect pairs named above are triggered by the way information comes in to a central assembly system through neural pathways. Essential to his system is the concept that it is the number and intensity of neural firings per unit time, which he calls the "density" of neural firing, that is responsible for affect activation. For instance, if information enters rapidly, with great intensity, and stops just as rapidly (what is called in mathematics a "square wave") as in the case of our response to a pistol shot, it activates the program for affects in the range of surprise and startle, affects that Tomkins views as clearing and resetting the central assembly system, allowing preparation for assessment of new information unfettered by whatever may have been going on previously.

A less rapid increase in stimulus density activates affects in the range of fear to terror, while a still less rapid increase in stimulus density activates interest or excitement, the response to novelty. Any decrease in stimulus density triggers the affects of enjoyment, as when hunger is reduced by eating, or an offending splinter is removed from a foot; sudden reduction in stimulus density produces laughter. Relatively constant levels of stimuli at a moderately uncomfortable level activate the affect distress, the crying response; while constant stimulation at a still more uncomfortable level activates affects in the range of anger to rage. Thus a group of quantitative messages can be understood as a quality, and by this system the human infant is equipped from birth with mechanisms allowing reaction to the variety of situations produced by any possible combination of stimuli.

Each program can recruit a host of bodily functions, including the circulatory system, voluntary muscles, and the exocrine system, accounting for the variety of odors, postures, and behaviors (including patterns of vocal expression) associated with emotion. Once activated, the subcortical program then begins to produce affect, which itself triggers more affect. It must be understood that the above description applies to what Tomkins calls the *innate* affects, that is, the affects as they appear in the neonate before any modification by learning. Each and every innate affect involves the activity of groups of voluntary muscles *taken over* temporarily by the affect program. The infant learns rapidly to arrange his or her face in the patterns initially formed by the innate affects, thus allowing affect display to be used as voluntary activity in addition to its innate function. Throughout life the human exhibits a complex combination of learned display of affect patterns with true innate affect; it is the rapidity with which the infant assumes control over these muscular activities that Tomkins feels may have led many investigators to ignore the face. Basch (1976) suggests that we use the term "affect" to refer to biological events, *feeling* to indicate awareness of an affect, and *emotion* for the combination of an affect with our associations to previous experiences of that affect. In this sense, affect and emotion are not matters of "brain" and "mind" but rather of biology and biography.

The affects comprise a system of action patterns with which the infant is genetically endowed, mechanisms that are called into play by a discrete group of activators, and that can be coassembled with any other neurophysiologic mechanism. Unless one understands the inherent plasticity of the affect system, the combinatorial variations made possible by the human ability to mix learned and innate affects, and the enormous range of intensity over which each moiety in such a mix may be elaborated, one may be tempted to describe such coassemblies as a "new" form of affect (e.g., Stern's [1985] "vitality affects"). The coassembly of an affect with any drive, with cognition, with memory, with another affect, or with any combination of the above, produces powerful amplification of the preexisting function. In other words, affect is the amplifier that brings motivation to drive, to memory, or to any human activity. Wherever there is urgency it has been achieved through such amplification. The affects can be intensely rewarding, as in the case of the positive affects, or intensely punishing, "but the biological effect of this amplification through affect is to make the organism care about quite different kinds of events in different ways" (Demos, in press, p. 8). As Tomkins says: "Affect either makes good things better or bad things worse" (1980, p. 148).

Tomkins states that the face is the *primary* site of action of the affect system. Demos (in press) summarizes this position as follows:

> Because the facial muscles in humans are more finely articulated and can change more rapidly than the correlated autonomic responses (three tenths of a second vs. one to two seconds), Tomkins argued that the face is the primary site of affect, and takes the lead in establishing and creating an awareness of an affective state, with the other correlated responses coming into play later.

It seems unlikely that the James–Lange (James, 1980) theory of emotion (postulating a sequence of events beginning with a global visceral response which is followed by an act of cognitive labeling, which in turn evokes an experienced affect) can be substantiated in view of much current research.

Most theories are based neither on new data nor on a radical reorganization of existing data, but rather on a selective inattention to what the creator of the theory considers extraneous. Such is the relationship of drive-based theories about emotion to this understanding that emotion shows on the face well before it can be expected to appear in consciousness. Tomkins was not the first to recognize the relationship between affect and the face, for Darwin (1872/1979) devoted much of his attention to the importance of the face as a display board. Where they differ, and the reason Tomkins can by no means be dismissed as "Darwinian" (Stern, 1985, p. 57) is that Darwin (as is implicit in the title of his book *The Expression of Emotions in Man and Animals*) saw facial affect display as the external expression of an internal emotional state, while Tomkins demonstrated that the affect system is *primarily* displayed on the face—information is fed inward from the face toward consciousness. Cross-cultural studies by Ekman (1972, 1977) and Izard (1968, 1971) have demonstrated the spontaneous elaboration and recognition of these expressions in a remarkable number of quite different cultures.

Until the development of speech as symbolic communication, facial affect display is the major means of information transfer between infant and caregiver; it remains a significant form of nonverbal communication throughout adult life. Recognizing this, Basch (1983a) pointed out that empathy, the sharing of emotional experience, involves the mirroring of facial affect display followed by inward feeding of that affect message as a feeling, and associations to that feeling, which produce a full-fledged emotion. The subsidiary role of nonfacial expressions of affect has been discussed by Stern (1985) as "cross-modal capacity" (p. 51) and "amodal perception" (p. 49), and constitutes another major moiety of affect as communication.

Broucek (personal communication, August 1985) has offered another possibility for the mechanism of affective resonance: "I don't agree that affect transmission is based on complex processes of inference (but rather) that the brain mechanisms involved in the production of affective expression are closely allied to the mechanisms for the recognition of affective expression. I believe they evolved simultaneously." He cites an ingenious experiment in which crickets were genetically altered to produce a new mating song. "The females of the new species were attracted exclusively to the new mating song without having previously heard any mating song. These experiments revealed that the production and recognition of crickets' mating songs were governed by the same genetic factor." Much work is needed to explicate the nature of human affective resonance.

Buck (1984) suggests that the emotions evolved in three phases. Arising first as subcortical mechanisms concerned with bodily adaptation and the maintenance of homeostasis, they operated out of awareness (Emotion I). In the second phase, the affects became expressed in externally accessible behaviors as spontaneous expressions of internal states, perhaps useful for the coordination of behavior in a species (Emotion II). The final phase of development (Emotion III) involves the direct subjective experience of the state of certain neurochemical systems. In view of the data quoted by Demos (in press) suggesting that the facial musculature can react with greater flexibility and at greater speed than humoral mechanisms, I agree with Tomkins that the inward feeding of facial kinesic information is at least as important, and possibly more likely to be the source of this subjective experience than the neurochemical. Nonetheless, it is this last adaptation that has allowed the linkage of the phylogenetically earlier subcortical affect mechanisms with higher cortical function to form the type of emotion with which we are most familiar in psychoanalytic thinking.

Affect theory is one of the most complex additions to psychoanalytic thinking yet attempted, offering the very links between neurobiology and intrapsychic process for which Freud searched so tenaciously. The reader even fractionally intrigued by my summary of this landmark work will be richly rewarded by study of the first nine chapters of Volume 1 (*The Positive Affects*) of *Affect/Imagery/Consciousness* (Tomkins, 1962).

## *THE AFFECT INTEREST*

In the path toward a new understanding of shame, I should like to focus attention on the specific affect that Tomkins calls *interest*, the infant's reaction to novelty. Tomkins defines individual affects as part of a dipole, with the least intensely experienced form of the affect given first, and the most intense form second. Thus interest is properly part of the *interest-excitement* affect pair. Most likely, the reason previous investigators had not viewed interest as a discrete emotion was just this matter of its graded relationship to excitement; Freud had misunderstood all excitement as derivative of sexual excitement, and nonsexual curiosity as neutralized sexual curiosity. Furthermore, Freud (using the physics of his day as the source of this analogy) attempted to explain such matters as the degree or intensity of interest associated with a person or possession in terms of the psychoeconomics of cathexis, as if there were a finite amount of interest energy to be invested.

The crackle of a leaf on a silent evening can garner our full attention; excitement at the sound of a waterfall in the distance mounts with increasing intensity as the falls are approached; investigative work that is nearing its conclusion can cause us to search for data at fever pitch; all these are manifestations of interest-excitement. Whole industries depend on novelty as an antidote to boredom, hoping to engage the buyer through this affect system: automobiles, fashion, home decorating, and a myriad of others. Our emotional investment in the changing of the seasons is partly a response to the need for change as a way of maintaining interest; vacation trips provide a change of venue with new challenges, new food, new discomfort, new anything. The anhedonia of depression may be a lesion in the realm of interest.

What links these phenomena is the presence of data entering a central assembly at a steadily increasing rate, activating an affect program that, in turn, makes the organism interested in these data, allowing it to focus with greater intensity, and rewarding this focus with excitement.

> One's sexual drive and one's hunger drive can be no stronger than one's excitement about sexuality or about eating. Anything which impairs such excitement strikes also at the heart of the drives. If an erection evokes fear or shame, then excitement may be inhibited, and with it the possibility of intercourse. If hunger is experienced with fear or depression, appetite and eating alike lose their urgency and their promise of reward. (Tomkins, 1962, p. 342)

> A domesticated animal such as the cat, once it has thoroughly explored its environment and if restricted to this environment, loses its characteristic curiosity and spends much of its adult life sleeping. *Interest is not only a necessary support of perception but of the state of wakefulness.* (p. 343; my emphasis)

What evidence exists for Tomkins's claim that interest-excitement is innate? Discussing the capacity for inner experience that may exist in early infancy, Sander (1969) and Wolff (1973) have defined *state* as any recognizable recurring organizational coherence that can be perceived in the organism. In a review of this work, Demos (in press) comments that "most attention has been paid to the cyclical states along the sleep-wake continuum, which have been given descriptive labels—regular sleep, irregular sleep, drowsiness, alert inactivity, waking activity, alert activity and crying" (p. 14).

Commenting on later work by Sander, Demos quotes him as saying "The ego begins as a state ego, rather than a body ego," and "the organization of state governs the quality of inner experience" (Sander, 1982, p. 20; 1985, p. 16). By comparing the descriptions of these states, as given by most investigators, to the well-known, carefully mapped standards of facial affect coding established by Ekman and Friesen (1975, 1978) and Izard (1979) on the basis of Tomkins's work, Demos draws compelling parallels. More recently, observing a 2-week-old baby react to sequential experiences with her mother and a stranger, Demos (personal communication, December 1986) noted that the infant began to squirm in distress while in the arms of this new person, finally closing her eyes and shutting out the sight of the stranger. When returned to the arms of her mother, the infant's body calmed considerably as she searched mother's face with lowered eyebrows, then relaxed with the face of enjoyment. One must work hard to resist the notion that the earliest behaviors of the infant are affect behaviors, and that the states of alert inactivity and alert activity are only the affect interest co-assembled with increasingly complex degrees of motor activity.

## *SHAME AFFECT PROPER*

Interest, says Tomkins,

> supports both what is necessary for life and what is possible, by virtue of linkages to sub-systems, which themselves range from concerns with the transport of energy in and out of the body, to concerns about the characteristics of formal systems such as logic and mathematics. The human being cares about many things and he does so because the general affect of interest is structurally linked to a variety of other apparatuses which activate this affect in ways which are appropriate to the specific needs of each sub-system. . . . If

> thinking had to wait on the slow moving and relatively inert and overly urgent demands of the hunger and sex drive, it would never be capable of much development. (1962, p. 345)

Interest is avidity, zest, excitement, curiosity. Essential to life, certainly. But the universal caution "curiosity killed the cat" seems to indicate a general cultural awareness that the affect interest needs a modulator, much as the drive hunger is served by the sentinels of smell and taste.

Using the model of disgust, wherein an organism's food intake is inhibited at a moment when the hunger drive is at its peak (for which reason he classifies disgust as a drive-auxiliary rather than an innate affect), Tomkins argues that shame is an auxiliary to the affects interest-excitement and enjoyment-joy much as disgust is an auxiliary to the drive hunger. In the saying cited above, the threat of death, as a punishment for the cat's uncontrolled interest, is presented as a cognitive modulator by calling on memorialized fear. Certainly there are many ways to inhibit adult interest, curiosity, excitement, avidity, zest, happiness, or joy. Yet none of them seems quite applicable to the earliest days of extrauterine life, when interest (taking on the all-pervasive aspect of a "state") seems to be a major organizer of the primitive ego.

Tomkins postulates that the trigger to shame affect is any experience that requires rapid decrease in the affects of interest-excitement and enjoyment-joy in situations where the organism wishes to maintain the pre-existing affect state. Failure ranks high as such a trigger, for inefficacy is a potent releaser of shame. Broucek (1982), reviewed experimental studies that dealt with the joy expressed by the 3- to 4-month-old child when s/he was able to exert some control over environmental events and recreate certain events at will.

> These studies also revealed a corresponding acute distress state associated with the inability to influence, predict or comprehend an event which the infant expected, on the basis of previous experiences, to be able to control or understand. The description of the behavioral and physiological characteristics of certain of these infantile "distress" states suggests a primitive shame experience. Infants in such states show signs of distress in facial expressions and vocalization,

> uncoordinated movements, autonomic changes consisting of intensified respiration and increases in pulse rate, perspiration, and blood flow to the skin. . . . The idea that such distress states may reflect primitive shame experiences is consistent with Tomkins' thesis that shame occurs in association with sudden decrements in any one of the interest-joy-excitement group. (p. 370)

Throughout life, the inability to carry out a plan that one has generated will activate inadequacy and shame.

Discussing the theme of this chapter at a recent meeting (of the American Psychoanalytic Association, New York, December, 1986), Demos gave her own personal interpretation of the "still face" experiment (Tronick, Als, Adamson, Wise, & Brazelton, 1978) in which interchanges between infants and their mothers are filmed under closely replicated conditions. In the first phase of this experiment, the mother is told to behave normally as she and the infant sit face-to-face in pleasant surroundings; slow-motion review of these films demonstrates the rapt interest with which they view each other, and the complex, rapidly shifting interplay of expressions between them. (This is what Stern [1985] calls interaffectivity.) Next, the mother is asked to leave the room for a few moments; on her return she is instructed to sit opposite her child as she had before, making eye contact, *but refraining from making any facial gesture.*

For a short time (reports Demos), the 2½- to 3-month-old child will exhibit a number of facial expressions in an apparent attempt to engage the mother in the mode of interaction normal for that dyad. After a while (the time varies for each child) the infant exhibits one of two characteristic behaviors. Some children will cry in distress, but many will slump down in the chair with a sudden loss of body tonus, turning the head downward and to the side, averting their eyes from the mother's face. Viewing such films in slow motion, Demos felt it was difficult to avoid the interpretation that this latter group of children was exhibiting a primitive shame response. Here was a situation that seemed to fit Tomkins's criteria: Shame affect operated to interrupt the affect interest that had been powering the child's attempted interchange with the mother, shame triggered by some signal related to the maternal refusal to participate in the expected interchange.

Just as the affect interest-excitement may be assembled with any other function to make it "interesting," so can events cause moment-to-moment decreases in stimulus density to add the innate affects of enjoyment and joy in a central assembly. The individual or interpersonal activities called "fun" or "pleasure," and described by such terms as "having a good time," are not experiences of the innate affects enjoyment or joy, but rather are the names we give complex situations characterized by oscillations between enjoyment-joy and anything that causes transient increases in stimulus density. The enjoyment of a meal can vary from the "animal" or "primitive" pleasure achieved through sudden relief of the high stimulus density of raging hunger, or the far more complex oscillations of hunger, interest, and aesthetic pleasure accompanying the many courses prepared by a great chef for a gourmet feast.

Whenever the organism is required to break off enjoyment-joy in a situation in which it wants to maintain the enjoyment, shame affect may be recruited to turn off enjoyment-joy in a manner analogous to the action of shame as a reducer of interest-excitement. Thus, when we commune with another person, this mutual enjoyment is a major force in socialization. But if we realize suddenly that our partner is no longer enjoying what had been a shared joke, we may turn away in shame.

It is important to note that not every infant exhibits a primitive shame response in the "still face" experiment, or in the experiments cited by Broucek (1982). One of the major themes emerging from this work of infant observation is that there does not seem to be any justification for the concept of rigid, specific, replicable schedules of growth and development. As Stern has stated,

> This last point highlights a more general conclusion. I question the entire notion of phases of development devoted to specific clinical issues such as orality, attachment, autonomy, independence and trust. Clinical issues that have been viewed as the developmental tasks for specific epochs of infancy are seen here as issues for the lifespan rather than as developmental phases of life, operating at essentially the same levels at all points in development. (1985, p. 10)

Everything in this chapter is meant to be taken as an enthusiastic amplification of this point. Despite the fact that I have entitled the chapter "A Timetable for Shame," the reader is encouraged to understand there is no validity to the idea of a rigid, "railroad-style" timetable, but rather a sense of flow over time. The mature emotion shame evolves from a myriad of life experiences, different for each developing child, summating eventually to form the particular kind of shame experience characteristic for each adult.

An analogy may be drawn from the language of atomic physics: Despite the later discovery of subatomic particles, the word "atom" was created from the Greek word meaning "incapable of further division"; that which cannot be cut further. The existence of the primitive shame experience suggests that one can treat an adult emotional situation as if it were a molecule, breaking it down and analyzing it to determine the specific combination of drives, cognitions, and affects coassembled to make this molecule, until you get a point where you can't "cut" any more. What emerges from our current study of shame is that there is a "proto" form of shame which acts as an auxiliary to the positive affects, and which can be shown to operate from infancy, but which does not require the presence of another person and thus cannot be said to be inherently related to interpersonal interaction or an attachment system of emotion. Proto-shame has no "meaning" because the infant does not as yet possess the neocortical connections required to form such concepts as "meaning." By the time the individual has matured to the point where we recognize shame as an emotion, much has been added to the original affect.

I have observed a 10-month-old become fascinated by a shiny bracelet, look to his mother for permission to inspect it, then do so with growing interest and excitement, and finally (responding to an unknown stimulus), tear himself away from his involvement with this wonderful object only with great difficulty *by covering his face with his hands and turning his head.* This form of shyness may be the innate affect shame functioning to reduce interest-excitement. It is not being suggested that this 10-month-old child is *embarrassed* by the bracelet or by his involvement with it, nor that the 6-month-old is embarrassed when turning away from not-mother in what has been called "stranger anxiety." Both can be seen as examples of proto-shame (shame affect proper) un-self-consciously utilized to interrupt interest in something from which the child cannot break away voluntarily due to the power of the affect interest and the child's reluctance to abandon the object of this interest. It is not unless and until an interaction carries meaning in terms of the self that this proto-shame mechanism becomes the core of what we call embarrassment. Only at this moment, and in such situations, has the molecule accreted to itself enough constituent atoms to be recognizable as the adult emotion shame. Perhaps it will be possible to explore this hypothesis by the direct observation of infants; more likely such data already exist but we have failed to perceive the existence of shame in infants because of our bias that shame cannot exist in the neonate.

On the adult level, some indication of this relationship between interest, enjoyment, efficacy, and shame can be exemplified by the game of golf. Golf is an intensely personal game, in which one loses by one's own actions rather than by those of an opponent; in that success or failure depend only on one's own attributes, golf is peculiarly suited for the study of shame. Noting that even a great golfer has "good days" and "bad days," a colleague of mine has described the sense of disappointment in himself that accompanies the combination of incorrect actions producing a "bad hole." Much of the humor generated about golf has to do with the humiliated fury experienced and expressed by golfers who find themselves suddenly unable to do what they thought they could do and be all they thought they could be.

When playing well, my colleague notes, one approaches each hole with a sense of mounting excitement. The combination of good holes leading to the experience of a great round produces intense and lasting pride, defining a new self with wished-for competence, to the extent that golfers will describe such a round in astonishing detail for years. Thus the game of golf provides opportunity for intensely rewarding affects if one is both competent and consistent. When playing badly, each hole, indeed each shot is approached with increasing anger—it is at this point that golfers will throw or break clubs—for the continued sequence of incompetent actions reduces the hope for a great round. This humiliated fury augments the increasing incompetence and continues until the golfer makes the cognitive decision that this is a "bad day," that because of indefinable factors this particular round is not representative of true ability (self), and that interest may thus be withdrawn. The decision that this particular day is "not important," or that the golfer doesn't "care" about this round, is immediately followed by a dramatic reduction in shame anger.

## *SHAME AND COGNITION*

Most writers on shame comment that the experience of embarrassment is usually associated with some alteration in cognitive function. In her landmark text, Lewis (1971) notes that patients in therapy frequently equate shame with feeling "lousy," or "tense," or "blank" (p. 197); she calls this ideo-affective complex the state of "overt, unidentified shame" (p. 197). Sartre describes shame as "an immediate shudder which runs through me from head to foot without any discursive preparation" (1956, p. 222), a disruption so powerful that it feels to him like "an internal hemorrhage" (p. 261). Darwin sees this "confusion of mind" as a basic element in shame: "Persons in this condition lose their presence of mind, and utter singularly inappropriate remarks. They are often much distressed, stammer, and make awkward movements or strange grimaces" (1872/1979, p. 332).

How shame manages to derail cognition and coordination is quite another problem. Since affect theory assumes that the affects are subcortical mechanisms, and that they have always existed in the "reptile brain" (MacLean, 1975, p. 214), I think it unlikely that shame (or any affect for that matter) is produced by a very complex mechanism. Let us consider the possibility that the innate affect shame involves circulatory changes.

In his attempt to explain blushing, Darwin (1872/1979) states:

> The hypothesis which appears to me the most probable, though it may at first seem rash [*an unconscious pun?*], is that attention closely directed to any part of the body tends to interfere with the ordinary and tonic contraction of the small arteries of that part. These vessels, in consequence, become at such times more or less relaxed, and are instantly filled with arterial blood. This tendency will have been much strengthened, if frequent attention has been paid during

> many generations to the same part, owing to nerve-force readily flowing along accustomed channels, and by the power of inheritance. Whenever we believe that others are depreciating or even considering our personal appearance, our attention is vividly directed to the outer and visible parts of our bodies; and of all such parts we are most sensitive about our faces, as no doubt has been the case during many past generations. Therefore, assuming for the moment that the capillary vessels can be acted on by close attention, those of the face will have become eminently susceptible. Through the force of association, the same effects will tend to follow whenever we think that others are considering or censuring our actions or character. (pp. 338–339)

Although Tomkins agrees with Darwin that blushing is an example of "heightened self-consciousness" (1963, p. 121), it might be observed that self-consciousness (as used in this sense) is a cognate for shame; in other words, it is shame that causes blushing, although shame is not synonymous with blushing. Nonetheless, it seems reasonable to assume that if shame can dilate arterioles in the periphery, it is because arteriolar dilatation is intrinsic to the mechanism of shame affect. It is possible that shame affect interferes with cerebral function by causing vasodilatation, perhaps through the release of an intrinsic humoral substance. Unlike the seven innate affects which are more easily linked to facial muscle contraction and which wane relatively rapidly (Tomkins speaks of affect contours), shame tends to linger for quite a long time until the subject recovers. The time variables for the elaboration and clearing of a humoral substance would be consistent with the universal observation that shame involves a "short fuse and a slow burn." Furthermore, the existence of such a substance might explain the peculiar ability of shame to act as a cognitive shock, derailing higher cortical function. Both sexual excitement and anger also involve facial vasodilatation, and both are commonly associated with decreased critical cortical function. One wonders if related mechanisms are involved.

It should be relatively easy to test this hypothesis using modern radiographic techniques for the assessment of cerebral blood flow. If the cognitive shock produced by shame affect can be associated with the action of a neurohumoral vasodilator it may be possible to isolate this compound for the treatment of symptomatic vasoconstriction, and to develop medications that counter the effect of shame in those who are oversensitive to it for developmental or genetic reasons.

Additionally, I suggest that this very confusion, this momentary lapse in the smooth, normal functioning of the organism, is a major factor in the development of the sense of self. The difference between the infant before the moment of shame (the infant in the moment of alert activity, of interest, excitement, or enjoyment) and the infant suddenly unable to function, this difference itself may be registered by the infant as a significant experience calling attention to and helping to define the self. In other words, I am suggesting that the physiological experience of the proto-affect shame is a major force in shaping the infantile self, and remains so throughout life. If this is true, then I suggest further that the adult experience of shame is linked to genitality, to self-expression, to physical appearance, to our entire construct of what it means to be lovable, initially and primarily simply because the episodes of shame experienced during the formative years (as these other psychic structures are established in the context of success and failure, of positive affect and of shame as the occasional accompaniment to failure) are crucial to the development of a sense of self.

A number of problems remain unsolved, most important among them the association of shame with laughter and with anger. I can offer some speculations about both, but they are speculations with the clear warning that clinicians who theorize about development without verifiable data from the laboratory, or at least from videotaped sessions with adults, are not to be taken with a fraction of the authority once accorded them. We have entered an era when theory can no longer be offered solely on the basis of a participating observer's memory of what went on during a particular session, a period of attention to the affects and their vicissitudes which requires the meticulous study of facial display and body motion during the interaction in question; that of the "patient" as well as the other person in the interaction. Every therapist, whether sitting face-to-face with the patient or behind the analytic couch, is always involved in affective interaction. Words (pure verbal reports) have had their day in the making of developmental theory, especially in the area of affect.

Tomkins suggests that the innate affect *anger* is activated when the stimulus density remains at a higher than optimal level for a critical period of time. If there is any connection between shame and anger at the level of innate affect, I suspect that the confusion produced by (normal to) shame produces anger when the organism's reaction to this confusion recruits memory in such density as to trigger anger on the innate level. Tomkins also notes that learned anger (the combination of innate anger and the learned display of anger) is used by the organism to alter the interpersonal field, usually by the instigation of negative affect in the other. Kaufman (personal communication, September 1986) believes that shame-anger represents a conscious shift of "scene," in which the person attempts to use the display of anger to alter the shaming interaction as well as the levels of dominance defined in that moment. This admittedly adult-centered explanation is capable of evaluation in the laboratory. My own view is that shame can produce an "overload" condition in many adults who learn to use anger to alter the interpersonal field (or what they assume is the interpersonal situation that had caused the shame) by becoming angry. Nevertheless, I do not believe that anger is intrinsic to shame, but that it is associated with it in the adult with such frequency that it has led many observers to assume a connection at the innate level.

Laughter, too, is so often associated with shame that some (Lewis, 1983) have actually suggested that shame is the innate stimulus for laughter. Yet there seem to be so many situations which comply with Tomkins's theory that enjoyment-joy is an innate affect triggered by reduction in stimulus density, and laughter by very sudden reduction in stimulus density, that I think it more likely that embarrassed laughter is rather the result of the sudden reduction of stimulus density following real or imagined relief of the shaming situation. In short, I suspect but cannot prove that both anger and laughter are common concomitants of shame because of the enormous stimulus density associated with the moment of embarrassment, and our variable response to that striking increase in stimulus density. Most important, however, is that these speculations (which are no better than the speculations they seek to replace) can be tested in the laboratory.

## *COMMUNICATION AND ATTACHMENT*

Noting that the first mode of communication is the sharing of facial affect display between infant and mother during the experience of mutual gaze (see Basch, 1983a; Nathanson, 1986; and Stern 1985) for recent confirmation and elaboration of this view); that this communication format is held in place by mutual interest; and that shame primarily involves removal of the face from this interchange, Tomkins suggests that the reason shame functions to interrupt affect communication is that it attenuates interest and enjoyment. "Such a barrier might be because one is suddenly looked at by one who is strange, or because one wishes to look at or commune with another person but suddenly cannot because he is strange, or one expected him to be familiar but he suddenly appears unfamiliar, or one started to smile but found one was smiling at a stranger" (1963, p. 123).

The infant is a registrar and comparator of images (Basch, 1975; Lichtenberg, 1983). Any experience is transformed into an image which may be stored and later retrieved for comparison. Winson (1985) suggests that the mental process of comparison, or pattern matching, is a hippocampal function and may be the neurophysiologic basis of the Freudian unconscious. It seems logical to assume that scanning the face of the mother produces a pattern match; scanning not-mother produces no-match which triggers an error signal, which in turn recruits shame affect to interrupt communication by removing the face of the infant from the interchange. The generality of the affect system allows each affect to be coassembled in many ways; shame, by reducing the affect interest (which at this moment is holding together the communication link between mother and child) has been used to break communication. For the purpose of our timetable for shame, I suggest that beginning in the period (3 to 4 months) when most observers believe the infant can determine the difference between mother and not-mother (Gaensbauer, 1982, 1985) and culminating at 8 months, the behavior of hiding is added to what will be the "molecule" of adult shame experience. Once again, in view of the evidence cited by Demos (personal communication, December 1986) suggesting that the 2-week old can make this distinction, we must allow for great variability in the timing of such linkages. At issue is not the matter of precise timing, but that such a linkage must form in order to produce the mature emotion we call shame.

Wurmser (1981), in the most eloquent and allusive description of shame ever to appear in psychoanalytic writing, attempts to retain the classical model of drives and inner conflict without calling on a separate affect system. Independent of the line of thinking that produced affect theory, of the red thread stretching from Darwin to Tomkins; thence on one hand to Izard and Ekman as observers of the face, and on the other to Stern, Emde, Lichtenberg, Demos, and other modern observers of the infant, Wurmser, in his independent explanation, suggested that shame operates at the locus of "the zone of perceptual-expressive interaction" (p. 156), which is defined in terms of the face and facial interaction.

> In this model, the zone is that of perceptual and expressive interaction with the environment. The two basic modes could be called attentional and communicative, and the corresponding social modalities could be described as "being impressed, " with its modifications of being attentive, curious, exploring, and fascinated, and as "expressing oneself," with its modifications of impressing, influencing, and fascinating others. Sexual scopophilia and exhibitionism would be narrower versions of these more broadly conceived partial drives. . . . It would then make sense to coin two broader terms, *theatophilia* and *delophilia*. (pp. 157–158)

Wurmser goes on to derive the former from the Greek *theasthai* (to see, watch, wonder, and admire) and the latter from *deloun* (to show, demonstrate, or exhibit). One cannot help but be struck by how close Wurmser comes to Tomkins's concept of the face as the primary site of affect display and affective interaction, to the idea of affective communication as a system of broadcast and resonance held together by the affect interest, and to the views of shame offered here.

The human being is not the only animal that displays shame affect. One of the reasons dogs have been the favored companion of so many people for so many generations is the general resemblance of the canine facial affect system to that of the human; Darwin drew many of his analogies from pictures of dogs. It is hard not to smile when a beloved dog, made aware of its transgression, responds to verbal censure with bowed head, averted eyes, generally decreased body tonus, and drooping tail. (People spend a great deal of time in face-to-face contact with their pet dogs, talking with them, "making faces" at them, mirroring, just as a mother might mirror the face of her infant. I believe that this mirroring accounts for the common observation that many people who choose a dog as an intimate partner, and who live in good affective communication with their dogs, seem to resemble their pets. The facial affect display of cats is far less dramatic than that of dogs—while other manifestations of affect, like body movement and posture, are described by cat-lovers as attractive and desirable attributes.)

Shame is more important to humans than to other animals, possibly because the cognitive powers bestowed by the cortical and neocortical brain make it possible for us to be interested in more aspects of the world, and in more complex matters than those species from which we descended; because communication as a basic link between humans is so much more important than between earlier life forms; and because shame, in its communication-sundering mode, is a powerful modulator of interpersonal relatedness. Why this should be is not immediately apparent, for the general reluctance on the part of most investigators of attachment to study the face, and to accept interest-excitement as the pivotal affect in attachment (Ainsworth, 1979; Bowlby, 1969; Sroufe, 1979) has led them to postulate that attachment comprises a separate emotion system.

Yet there can be no attachment without interest. What powers the rapt mutual attention of mother and neonate, the excitement of a dating couple (despite the role of libidinal drive forces), of partners in any venture, is interest-excitement. Indeed, in our clinical work with adults we see good evidence of the primacy of interest-excitement in close relationships. Couples living together so long that neither partner is able to act as a source of novelty for the other (the "seven-year itch") may seek novelty outside the relationship. A "good marriage" generally includes some balance of "interests" as well as a good fit of ongoing mutual interest.

I would agree with Lewis (1981) that shame and guilt act to modulate attachment; the former by governing the interpersonal effect produced when one member of a dyad assumes a *self-image* unjustified by what can be validated consensually or accepted within the bounds of the relationship as previously agreed, the latter governing the effect on the dyadic relationship of untoward *action*. As such both are complex emotional states in which the basic affect of shame (as a modulator of interest-excitement and enjoyment-joy) is coassembled with varying cognitive structures. Attachment itself is a complex multivariant assembly of affects, images, beliefs, memories, and drives. It is not necessary to postulate the existence of a whole new emotion system when we have adequate building blocks from the present model. To postulate attachment as a "new" emotion is to declare the existence of a word that uses no letters from the alphabet. Further, to postulate that the *inherent* (rather than the derived) function of shame is to modulate attachment violates the concept of the plasticity of the affect system.

Many would argue that one may not postulate the existence of shame before the development of the superego, as if the previously amoral toddler, like an adult consumer, were suddenly to take delivery of a fully built, new-model, superego machine which (upon installation) then began to attack its new owner with its weapons of shame and guilt. Such an understanding of the superego is another example of an adultomorphic and perhaps pathomorphic restriction of analytic thinking. It is not true that there is an entity called superego that forms and produces shame, pride, and guilt after the secure development of a compartment called "the ego ideal." It seems far more likely that a myriad of linkages between behavior and affect becomes structuralized. The growing child accumulates and stores experience as an image colored by the affect that accompanies it. This leads to the clustering of memories linked by their relationship to specific affects, thereby providing the reference standards that form the ego ideal, the library of the primitive superego.

Wurmser (1986) has offered a map of the ego ideal based on the earlier work of Sandler, Holder, and Meers (1963), suggesting four separate but related realms:

1. The *ideal object* incorporates all the attributes of the idealized, all-powerful person who is admired.
2. the *ideal child* is "the parents' ideal of a desirable and loved child as perceived by the child, their expectation of the child which determines their approval or criticism" (p. 8). These first two categories are the nidus of the idealized self.
3. The *ideal self* is that configuration of attributes and behaviors which would maximize positive affect and minimize negative affect.
4. The *ideal relationship* is that which is currently wished and is dependent on ideal behavior—that which conforms to "a system of actions that either ought to be done or ought to be avoided if such a desired relationship should prevail" (p. 8). Violation of the codex implied in this latter system of actions, prohibited or ideal, produces the emotion guilt, "just as the ideal self serves as the measure failing which one would experience shame" (p. 8).

Whereas in the treatment of adults it is useful to accept the adult image of guilt and shame as a discorporate "inner judge" (Wurmser, 1981), a reification of the aforementioned cluster of affects and memories, I suspect that the concept of the superego as a true psychic structure has restrained as much as it has assisted the growth of our thinking. More and more I have come to believe that shame is an innate affect; that guilt derives from it as relationships become more complex, and veers off onto its own developmental track; that pride (as will be discussed below) can be explained on the basis of certain specific coassemblies of affects, drives, and behaviors; that development consists of learning to handle the astonishingly varied possible coassemblies of drives, affects, behaviors, and memories; that the id is not a structure but the coassembly of drives and affects seen in the neonate; and that the superego is best viewed not as a structure but as a device created by us for its heuristic value in psychoanalytic therapy.

## *SHAME AND THE SELF*

In the passages above I have tried to sketch some of the ways shame can be understood in terms of Tomkins's affect theory, and how this understanding can help to link a quite disparate group of observations. I have demonstrated a logic for the relationship between shame and attachment, between shame and communication, and for the effect of shame affect on cognition. The innate affect shame may be taken as a mode of interference with the affect interest, to which the behavior of hiding accretes when the infant finds itself using proto-shame in order to terminate affective communication with not-mother. Now I should like to turn to the aspect of shame that occupies us most in our clinical work, and in our personal lives—the matter of shame and the self. If the foregoing is correct, one must ask how shame affect gets attached to the concept of self; and beyond that, the concept of bad-self.

Commenting on the behavior of the 4-month-old child, Broucek (1982) notes that: "There appears to be a clear relationship between joy, efficacy experience and the formation of the sense of self. In a complementary way, inefficacy, if occurring in the context of the activation of any affect in the interest-joy-excitement group, may result in a primitive shame experience with a (consequent) disturbance of the sense of self" (p. 370). Our name for the happy confluence of excitement or joy and the experience of personal efficacy is pride, which by its nature is always linked to the emotion shame in reciprocal fashion. At this phase in development we may assume that pride forms as a complex assembly of enjoyment-joy with the primitive evaluation of successful personal activity; pride is intrinsically linked to a concept of self. Conversely, it seems likely that shame affect (in addition to the accretion of the hiding behavior now embedded in the cessation of affective communication) is used by the organism to reduce the interest-excitement associated with the infant's personal activity, and thus adds the atoms of self and failure to the steadily building molecule of shame emotion.

The derivation of the specific cognition "bad self" is far more complex and speculative; in order to answer this question we must digress a moment to discuss some evidence for the inherent plasticity of the affect system, and for the lack of inherent connection between affect and any specific complex of drives and/or cognitions. My attention was first drawn to this concept in 1957, when (lecturing to our second year medical school class) the professor of pharmacology discussed his (rather risky and unscientific) use of reserpine, a derivative of the rauwolfia serpentina plant then under investigation for the treatment of hypertension. Ingesting a small dose one morning, he recalled that some 15 minutes later he found himself standing in front of his shaving mirror, uncharacteristically paralyzed into inaction, unable to decide where and how to start shaving. After some minutes he began to *feel guilty*, and then watched with some detachment as he began, in what he described as an experimental way, to *attach* this guilt to one or another of his past experiences. He had the clear feeling that the guilt was searching for a source; when he was able to *assign a reason* for this guilt he felt able to go on with his day, although somewhat preoccupied with what had by now become a *guilty memory*; when, in a few hours, the drug effect cleared, he had neither further experience of guilt, nor any concern about the memory to which it had been tentatively attached.

The catecholamine hypothesis of depression was in its infancy then, and we all recognized that there had to be some connection between the ability of reserpine to block the peripheral effects of epinephrine/norepinephrine and its effects on those chemicals in their role as neurotransmitters responsible for the maintenance of mood. We knew that guilt involved both neurology and biochemistry, notwithstanding the fact that we experience it as a feeling. To a medical student reared in the climate of chemical reactions operating in dynamic equilibrium, moving in either direction depending on ambient circumstances, it seemed quite natural that guilt involved chemicals; that the production and transmission of guilt involved chemicals and nerves; and that it could be produced by those same chemicals introduced for other reasons. Similarly, guilty thoughts and guilt chemistry must operate in a dynamic equilibrium: If the neurochemical experience of guilt were to be produced without antecedent personal action, some mechanism might search through memory to assign the responsibility for this guilt to a past experience.

During the years I have listened to the "confessions" of depressed patients I have noticed that none has seemed to profit much from this assignment of early "crimes" to the current experience of guilt. An inescapable image has claimed my attention, for each of these people seems to be searching through a file system, one much like the ubiquitous Rolodex of today's business world, a rotating vertical file filled with small cards containing the information necessary for us to make contact with someone. "Chemical" guilt makes people look through their file cards for experiences that have in the past produced the amount of "experience" guilt that matches the current feeling state. In my clinical experience such a situation provides fertile soil for the maximal frustration of an analytic psychotherapist. It brings to mind the *New Yorker* cartoon depicting an African village with a tribal dance going on in the background, the sorcerer and his apprentice walking through the mid- and foreground; the sorcerer saying, "I danced the best I could, but that guy has an iron-deficiency anemia." Unlike situational guilt, chemical guilt does not respond to psychoanalysis. Today many psychotherapists work with guilt-laden associations as long as they prove useful, but add one or another of the antidepressants when analysis of these associations does not yield clinical improvement, particularly when the supply of such associations seems limitless.

Affect can produce or trigger memory just as memories can produce affect. Tomkins's concept of an affect system provides a competent mechanism for this phenomenon. But the Rolodex contains more than our memories of guilt alone. Stored in our filing system, easily retrieved for linkage in a central assembly when needed, are memories of a myriad of situations in which we felt alarmed, anxious, startled, distressed, angry, excited, fascinated, disgusted, frightened, or embarassed. If an affect is produced and we cannot immediately assign it a source, the natural operation of what Tomkins calls the "central assembly system" is to search through memory and locate a scene that matches the "unattached" affect. The assignment of a "cause" for the ambient feeling seems to satisfy some basic need.

Affect unbound by cognition can present in many situations. When we mistake the adrenergic effects of nasal decongestants for anxiety we have formed an emotion out of an affect by this process of association; similarly the hyperthyroid patient more frequently presents for evaluation of emotional, rather than medical problems.

One of the ways the individual can split off affect from its apparent connection to the triggering incident is through the mechanism of denial, more properly called disavowal, which Basch (1983b) describes as an alteration in the perception of reality through the disavowal of meaning. The mechanism of disavowal allows us to prevent "the union of affect with percept, without, however, removing the percept from consciousness" (p. 147). Similarly, the affect (now stripped of its "real" meaning, the association with the triggering event) hovers in the intrapsychic and interpersonal fields, creating discomfort until it can be attributed.

Such an understanding of the generality of affect and the way it can be moved from one assembly to another permits a new understanding of the concept "bad self." Recall (from our discussion of the action of shame affect in interrupting affective communication) that the infant responds with what I have called an early or incomplete form of shame to the recognition of not-mother. Further, it is understood that mother cannot remain always centered, calm, and available to the child; thus the disappearance of the receptive mother and her "replacement" by a person with a facial affect display that makes her look like not-mother may force the child to break communication by the shame mechanism. Broucek (1982) summarizes this situation by noting that here shame still arises from a disturbance in recognition, in which the child withdraws from making a response of familiarity to an unfamiliar person, as long as we understand that the "unfamiliar" person is the now-different mother. "That a mother (even a 'good-enough' mother) can be a stranger to her own infant at times is not really surprising since the mother's moods, pre-occupations, conflicts and defenses will disturb her physiognomy and at times disturb her established communication patterns" (p. 370).

If we can accept for the moment that the infant responds with shame affect to transient disturbances in the physiognomy of mother, one may ask what cognition might accompany such an experience of affect. The relationship with mother is so critical for survival that it is unlikely that the infant could accept a definition of the suddenly unfriendly, unloving, unacceptable mother as "bad." So terrifying is the very idea of abandonment by mother, or the possibility of evil at her hands that the child must use any available mechanism for protection from the affective meaning of the "bad mother" percept. Disavowal allows the infant to unbind the perception of mother-as-bad from the shame affect that was used to "escape" her, reducing the toxicity inherent in the idea of a dangerous caregiver but leaving shame affect unbound and the image of "badness" split off from it. Shame unbound is like guilt unbound—it needs an acceptable precipitant.

Demos (1983) states that "the child's capacity to experience positive self-esteem rests on the degree to which she feels competent, reliable, and related to others" (p. 56). The sudden *unrelatedness* accompanying shame-mediated sundering of the infant–mother communication dyad in the specific condition of maternal affective transformation produces an experience of incompetence in the context of which the child attempts to form a safe linkage for the unbound shame affect and the unbound image of badness and dangerousness. The resultant ideo-affective complex is what Klein (1957) termed "bad-me"; following the establishment of this linkage any experience of shame now brings with it images defining one as defective, weak, or inadequate. Future considerations of the Kleinian split must take into account that the infant may respond with shame to the unexpected replacement of mother; this despite the fact that the word shame does not appear in *Envy and Gratitude*. Although the foregoing is admittedly speculative, it offers certain advantages for study over Klein's original construct because of the general visibility of shame-linked behavior and the general invisibility of cognition. Undoubtedly a myriad of other experiences characterized by the actual or fantasized rejection by mother will assume variable significance in the linkage between proto-shame (pure innate shame affect) and the concept of "bad self." Only through the careful analysis of data from the direct observation of children can the validity of such statements be established.

## *SHAME AND CONTROL OF EXCRETORY FUNCTION*

So much has been written about the relationship of shame to urination and defecation that it seems almost redundant to add to this literature. Despite the general absence of observational data confirming what has long been assumed by psychoanalysts, Lichtenberg (1983) believes that there is an increase in perineal awareness and sensitivity occurring during the second year of life. There is less controversy about the pride which accompanies excretory activity. It seems likely that excretion is viewed by the child as another form of activity that produces a definable product (action with a result) and is therefore a prime candidate for linkage with both pride and shame. Clearly, parental schedules for the accomplishment of control will largely determine the importance of this control in the geometry of the shame/pride axis.

## *SHAME AND SEXUALITY*

Until recently it has not been clear why shame is so intimately involved with sexual themes, and why Lewis (1971) finds such gender-specific differences in the adult perception and experience of shame. Two separate bodies of work deriving from the study of infants and children, both emerging quite recently, help solve this puzzle and provide fertile material for further investigation. To do this I will sketch the evidence that the earliest manifestations of genitality and gender identity are exactly contemporaneous with the period during which shame takes on its deepest significance in terms of the self, forming an extraordinarily powerful linkage between shame and genitality.

It seems logical to assume that since shame attaches to the concept of the self, the intensity and significance of the shame experience will increase in proportion to the firmness of the child's growing self-concept. Amsterdam and Levitt (1980) define shame as a painful form of self-awareness, and demonstrate that between 18 and 24 months of age the infant becomes capable of painful self-awareness on exposure to a mirror. Broucek (1982) extends our understanding of this period by introducing the term "*objective self-awareness* . . . the awareness of oneself as an object of observation for others and, through identification with the observing others, taking oneself as an object of observation" (p. 371). Lichtenberg (1983) describes this as "the increasingly discrete awareness of the self as a whole"

(p. 107). Kinston (1983) quotes Lynd (1958) as saying, "When you look at yourself in the mirror, someone stares at you who is not you and yet it is—this is the form of exposure in the shame experience."

Broucek continues:

> When the child achieves objective self-awareness, the oscillations between sense of self (as indwelling) and objective self-awareness (as an outside looking-on experience) will become gradually regulated into a pattern unique to that individual. A weakened sense of self and strong shame propensities may tip the balance toward the dominance of objective self-awareness over the subjective sense of self. (p. 371)

Broucek adds, "Objective self-awareness . . . brings with it a shame crisis" (p. 376). Where previously attention had been drawn to the self by one's own activities, and shame therefore triggered by self-awareness, now shame is linked to awareness of self by other, as well as the internalization of self-as-other.

Discussing the prototypes of shame, Wurmser (1981) notes that "shame about exposing one's sexual organs, activities, and feelings . . . is of such cardinal import that in most Western languages shame is practically synonymous with sexual exposure and the sexual organs themselves" (p. 32). Why should this be so? It seems that the development of objective self-awareness predisposes the child to take "more personally" parental criticism or censure; whatever is important to the child during this era can be linked to this newly amplified sense of shame.

Tabin (1985) reviews the tasks faced by the toddler in terms of Mahler and Freud: mastery of separation/individuation, psychosocial cueing, oral dependency, anal phase conflict, sphincter maturation, control of large muscle groups—with a brain as yet capable only of categorical thinking. The development of the internal reference library contemporaneous with this era of struggle and turmoil splits images and experiences into sharply delimited categories of "good" and "bad." Intrinsic to the development of a sense of self are these powerful shame and guilt states, which we have called the primitive superego. Mahler *et al.* (1975) identified the task of the second year of life as a phase of learning voluntary separation from mother on the way to becoming an independent self, activities that are relatively gender nonspecific. As Tabin points out, the meticulous work by Stoller (1968) and by Money and Ehrhardt (1972), placing the formation of gender identity in this period, forces us to reject Freud's stubbornly held conviction that 3-year-old girls are but little men.

Tabin assembles convincing evidence from a vast array of material published by others to demonstrate that the toddler can experience genital excitement in the presence of the opposite gender parent. Further she suggests that it is precisely this excitement that draws the child to examine its genitals and thus to develop gender identity. The little boy feels his penis in a new way, sees his erection, feels something in his penis that defines him as a boy. The girl feels something "up inside" that calls attention to clitoris and vagina and defines her as a girl. Tabin's interpretation of the data is compelling—a significant portion of gender identity derives from genital excitement; the toddler's sense of self contains a gender label.

In Tabin's cases, this gender label is achieved in the context of genital excitement, excitement in the presence of the parent of the opposite gender; parents who are unlikely to be prepared for childhood genitality. It was difficult enough for the public to accept Freud's assertion that between 4 and 5 years of age children are sexual and competitive with parents. Here is a new complex, a "primary" oedipal complex (to be differentiated from the classical oedipal complex), one that makes the world of the toddler triadic rather than dyadic. There are other explanations of the data cited by Tabin, interpretations which focus on parental seductiveness as the cause of toddler sexuality. Further, it may be said that some of her statements (about the inner experience of the children described in her work) are inherently biased by her belief in the schemata of Mahler and Freud; yet there is much to be gained from her understanding. The earlier a child experiences sexual excitement, the earlier and the more forcefully will this excitement, and the organs in which this excitement is experienced, be capable of linkage with both shame and pride.

It will be clear from the foregoing that genital excitement in the toddler era affects boys and girls quite differently, for the desire to be close to the source of this excitement pulls the female child away from mother and male child toward her. In striving toward mother, the primary oedipal boy is threatened with engulfment just at the time he is learning separation; heading for father the primary oedipal girl is threatened with maternal abandonment before she has mastered individuation. Until the primary oedipal phase, external psychosocial cueing has been the only force shaping gender identity—the child described by Tabin must now balance the implications of parental attitude and conscious parental gender assignment against new information derived from the experience of genital excitement.

The second observation drawn from Tabin's work is that we must reinterpret what has until now been taken as "childish exhibitionism." Amsterdam and Leavitt (1980) believe that a major source of shame during the toddler period is "the negative reaction of a parent who looks on the infant anxiously when the child is engaged in genital exploration or play" (p. 78). Before this phase I suspect that the infant may be involved in fairly neutral exploratory activity with little dynamic significance. But the child who has achieved objective self-awareness is neither merely demonstrating its genitals nor idly exploring. It is in the throes of real genital excitement. Rejection, or censure by the (unwittingly) exciting parent must come as a powerful stimulus to shame. When as adults we experience the sting of shame at the rejection of our sexual desires (surely one of the universal humiliations of adolescence) it is with a superego lodged in a brain that can process minute gradations of self-esteem. The toddler, equipped only for categorical thinking, is left to defend against global shame states only by the most primitive of defenses.

Here then is a possible answer to two important questions surrounding the study of shame. Tabin's demonstration of the divergence between male and female development at the period of the primary oedipal complex (at least in children for whom such sexual excitement can be demonstrated) may lead to work explaining Lewis's (1971) finding that women are field dependent and more sensitive to shame than men. And finally we have a logic that ties shame affect to genital issues.

In considering the interaction between a parent and a sexually excited infant, it may be useful to discuss the implication of excitement in the interpersonal field. I have long been interested in the communication of emotion; actually communication by emotion (Nathanson, 1986). What forced my attention to this subject was an occasional helplessness to avoid experiencing as my own the emotion of the person with whom I was at that moment in contact. When doing psychotherapy it is convenient to call this "empathy" and be proud of it, and when in a public auditorium such emotional resonance is essential to enjoyment of an entertainment; but it is frequently less than useful to be caught up in the anger or lust of a stranger. When infectious disease was the frontier of science, such transmission was called "contagion of affect" (Scheler, 1913/1970; Sullivan, 1954). One has only to watch dispassionately the flow of laughter through an audience, or the flow of anger through a mob to wonder how the normal human develops immunity to this contagion; how do we learn to maintain our sense of self in the presence of the affect of the other?

Freud (1921) postulated that the reception phase, or the resonance necessary for the communication of emotion, is accomplished by a subtle mimesis, an automatic imitation of the bodily position and facial display of the other. Ekman, Friesen, and Levenson (1983) demonstrated that actors, asked (without any reference to emotion, and with no access to a mirror) to contract and relax their facial musculature in the pattern of specific affects, reported "feeling" the emotions normally associated with that facial display. As Freud predicted, subtle mimesis feeds information inward to produce affective resonance. Basch (1983a) points out that while it is affect that is transmitted in empathy, we experience this empathic perception as emotion because of our associations to the particular affect so produced in us.

It is to describe such resonance that I have introduced the idea of an "empathic wall," an ego mechanism that monitors and modulates the flow of broadcast affect, allowing us to determine whether the affect of the moment is generated from within or without, thus helping to define the difference between self and other. It may be the root mechanism for a host of normal and pathologic defenses of the ego (Nathanson, in press). For the moment, however, let us reexamine in terms of affect transmission the dyad formed by the sexually excited toddler and the parent of the opposite gender.

What Emde, Gaensbauer, and Harmon (1976) called affective attunement, the empathic link between infant and caregiver, and which is so beautifully described by Stern (1985), implies that intrinsic to one's role as parent is the risk of being taken over by broadcast affect. The very attunement that makes for good parenting demands that a child in the throes of sexual excitement will broadcast this excitement at, and forcefully affect a parent quite poorly prepared to experience his or her own sexual excitement over an infant. Discussing a similar example of affective tension, Gaensbauer (1985) writes: "Intense affect generated in the caregiver in these situations becomes a critical determinant for the quality and intensity of affect generated in the infant. . . . In my opinion, the potential for intrapsychic conflict is greater in contexts wherein affect based on the caregiver's attitudes is mobilized rather than to particular erogenous zones and intrinsic physiological drives per se" (p. 521). I suspect that such parental sexual excitement is accompanied by both guilt and shame, which is transmitted to the infant in the form of anger and rejection, as well as the affective transmission of guilt and shame proper.

The occurrence of this complex and highly charged series of interactions during the development of objective self-awareness might link the affect shame to any or all issues concerned with genitality. Shame, of course, turns off the excitement part of sexual excitement, and (for the moment) resolves the parent's difficulty. As Lewis (1981) points out, parental awareness of the child's blush (the "all clear" signal for the reduction of sexual excitement) allows resumption of the preexisting state of affectionate bonding. Actually, shame turns off all affects. Shame can bind, or it can prevent the expression of any individual emotion, or of the expression of emotion itself (Kaufman, 1985; Tomkins, 1963). But for our purposes here, shame has taken on the last major accretion necessary to characterize the full-fledged emotion that we will recognize throughout the remainder of development and throughout adult life.

The relationship between sexuality and shame, and between the genital organs and shame is too variable across cultures to be capable of any simple position on a timetable. As in so many matters once thought to be part of a rigid developmental sequence, the relationship of shame to genitality is one of a number of developmental issues to be negotiated in the first 3 years of life. Sexual assertion is part of self-assertion; with each increase in the intensity of self experience comes an increase in shame. In her attempt to derive a sound treatment program for adult sexual dysfunction, Kaplan (1979) separated out three phases of sexual activity—desire, excitement, and orgasm—and suggested approaches to problems occurring in each. Her useful introduction of the concept "inhibited sexual desire" draws attention to desire phase activity. One is struck by the frequent reference to "anxiety" stemming from early trauma and causing interference with desire, despite the absence of reference to the shame family of emotions. The real name for this "anxiety" is shame, and treatment may be more effective when initiated with the understanding that shame is a reducer of interest-excitement (and therefore desire), and that one of the earliest manifestations of mature shame may be the reduction of sexual excitement during the primary oedipal phase of development. I have never seen a case of inhibited sexual desire in which parental control by shame was not a major factor.

Wurmser (1981) offered a view of shame as a layered emotion, and presented a number of cases demonstrating the nature and significance of these layers. By interpreting in the language of Tomkins's affect theory I have attempted to reconcile the large body of data offered by the field of infant observation with the information about shame derived from the analysis of adults; the result is a schematic diagram showing how the layers are built up and how they interrelate. It is hoped that these interpretations may lend themselves to experimental validation.

## *GUILT*

There seems to be no evidence for the existence of a predecessor emotion specifically linked to guilt in the way protoshame (Tomkins's innate "shame affect proper"), as a reducer of interest-excitement, operates for shame; a predecessor emotion that would allow the definitive separation, at all levels of infant development, of these two emotions that appear so different in the adult. Might not guilt and shame be considered as related "molecules" built of similar atoms, yet through specific variation in development appearing in the adult as quite different emotions? Both involve the reference library stored as the ego ideal; both involve withdrawal and limit activity; both emotions monitor and limit social behavior.

As mature emotions shame and guilt differ, of course, in that guilt limits action, especially action that may be harmful to another; while shame guards the boundaries of the self (Alexander, 1938; Lewis, 1971; Wurmser, 1981). In order to experience guilt the child must *know* that s/he has *performed an action* and that this action has *caused harm* to *another person*. Indeed, the child must know a great deal about the inner life of this other person in order to understand that harm has been done; and, finally, the child must understand the nature of harm. This series of cognitions is possible only quite late in development, considerably later than the period at which innate shame develops and with it the elements from which adult shame is assembled.

The geometry of the ego ideal offers a clue to this branched development. Although the "ideal self" is the reference source acting as the yardstick for shame and pride, the "ideal relationship," incorporating as it does a codex of behavior, acts as the reference source for guilt in terms of attachment. To find the origin of guilt one must determine at what point in development the infant is able to understand that the object is also a person with a self, and that this person is capable of experiencing discomfort much as does the infant. If we are to accept that the reference standard for guilt is the ideal relationship, then guilt cannot appear in development until the child masters the concept of a relationship.

If guilt derives from shame, why is there no blush in guilt? Recall that Darwin (1872/1979), as quoted above, suggested the blush is produced by vascular reaction to specific *attention to the self*. Guilt, as discriminated from shame by Lewis (1971) and Wurmser (1981), rather than forcing attention to the self, focuses on action and cognition, neither of which carries the implication of being purely "self." I suspect that inherent to the emotion guilt is *fear* of reprisal, as in the biblical injunction "an eye for an eye, a tooth for a tooth." The coassembly of shame with the affect fear, with memories of prior punishment, and with certain drive-related complexes associated with castration as punishment for oedipal fantasies, may account for the perceived or experienced difference between shame and guilt. It seems likely that experimental situations could be devised to check this hypothesis.

In my own clinical work, one observed difference between shame and guilt has led me to design a prospective study involving a large patient population. If the catecholamine hypothesis of depression is correct, and the symptomatology of depression is due to alterations in the level of circulating neurotransmitters, or at least in the concentration of neurotransmitter substances in the interneuronal clefts, why do patients differ in their response to the various tricyclic and monoamine oxidase antidepressants? The same digitalis preparation works on any failing myocardial muscle, the same insulin works in any diabetic, and any benzodiazepine tranquilizer will quell anxiety. But the commercial availability of dozens of antidepressant medications differing only slightly in molecular structure but greatly in their effects on individual patients, and the general acceptance of a "stepladder" technique in which the clinician switches from one antidepressant to another according to a predetermined schedule until a particular patient achieves benefit, suggest that humans are not fungible in this regard and that depression is not the same in everybody.

One way of looking at the population of depressed patients is to divide it on the basis of expressed symptoms into the group complaining mostly of guilt, and the group complaining mostly of shame. Guilt-loaded depression is characterized by confession of wrongdoing over a wide range of behavior. As I commented above, it is my impression that in clinical depression the experience of guilt precedes the attribution of behavior, with the attributed "crime" chosen carefully from a card file to match degree of gravity to the degree of experienced affect. We tend to rank the degree of illness on a basis of the crime chosen; thus a patient who recalls, and attributes symptoms to a history of filching candy or cheating on a high school test is labelled as having a neurotic depression, while one who is guilty about crimes that could not have been committed but are chosen as metaphorical representations of huge amounts of guilt ("I am a murderer" or "I have done something that will wreak havoc in the world for all time" or "God has punished me by turning my insides to rot") is designated as having psychotic or delusional depression.

Shame-loaded depression is characterized by complaints about the self. These patients admit only with great reluctance and evident painful self-awareness that they are defective, inadequate, damaged, or incompetent. Here too one sees the patient searching for a metaphor that quantifies the amount of experienced affect, in this case shame. The content of shame-loaded and guilt-loaded depression differs on the basis of our discrimination between shame and guilt. Although the degree of "depression" may appear to be similar, it has been my experience that shame-loaded and guilt-loaded depression function as two quite different forms of illness.

In general, neglecting for the moment the entire debate over the efficacy of insight-based treatment versus medication, guilt-loaded depression responds to tricyclic antidepressants—the choice of medication seems related to the balance between agitation and somnolence. Shame-loaded depression is more likely to involve withdrawal, and is in general refractory to treatment with tricyclic antidepressants (with the frequent exception of protryptiline [Vivactil, Merck]) but generally responsive to the monoamine oxidase group of antidepressants. In the literature of psychopharmacology this latter group is referred to as "atypical depression" and is characterized by such typical stigmata of shame as social phobia, rejection sensitivity, hysterical features typical of shame conflict, and withdrawal characterized by hypersomnia.

Shame is rarely mentioned in psychopharmacologic studies of depression. It would, however, seem logical to implicate shame in a patient complaining of a morbid fear of being seen as deformed. In "A Case Report of Successful Treatment of Dysmorphophobia With Tranylcypromine" (Jenike, 1984), a young woman (initially treated with "psychodynamic psychotherapy" for "feelings of low self-esteem, shyness and inadequacy") developed a terrifying feeling that she looked like a "monster" 2 days before her therapist was due to go on vacation.

She translated this feeling into the language of the body, claiming that her face had swollen to monstrous proportion, despite the inability of competent observers to see anything unusual. According to Jenike, "EEGs with nasopharyngeal leads were within normal limits," and she was treated for depression with a correctly managed stepladder technique involving a series of medications of increasing potency. One tricyclic medication made her feel less depressed but more "crazy," while she achieved complete resolution of all symptoms within 4 days of taking her first monoamine oxidase inhibitor. This published case, and a number of my own, lead me to suspect that there is a neurochemistry of shame that differs from that of guilt. Clearly, further study is needed to determine the implication of these clinical observations. Eventually, I hope to design a simple questionnaire that will enable the clinician to assign a particular depressed patient some position on the continuum between shame and guilt, and thus facilitate the earlier choice of an effective medication. At this juncture, however, I wish to stress my point that careful identification of affects, the specific naming of emotion states, may lead to greater clinical efficacy.

Throughout this current study I have been struck by the difference between the derived infant and the observed infant. Working backward in time, using the powerful tools of psychoanalysis, working within the transference, we derived a concept of shame and guilt as vastly different emotions, emanating from a distinct locus called the superego, and used by the organism to limit the narcissism and tame the misbehavior caused by an unruly id. Observing children from birth through and into toddlerhood one is struck by the clarity of the innate affects; by the rapidity with which the infant learns to modulate affect, to mimic affect display, to use both innate and learned affect as a communication system; and by the astonishingly varied coassemblies of affect with cognition, memory, drives, and other affects that characterize human development. We can trace the development of both shame and guilt from an innate affect that acts as an auxiliary to the affects of interest-excitement and enjoyment-joy and is related to their appearance as mature emotions in the adult. It is unnecessary to postulate that shame and guilt are intrinsically different despite the fact that the ideo-affective complexes from which they are formed make them "feel" different to us. Shame observed is quite different from shame derived; the affect shame may well be the nidus from which the organism forms the emotion guilt.

What happens to psychoanalysis if we discard the structural

hypothesis in favor of an affect-loaded system, analogous to what Slap (1986) has called the schema model? Very little, I suspect. Transference will go on quite as usual, yielding its rich harvest of information about the inner life of the human being, yet these new data about affect and the scripts within which it is embedded will allow interpretation at increasingly deep levels with increasing accuracy. Careful analysis of the defenses will be made more rewarding by integration of affect theory with drive theory. What we have called intersystemic conflicts will be renamed in terms of the ideo-affective complexes actually involved; what we have defined as intrasystemic conflict will be seen as specific complexes of affects and drives occurring along a maturational line of development. What we cannot afford to do is claim that affect theory and the associated data of infant observation are "not psychoanalysis" and therefore can be ignored by those to whom developmental theory is central to an understanding of the human condition.

## CLINICAL APPLICATIONS

Psychoanalytic inquiry is a dialectic juxtaposing the study and treatment of the adult with the study of the child. Despite the fact that most of our understanding of psychopathology comes from analytic investigation of the adult, it must be remembered that this same investigation of the adult became a vantage point from which to make suppositions about infant development, and that these suppositions about the infant were then treated as immutable natural law *and reentered into our clinical investigation in the form of observational bias*. It is now possible for us to reevaluate our experience with adults in terms of the new information about early life, particularly the observations and ideas about affect initially presented as a theoretical system by Tomkins and now so often confirmed by infant observation. It is my belief that an orientation based on a solid theory of affect, of affect modulation, and of affective development should assist in our investigation of affective illness. In the brief passages that follow I should like to demonstrate the possible utility of the theoretical material discussed above, and sketch an outline for further study. For this purpose I will discuss manic–depressive illness, a specific affective illness known for centuries and about which there is a wealth of generally accepted clinical data.

As a physician trained initially in internal medicine and endocrinology, and who entered psychiatric residency after some years of medical teaching, practice, and research, it seemed strange to me that psychoanalytic psychiatry recognized no diseases. I had been in personal analysis during those medical years and had been powerfully affected by my understanding of the unconscious. In particular, Groddeck's (1923/1961) *Book of the It* convinced me that the unconscious could manifest itself through any organ system in whatever way might capture attention. That so many emotional disorders could be explained by the many possible and varied combinations and interactions of the normal mental mechanisms seemed wonderful, then as now. Nevertheless, throughout my training and years of practice I remained unconvinced of two staunchly held psychoanalytic positions—that the emotions were derivative of the drives, and that all humans carried pretty much the same equipment. My long investigation of the direct transmission of emotion, culminating in a description of the ego mechanism I have called the empathic wall, and my recognition of the contributions to our field made by Tomkins, speaks for my opposition to the former position. It is to the latter position, the psychoanalytic belief that patients with emotional illness are physically healthy and essentially fungible, that I now wish to address our attention.

To start by drawing an example from the world of medicine, it is well recognized that gout is not a primary disorder of the joints. The acute arthropathy that has been known for ages and that is associated with such disorders-in-living as overindulgence in food and drink is now understood as a disorder of purine metabolism. Instead of being converted to urea, which is highly soluble and easily excreted in urine, purines are metabolized to uric acid, which is only weakly soluble, which builds up in the body, and which accumulates in the joint spaces. Uric acid forms spiky crystals that irritate the lining of the joints; the pain and swelling caused by this irritation is called gout. We can create the symptoms of gout by artificially increasing the amount of uric acid in the body, or by injecting uric acid crystals into the joint space, but this is not the disease gout. Many normal mechanisms, present in every human being, are involved in the inflammatory reaction to uric acid crystals, but true gout stems from an inherited abnormality in metabolism present only in those so afflicted.

Might not there be psychiatric illnesses characterized by the attempt of normal mental mechanisms to deal with disorders of neurophysiology? I wish to offer the hypothesis that manic–depressive illness, better known today as bipolar affective disorder, is the clinically observable manifestation of disturbance in the neurophysiology of, and therefore the *expression* of the subcortical mechanism we call the affect interest-excitement. I will demonstrate a logical connection between interest-excitement and the phenomenology of this illness, and suggest that a significant portion of the symptom complex familiar to us in clinical psychiatry derives from the role of shame as an innate modulator of interest-excitement. In order not to distract from the theme of shame around which I have organized this present book, I will present my hypothesis only in detail adequate to introduce a concept that I will expand in later communications.

Let us first address the primary symptoms of the manic phase of this illness as it presents clinically. Cardinal features include an elated but unstable mood, pressure of speech accompanied by the subjective experience of "racing thoughts," and increased motor activity. It is not unusual for the hypomanic to exhibit remarkable facility in garnering the support of others for his or her activities, whether in the form of business ventures, political ambitions, or sexual seduction. So rapidly does the hypomanic make or assume entry into the personal system of a stranger that behavior initially appearing to be warm and friendly blends imperceptibly into the intrusively intimate. Interference with any of the above processes is likely to be met with impatience, intolerance, quarrelsome irritability, and an absolute form of personal dismissal quite in contrast with the preceding assumed intimacy. Should the illness move from hypomania toward full-fledged mania, all of the above-listed symptoms are amplified to "psychotic" levels. While some degree of hypersexuality is common in hypomania, it is not unusual for a fully manic patient to masturbate nearly continuously until restrained by genital injury.

It will be recalled that Tomkins described the affects as *analogic* amplifiers, essentially neutral with respect to the functions amplified, but amplifying in a mode *analogous* to the stimulus that triggered the specific affect. Thus enjoyment-joy, which is triggered by any decrease in stimulus density, produces further decrease in stimulus density; as exemplified by the quietus following orgasm and the feeling of calm and pleasure attending our laughing response to a joke. Interest-excitement, the affective response to a steadily increasing input of data, works by further increasing cognitive, motor, and affective activity, thus further increasing stimulus density and producing excitement. And shame, acting to decrease interest-excitement that the organism must halt (but cannot volitionally) magnifies shame by calling attention to itself and further reducing the positive affect of interest.

Such an understanding of the affect interest facilitates a new interpretation of hypomania. Each of the above-mentioned symptoms can be seen as a specific coassembly of interest-excitement with a particular assortment of drives, cognitions, and other affects. Racing thoughts and pressured speech involve analogic amplification of cognition and verbalization, which have been augmented by interest to a degree inappropriate to (out of synchrony with) the ego structure of the individual. Although it has been accepted without question that manic excitement occurs as an attempt to reverse "opposite attitudes . . . not a genuine freedom from depression but a cramped denial of dependencies" (Fenichel, 1945, p. 410), I tend to believe that the excitement (this physiological alteration of affect mechanisms) is the primary illness, and the well-known findings of psychoanalytic investigation a group of secondary, or derived phenomena.

Anybody who lives in the world of creative endeavor knows the heady feeling that accompanies the rush of new ideas and images that will become the next new work. In an era when psychoanalytic theory toyed with the idea that all creativity was based in neurosis, therapists were somewhat reluctant to treat artists, fearing that treatment might reduce creativity. Now we are certain that neurosis only interferes with the expression and elaboration of all forms of ideation, and that treatment enhances artistic productivity. I doubt that there breathes one creative soul who has not lain awake at night, brain racing at fever pitch as ideas rush here and there, cognitions seeking a match with previously established patterns, templates forming and templates checking. Books, films, businesses, experiments, hypotheses, and concepts emerge from such sessions, for after the work of idea-formation lies the work of realization into the transmissable form that we recognize as the product of this mentation.

I believe that normal creativity differs from manic production in one major aspect: In normal creativity the affect interest-excitement is triggered by the increasing flow of ideas produced by a mind that has come on something new, this novelty (presented in neurophysiologic language as increasing stimulus density) acting as the trigger for interest, which analogically amplifies the flow of ideas and the process of searching through memory—ideas first, then affect, then more ideas. In hypomania the situation is reversed, for the amplifying affect interest-excitement is produced first, not by the flow of new ideas, but by some as yet unknown aberration in neurophysiology triggered sui generis by alterations in biochemistry, or perhaps triggered by a nonordinary stimulus, and/or maintained by mechanisms that are aberrant. The central assembly searches for memories and cognitions that can be attached to this affect, much as described above for "chemical" guilt and shame, resulting in the type of thinking we call hypomanic—affect first, then ideas to "explain" it.

The dependence of attachment on interest, as the binding affect that holds together the involved dyad, explains the ease with which the hypomanic is able to penetrate the personal space of strangers. It is rare for someone to act truly interested in us; the intensely experienced and unabashed broadcast interest that characterizes the interpersonal behavior of the hypomanic makes the patient charismatic. Such a degree of interest unchecked by normal shame, or by the boundaries spelled out in the codex of the ideal relationship embedded in the ego ideal, tend to make the patient unconventional by definition. Further, in the language of my work on affect transmission and affective resonance, one can see that the degree of interest broadcast by the hypomanic breaches the empathic wall of the normal person, transforming hypomanic excitement into the *shared* enthusiasm that is the source of much of the socioeconomic and interpersonal trouble created by these patients. No one can influence, even take over the mood of others like the hypomanic patient.

The role of sexuality in manic symptomatology may be explained by reference to the affect enjoyment-joy, the reaction to decreases in stimulus density. Sexual behavior, in addition to the pride associated with conquest, is enjoyable to the degree that it is rewarded by positive affect—orgasm provides a rapid decrease in stimulus density, triggering the affect enjoyment which turns off the preceding excitement and analogically amplifies the sense of calm and peace. If sexual activity can do this for the normal person, it certainly offers a way for the hypomanic to achieve some decrease in whatever discomfort might arise from a constantly rising level of stimulation. In this sense, masturbation and seduction share with manic humor (puns and joke-telling) the goal of temporary stimulus reduction. Seduction is characterized by interest used in the service of sexuality rather than in the service of attachment, as seen in romance.

Where there is unchecked interest we should be able to find shame as its innate reducer, and manic–depressive illness provides a rich source for the study of shaming interaction. (Morrison [1983] makes a similar observation.) The quarrelsomeness and tendency toward anger that occurs whenever the hypomanic person feels thwarted, and which has been described since the days of Hippocrates, derive from the equation of shame with halted interest. Manic anger is humiliated fury, as can testify any clinician who has listened to claims that "They can't do that to *me*!" or who has watched helplessly the increasing spiral of litigation and/or the barrages of letters and telephone calls made by the hypomanic who has become suddenly and irrevocably indignant over a minor or even an imagined slight. Working in therapy with such patients one is constantly alert to the sudden stiffening of posture that precedes an angry defense against such anticipated shame; indeed, hapless therapists often adopt the placating style utilized by the families of such patients.

The depressive swing of this illness encompasses the full spectrum of shame- and guilt-loaded cognitions, accompanied by varying degrees of decrease in interest. Patients complain that nothing interests them, and that there is no joy in life. The intensity of all relationships is decreased, and the patient has no interest in new ventures. The classical triad of depressed mood, difficulty in thinking, and psychomotor retardation occurs in direct relationship to the severity of illness. If one were to devise an experimental protocol to determine the effect of reduction and eventual abolition of the affect interest-excitement, I suspect that it would replicate the depressive phase of uncomplicated manic–depressive illness.

In the pre-lithium era it was generally understood that a psychoanalytic approach to manic–depressive patients was contraindicated, for not only did the patients seem to get worse, but the analyst frequently reported an intense and growing dislike for the patient (Fromm-Reichmann, 1950). Anthony (1981) has commented that psychoanalysis is an arena of shame, wherein that analysis of defense which facilitates inner looking and which produces sudden exposure (if "only" to self-scrutiny) must produce noxious degrees of shame. It is difficult enough to hold within the transference a patient with normal neurophysiologic mechanisms who is experiencing shame courtesy of the analytic process, and nearly impossible to do so with a bipolar patient whose tendency toward shame has been augmented physiologically. Not all patients are grateful for the boon of lithium. Many mourn the loss of the degree of interest-excitement that infused their lives from time to time, and are willing to risk the periods of anergia that accompany the states of reduced interest in order to experience occasional hypomanic augmentation of mental function. Nevertheless, the experience of treating in psychoanalytically oriented psychotherapy a great many patients before and after treatment with lithium, which does seem to modulate the wide swings in the affect interest-excitement, serves to confirm my belief in the relationship between interest, shame, and anger.

One final speculative note. After more than 20 years of experience in treating patients with lithium and with antidepressants, both in the context of analytic "uncovering" therapy and occasionally in the traditional medical mode of merely providing access to medication while watching the progress of the patient, I have come to the conclusion that affective illness does not start anywhere near the time we get to see the patient. Unless we are to ignore the overwhelming mass of evidence that this group of illnesses has a genetic origin, we must consider the likelihood that affective illness must exist in some *forme fruste* long before becoming a clinical entity. The person who will develop any of the group of illnesses that we now treat with lithium (or any of the other "antimanic" medications now entering the pharmacopoeia) has experienced "mood swings" for years before coming to our attention.

If I am correct in suspecting that at the core of these affective illnesses lies a primary defect in the neurophysiologic system for the production and modulation of the affect interest-excitement, we might do well to extend backward in time our understanding of both the clinical illness and of infant and child development. Demos (1983) states my position eloquently:

> If the self is understood as an organizing structure, then it too probably consists of a combination of affective and cognitive components that have formed on the basis of at least the three following aspects of experience: judgements of one's competence versus incompetence; trust in one's inner states versus mistrust; and judgements of one's relatedness to others versus one's isolation. . . . To the extent that the self is experienced as relatively competent, trustworthy, and related, positive self-esteem can be maintained. (pp. 47–48)

What happens to the developing self-structure of a child in whom affective experience is linked *not* to the normal stimuli ordinarily producing affect, but to some aberrant mechanism unassociated with or produced by his or her own activity?

It seems logical to assume that such children would grow up with an intrinsic mistrust of their affective experience, and live in a world of reduced self-esteem, reduced self-confidence, and reduced relatedness. My experience with lithium-responders seems to bear this out. During the first 2 years that a patient takes lithium I notice almost universally an improvement in the patient's ability to process emotional data, *whether or not the patient remains in psychotherapy*. In general this is accompanied by a distinct improvement in interpersonal relatedness. I feel certain that the future patient is burdened throughout childhood by bursts of interest-excitement, affect that cannot be "explained" on any relational or experiential basis, and that makes the young person unusually sensitive to shame/depression/withdrawal and/or unusually likely to become angry.

Using the inferences made here it may be possible to derive clues for the early detection of patients with what I believe should be called "affect illnesses" in order that proper treatment can be established. Not that this treatment need be entirely medical, however. During the period of my experience treating patients with lithium—a full generation—I have seen a significant number of patients with bipolar affective disorder stop their medication after many years of successful treatment and go on to live full lives without recurrence of clinical illness. These patients, especially the women among them, inform me that they continue to experience periodic shifts in the degree of interest-excitement infusing their lives, but that they now feel competent to handle these shifts much in the manner of a woman grown accustomed to the cyclic alterations in mood that accompany menstrual function. If we can isolate the children who are subject to the sort of shifting affect states that I have described, and teach them how to live with these inner experiences, we may avoid the later development of significant adult illness.

## REFERENCES

Ainsworth, M. D. (1979). Attachment as related to mother–infant interaction. In J. B. Rosenblatt, R. A. Hinde, C. Beer, & M. Bushel (Eds.), *Advances in the study of behavior* (pp. 1–51). New York: Academic.

Alexander, F. (1938). Remarks about the relation of inferiority feelings to guilt feelings. *International Journal of Psychoanalysis, 19*: 41–48.

Amsterdam, B., & Levitt, M. (1980). Consciousness of self and painful self-consciousness. *Psychoanalytic Study of the Child, 35*: 67–84

Anthony, E. J. (1981). Treatment of the paranoid adolescent. *Adolescent psychiatry: Developmental and clinical studies, 9*: 501–527. Chicago: University of Chicago Press.

Anthony, E. J. (1984a, May). *On the development of shame in childhood and adolescence.* Paper presented at symposium on Shame: New Clinical and Theoretical Aspects, American Psychiatric Association, Los Angeles.

Anthony, E. J. (1984b, February). Presentation at Institute of Pennsylvania Hospital.

Basch, M. F. (1975). Toward a theory that encompasses depression: A revision of existing causal hypotheses in psychoanalysis. In E. J. Anthony & T. Benedek (Eds.), *Depression and human existence*, (pp. 485–534). Boston: Little, Brown.

Basch, M. F. (1976). The concept of affect: A re-examination. *Journal of the American Psychoanalytic Association, 24*: 759–778.

Basch, M. F. (1983a). Empathic understanding: Review of the concept and some theoretical considerations. *Journal of the American Psychoanalytic Association, 31*: 101–126.

Basch, M. F. (1983b). The perception of reality and the disavowal of meaning. *Annual of Psychoanalysis, 11*: 125–153.

Bowlby, J. (1969). *Attachment and loss: Vol. 1. Attachment* (2nd ed.). New York: Basic Books.

Broucek, F. (1982). Shame and its relationship to early narcissistic developments. *International Journal of Psychoanalysis, 65*: 369–378.

Buck, R. (1984). *The communication of emotion*. New York: Guilford.

Darwin, C. (1979). *The expression of emotions in animals and man*. London: Julian Friedmann. (Original work published 1872)

D'Aulaire, I., & D'Aulaire, E. (1962). *D'Aulaires' book of Greek myths*. Garden City, NY: Doubleday.

Demos, E. V. (1983). A perspective from infant research on affect and self-esteem. In J. Mack & S. Ablon (Eds.), *The development and sustaining of self-esteem in childhood* (pp. 45–78). New York: International Universities Press.

Demos, E. V. (1985, October). Affect and the development of the self: A new frontier. Paper delivered at Self Psychology Conference, New York. to appear in A. Goldberg (Ed.), *Progress in self psychology* (Vol. 3). Hillsdale, NJ: Analytic Press.

Demos, E. V. (1986, December). Discussion of this chapter presented at the meeting of the *American Psychoanalytic Association*, New York.

Ekman, P. (1972). Universal and cultural differences in facial expression of emotion. *Nebraska Symposium on Motivation, 19*: 207–283.

Ekman, P. (1977). Biological and cultural contributions to body and facial movement. In J. Blackburn (Ed.), *Anthropology of the body*. London: Academic Press.

Ekman, P., & Friesen, W. V. (1975). *Unmasking the face*. Englewood Cliffs, NJ: Prentice-Hall.

Ekman, P., & Friesen, W. V. (1978). *Manual for the facial affect coding system*. Palo Alto, CA: Consulting Psychologists Press.

Ekman, P., Friesen, W. V., & Levenson, R. W. (1983). Evidence for autonomic reactions in specific emotions. *Science, 221*: 1208–1210.

Emde, R. N., Gaensbauer, T., & Harmon, R. (1976). Emotional expression in infancy: A biobehavioral study. *Psychological issues* (Monograph 37). New York: International Universities Press.

Erikson, E. (1950). *Childhood and society*. New York: Norton.

Fenichel, O. (1945). *The psychoanalytic theory of neurosis*. New York: Norton.

Freud, A. (1966). *Writings of Anna Freud*. New York: International Universities Press.

Freud, S. (1914). On narcissism: An introduction. *Standard Edition, 14*: 67–102. London: Hogarth Press.

Freud, S. (1921). Group psychology and the analysis of the ego. *Standard Edition, 18*: 67–143. London: Hogarth Press.

Fromm-Reichmann, F. (1950). *Principles of intensive psychotherapy*. Chicago: University of Chicago Press.

Gaensbauer, T. J. (1982). The differentiation of discrete affects. *Psychoanalytic Study of the Child, 37*: 29–66.

Gaensbauer, T. J. (1985). The relevance of infant research for psychoanalysis. *Psychoanalytic Inquiry, 5*: 517–530.

Groddeck, G. (1961). *The book of the it* (Authorized translation by V. M. E. Collins of *Das Buch vom Es*). New York: Vintage Books. (Original work published 1923)

Harlow, H., Harlow, M., & Hansen, E. (1963). The maternal affectional system of rhesus monkeys. In H. Rheingold (Ed.), *Maternal behavior in mammals*. New York: Wiley.

Izard, C. E. (1968). The emotions and emotion constructs in personality and cultural research. In R. B. Cattell (Ed.), *Handbook of modern personality theory*. Chicago: Aldine.

Izard, C. E. (1971). *The face of emotion*. New York: Appleton-Century-Crofts.

Izard, C. E. (1979). *The maximally discriminative facial movement coding system*. New York: Plenum.

James, W. (1890). *Principles of psychology* (Vols. 1 & 2). New York: Holt.

Jenike, M. A. (1984). A case report of successful treatment of dysmorphophobia with tranylcypromine. *American Journal of Psychiatry, 141*: 1463–1464.

Kaplan, H. S. (1979). *The new sex therapy: Vol. 2. Disorders of sexual desire*. New York: Brunner/Mazel.

Kaufman, G. (1985). *Shame: The power of caring* (Revised edition). Boston: Schenkman.

Kinston, W. (1983). A theoretical context for shame. *International Journal of Psychoanalysis, 64*: 213–226.

Klein, M. (1957). *Envy and gratitude*. London: Tavistock.

Kohut, H. (1971). *The analysis of the self*. New York: International Universities Press.

Landauer, K. (1938). Affects, passions and temperament. *International Journal of Psychoanalysis, 19*: 388–415.
Lewis, H. B. (1971). *Shame and guilt in neurosis.* New York: International Universities Press.
Lewis, H. B. (1981). Shame and guilt in human nature. In S. Tuttman, C. Kaye, & M. Zimmerman (Eds.), *Object and self: A developmental approach.* New York: International Universities Press.
Lewis, H. B. (1983). *Freud and modern psychology: Vol. 2. The emotional basis of human behavior.* New York: Plenum.
Lichtenberg, J. D. (1983). *Psychoanalysis and infant research.* Hillsdale, NJ: Analytic Press.
Lynd, H. M. (1958). *On shame and the search for identity.* New York: Science Editions.
MacLean, P. D. (1975). On the evolution of three mentalities. *Man–Environment Systems, 5*: 213–224.
Mahler, M. S., Pine, F., & Bergman, A. (1975). *The psychological birth of the human infant.* New York: Basic Books.
Money, J., & Ehrhardt, A. A. (1972). *Man and woman, boy and girl.* Baltimore: Johns Hopkins University Press.
Morrison, A. P. (1983). Shame, ideal self, and narcissism. *Contemporary Psychoanalysis, 18*: 295–318.
Nathanson, D. L. (1986). The empathic wall and the ecology of affect. *Psychoanalytic Study of the Child, 41*: 171–187.
Nathanson, D. L. (in press). Denial, projection and the empathic wall. In E. Edelstein & D. L. Nathanson (Eds.), *Denial: A theoretical clarification of concepts and research.* New York: Plenum.
Piers, G., & Singer, M. (1953). *Shame and guilt.* Springfield, IL: Thomas.
Robson, K. (1967). The role of eye-to-eye contact in maternal–infant attachment. *Journal of Child Psychiatry and Psychology, 8*: 13–25.
Sander, L. (1969). Comments on regulation and organization in early infant–caretaker system. In R. J. Robinson (Ed.), *Brain and early behavior* (Vol. 1). New York: Academic.
Sander, L. (1982, May). *Toward a logic of organization in psychobiologic development.* Paper presented at the 13th Margaret S. Mahler Symposium, Philadelphia.
Sander, L. (1985, January). Toward a logic of organization in psychobiological development. American Psychological Association Monograph.
Sandler, J., Holder, A., & Meers, D. (1963). The ego ideal and the ideal self. *Psychoanalytic Study of the Child, 18*: 139–158.
Sartre, J. P. (1956). *Being and nothingness: An essay on phenomenological ontology* (H. E. Barnes, Trans.). New York: The Philosophical Library.
Scheler, M. (1970). *The nature of sympathy* (P. Heath, Trans.). Hamden,

CT: Archon Books, The Shoe String Press. (Original work published in 1913)

Slap, J. W. (1986). Some problems with the structural model and a remedy. *Psychoanalytic Psychology, 3*(1): 47–58.

Spitz, R. (1965). *The first year of life.* New York: International Universities Press.

Sroufe, L. A. (1979). The coherence of individual development. Early care, attachment, and subsequent developmental issues. *American Psychologist, 34*: 834–841.

Stern, D. (1977). *The first relationship.* Cambridge, MA: Harvard University Press.

Stern, D. (1985). *The interpersonal world of the infant.* New York: Basic Books.

Stoller, R. J. (1968). *Sex and gender: On the development of masculinity and femininity.* New York: Science House.

Sullivan, H. S. (1954). *The psychiatric interview.* New York: Norton.

Tabin, J. K. (1985). *On the way to the self: Ego and early oedipal development.* New York: Columbia University Press.

Tomkins, S. S. (1962). *Affect/imagery/consciousness: Vol. 1. The positive affects.* New York: Springer.

Tomkins, S. S. (1963). *Affect/imagery/consciousness: Vol. 2. The negative affects.* New York: Springer.

Tomkins, S. S. (1980). Affect as amplification: Some modifications of theory. In R. Plutchik & H. Kellerman (Eds.), *Emotion: Theory, research and experience: Vol. 1. Theories of emotion.* New York: Academic Press.

Tomkins, S. S. (1981). The quest for primary motives: Biography and autobiography of an idea. *Journal of Personality and Social Psychology, 41*: 306–329.

Tomkins, S. S. (1982). Affect theory. In P. Ekman (Ed.), *Emotion in the human face* (2nd Ed.; pp. 353–395). Cambridge, England: Cambridge University Press.

Tronick, E., Als, H., Adamson, L., Wise, S., & Brazelton, T. B. (1978). The infant's response to entrapment between contradictory messages in face-to-face interaction. *Journal of Child Psychiatry, 17*: 1–13.

Winson, J. (1985). *Brain and psyche: The biology of the unconscious.* Garden City, NY: Anchor Press/Doubleday.

Wolff, P. (1973). Organization of behavior in the first three months of life. *Early Development, 51*: 132–153.

Wurmser, L. (1981). *The mask of shame*. Baltimore: Johns Hopkins University Press.

Wurmser, L. (1986). Glossary entry for "Ego Ideal." Glossary of the *American Psychoanalytic Association*. Manuscript submitted for publication.

# 2

# Shame: The Veiled Companion of Narcissism*

LÉON WURMSER

*It was Wurmser's book* The Mask of Shame *that persuaded me that concerns and conflicts about shame were of central importance in the lives of our patients. Each of us builds a personal therapeutic style embedded in a belief system, itself formed out of the matrix of our training. When we find a major defect in this training (for the relative absence of information about shame pathology and the general ignorance of the alterations in therapeutic technique it demands is just that) we are forced to make major shifts in therapeutic technique.*

*Wurmser's message is simple: Most needed is meticulous attention to the mechanisms of defense. Only then can we find the pain that lies at the heart of the human being, only then can we offer healing balm. But if shame is the emotion experienced when we are uncovered, then the very act of analytic exploration must produce shame, against which the patient must defend again and again. Here is a requirement for infinite patience. Also, most important is tact, defined herein as awareness of the patient's nearness to shame. "Psychoanalysis," Wurmser says, "at its essence is* teaching of self-observation." *The patient must be*

*I am very grateful to Dr. Paul Gray for many suggestions and contributions to this chapter.

Léon Wurmser. Clinical Professor of Psychiatry, University of West Virginia; Lecturer on Psychiatry, Harvard Medical School.

*taught to observe self but not to loathe and disvalue what is observed. This understanding of the relationship of shame to psychoanalytic and psychotherapeutic technique is in itself a major contribution to our literature.*

*The clinical examples used by most of the great writers on shame are truly terrifying—most of my colleagues have admitted to experiencing nightmares after beginning the study of shame. Why are we therapists, all of us inured to the drama of the human condition, so shocked by these particular revelations of human suffering?*

*As Wurmser points out so carefully, just as the one who is exposed feels shame, so do we (the observers) experience shame when we have seen too much, when we have intruded too deeply into the hidden. Our own ("countertransference") defense against this noxious experience is complex: We may exercise denial and fail to follow the trail of pain back to the initial wound; we may become angry at the patient and use pejorative labels like "borderline," "superego lacunae," or "psychotic" to create distance between the patient and ourselves; or we may become so alarmed at what is uncovered when we begin to analyze shame and the defenses against it that we may reel in fright from further exploration and leave covered what might otherwise be cleansed.*

*Psychoanalysis is about uncovering layers. No matter what your school or style of therapy, if you follow the leads and methods offered here you will be able to travel into the world of the patient at greater depth, with greater understanding of the layers involved.*

In the "Laws," Plato writes:

> Do we not distinguish two kinds of fear which are opposite. . . . On the one side we are afraid of some evil that we anticipate might happen—and on the other side we are often afraid of opinion, namely that we believe to be judged evil because we do or say something that is not honorable. We call, and I believe everybody else calls, this fear shame—*aischyne*. . . . This fear now is opposed to all the other fears and pain as well as it is opposed to most and the greatest pleasures. . . . And isn't it so that both the legislator, and everybody else who is worth anything, respects this fear and holds it in the greatest honor, calling it *aidos*—shame or reverence or awe—and the audacity opposed to it he dubs shamelessness, *anaideia*, and he holds it the greatest evil to

> everybody privately or publicly. . . . And isn't it further so that this fear saves us in many important ways. . . . There are two things which give victory—courage before enemies and fear of cowardly disgrace with friends. . . . Hence it is necessary for each one of us to be both fearless and fearful.

In Euripides' tragedy *Medea*, Medea tells her faithless common law husband: "What you do is neither overconfidence nor boldness—no, it is the worst of all human diseases—shamelessness—*anaideia*."

Hesiod says about the time of anarchy, the fifth age:

> Justice will lie in the hands, and *aidos*, shame, will not be. The spirit of Envy, Zelos, with grim face and screaming voice, who delights in evil, will be the constant companion of wretched humanity, and at last Nemesis and Aidos—the sense of justice and retribution, and the sense of shame and awe—shrouding their bright forms in pale mantles, shall go from the wide-wayed earth back on their way to Olympos . . . all that will be left by them to mankind will be wretched pain, and there shall be no defense against evil.

The Talmud tractate Shabbath says: "Jerusalem was destroyed because its people had no shame" (Baron, 1965).

Thus, the message is that shame is a fear of disgrace, but shame is also an attitude of awe or respect about the values central to culture and to all human interaction (cf. Carl D. Schneider, 1984; Helen M. Lynd, 1961).

Still, shame is even more than that. Edith, "bought" to be married by Mr. Dombey, is described by Dickens as follows:

> Compress into one handsome face the conscious self-abasement, and the burning indignation of a hundred women, strong in passion and in pride; and there it hid itself with two white shuddering arms [p. 414]. . . . Have I been hawked and vended here and there, until the last grain of self-respect is dead within me, and I loathe myself? . . . "Who takes me, refuse that I am, and as I well deserve to be" she answered, raising her head, and trembling in her energy of shame and stormy pride, "shall take me, as this man does, with no art of mine put forth to lure him. He sees me at the auction, and he thinks it well to buy me." (p. 415)

Later on, Dickens states that Mr. Dombey might have read in her expression of scorn and defiance "that, ever baring her own head for the lightning of her own contempt and pride to strike, the most innocent allusion to the power of his riches degraded her anew, sunk her deeper in her own respect, and made the blight and waste within her more complete" (p. 522). Shame is the degradation that has already occurred and the enduring sense of self-contempt and unreality that ensues from such humiliation and mortification.

Thus the word shame really covers three concepts: Shame is first the *fear* of disgrace, it is the *anxiety* about the danger that we might be looked at with contempt for having dishonored ourselves. Second, it is the feeling when one is looked at with such scorn. It is, in other words, the *affect of contempt* directed against the self—by others or by one's own conscience. Contempt says: "You should disappear as such a being as you have shown yourself to be—failing, weak, flawed, and dirty. Get out of my sight: Disappear!" One feels ashamed for *being exposed*, exposed as one who has acted in a way that reflects poorly upon oneself, by treachery, by bedwetting, by being a tattle tale, by having failed in school or life—in short, of failing someone else's expectations or failing the demands of performance by one's own conscience, standing under the glare of one's own mind's eye. To disappear into nothing is the punishment for such failure. At least originally there is a particular significance of seeing and being looked at, that is of exposure, in shame. As Fenichel says:

> "I feel ashamed" means "I do not want to be seen." Therefore, persons who feel ashamed hide themselves or at least avert their faces. However, they also close their eyes and refuse to look. This is a kind of magical gesture, arising from the magical belief that anyone who does not look cannot be looked at. (1945, p. 139)

From this it is evident that the eye is the organ of shame par excellence.

The aim in this second form of shame is the goal of wiping out that disgrace. How? "I want to be seen as different from the way I have been exposed." And more radically: "I want to hide, or to disappear."

Third, shame is also almost the antithesis of the second one, as in: "Don't you know any shame?" It is an overall *character trait* preventing any such disgraceful exposure, an attitude of respect toward others and towards oneself, a stance of reverence—the highest form of such reverence being called by Goethe (1829) "die Ehrfurcht vor sich selbst," reverence for oneself. This third form of shame is discretion, is tact, is sexual modesty. It is respect and a sense of awe—a refusal "to touch, lick and finger everything, a nobility of taste and tact of reverence," as Nietzsche calls it in *Beyond Good and Evil* (1885/1976, p. 211).

In short, we can discern three forms of shame: shame anxiety, shame affect as a complex reaction pattern, and shame as preventive attitude. "I am afraid that exposure is imminent and hence terrible humiliation"—shame anxiety. "I have been exposed and humiliated, I want to disappear as this being"—shame affect in the broad sense (shame as complex affect). "I must always hide and dissemble, in order not to be exposed and disgraced"—shame as preventive attitude, namely, as reaction formation. In all three forms we can discern an object pole, *in front of whom* one feels ashamed, and the subject pole, *for what* one feels ashamed.

Let me turn now to a more dynamic view of shame, its depth perspective, the layering of shame feelings. In this I'll focus upon the *inner* sense of shame, the inner version of all three forms. Jaeger said in the *Paideia* that it was Democritos's shift from the social meaning of shame, the shame felt in front of others, to the inner sense of shame, the one felt within oneself, that represented an ethical breakthrough in ancient Greek consciousness. Both poles of shame become internalized; the conflict is reenacted in ever greater complexity on the inner stage. I will select observations from several patients currently in treatment—to illustrate, rather than prove, these differentiations.

A young man with a phobic character structure—the younger of two sons—who had sought psychoanalysis because of generalized and severe anxiety and depression, an almost complete blocking of his love life, and grave concerns about homosexual propensities, took stock of the improvements brought about by 4 years of analysis. While depression, work inhibition, and overall submissiveness had ceded remarkably to our work, his social and especially his sexual anxiety had not:

I still have a strong sense of shame, especially about the

> sexual feelings I spoke about a few days ago. It's almost impossible to talk about them. I ignore them, I deny them, I fight against them, like with these long silences here." He referred to his shame (shame as preventive attitude) about sexual desires—both hetero- and homosexual ones: "I would lose control—let the wishes take over, be free of any constraint; I would run wild," but also that he would be overwhelmed by violent aggressive impulses, to "break windows, throw or smash things.

As if to confirm his lack of progress in that regard he had a severe anxiety attack the evening following the hour of therapy when he tried to participate in a radio talk show. "I feared I would make a fool of myself in front of many people or not measure up in competitive situations" (shame anxiety). Then he reported a dream in which he was with his father. When he pulled the curtain from the windows, he discovered that a lot of snow had fallen. He was very surprised, but the father dismissed it: "It's nothing." He replied: "How can you say a thing like that; just look at it!" Then he was walking again with his father through the city of Washington, looking at the landmarks, going on a long boatride, and then walking up the steps of the Washington Monument.

He commented on his father's wholesale denial—a downplaying of any adversity, and his own opposition to it in the form of the wish to discover something shocking. He tried to tie it together with a reconstruction of having observed his parents in intercourse. Though a likely construct, at this moment it was too intellectual, not at the edge of affective insight. Instead I commented upon what I saw as the surface of avoidance, by comparing myself with his father. Wasn't I the one who could have been seen as emphasizing in the previous hour only the positive, just like his father? He responded: "And today I come in stressing the negative, the wish to be critical. I begin the therapeutic hour by saying: here is a perfect example of where we have failed. It proves how in a very large aspect we have not succeeded." I stated that he had wanted to tell me, as he had done to his father in the dream: "You are a fool to deny the obvious. This is absurd!" (This is treating shame by reversal: "You should be ashamed, not I!")

In the anxiety attack he was terrified that *he* would be

ridiculed by an anonymous audience (shame anxiety). In the typical phobic fashion he thus warded off the dreaded wish to ridicule me and his father (by the complex sequence of repressing, projecting, reversing, displacing, and condensing).

In the following session he talked about his contempt against his equally phobic, pervasively superstitious mother and how the Washington Monument resembled a defiant gesture: "You have no penis, but look at that giant phallus!" Similarly his homosexual fantasies and desires expressed the sentiment: "I prefer the erect penis over the pussy"—an undercurrent of contempt and panic with women. The wish for expression of such contempt is responded to by shame: to be treated with similar contempt in return. His warded-off curiosity, his fear and disgust about the intrusive mother, and his view of her genitals as mutilated had already early on been contained by a phobia of cockroaches and spiders. These insects (as well as rats) still make a frequent and frightful appearance in his dreams. But he too is, like Gregor Samsa in Kafka's "Metamorphosis," identified with such a bug—numb, depersonalized, degraded, and helpless (shame as complex affect). Revulsion against the female genital as mutilated and dirty served as a regressive distortion of his feared attraction to women, and especially to his mother. "I don't love—that's too dangerous; instead I despise. But such contempt is also too frightening, so I project it: I am not the one who ridicules, it's they who treat me with scorn. And my loathing of the feared female genital is displaced onto the insects and rats which I want to exterminate."

Shame plays a role on a number of layers that I will try to summarize in a sequence from surface to depth. Some of this material has been easily accessible to consciousness all along while some has only gradually and grudgingly become available. I will state them in quasi-quotes, with interspersed editorial comments.

First: "I am ashamed to express my feelings and possible wishes. I might lose control over them, and I would be ridiculed. To express feelings and desires leaves me exposed and vulnerable to contempt, rather than excited and erect" (shame as preventive attitude). All excitement is dangerous, would rapidly get out of control, and has to be prevented. Almost from the beginning of the analysis his castration anxiety had been prominent and not deeply repressed at all. It was an attitude: "Please, don't cut me down. I don't want to cut you down. And anyway, I have already cut myself down."

Second: "My homosexual inclinations are a cause for social disgrace" (shame as complex affect).

Third: "I show my weakness and the failure inherent in my overall passivity and whining dependence, by submission and subservience. I have retreated from all competition with other men. Not competing means being not competent. I've lost out a priori, I am a born loser" (shame as complex affect). All his relationships have the tinge of his victimhood. In bitterness he blames others and blames himself as a failure. No one has helped him, everything is worthless (turning passive into active). There is a sexualized quality to this position of victim and blame. Such a masochistic attitude is a very potent reason for shame in him, and more generally one of the most frequent ones.

Fourth: All expression is equated with excretion: "What I show of myself may overwhelm and flood me; I am not sure whether I can hold it back once I start." This is the anal or urinary view of emotional expression and of releasing some of the inhibitions about drives: "It's dirty to express myself." (He shifts from phallic to anal conflicts, defense by regression [shame as preventive attitude].)

Fifth: "My own defiance and rebellion against my parents is reciprocated by everybody. Therefore I can remain safe only if I am largely inhibited. But because of this overall inhibition of feelings and actions, my overall inauthenticity and self-consciousness, I am not a real human being, but more like a loathsome insect, caged in by numbness and unreality." Insects are paradigms for such contempt (defense by depersonalization against shame anxiety and shame as complex affect).

Sixth: "I am ashamed of my parents—my mother's social ineptitude and superstitiousness, my father's dismissal of anything serious; I am ashamed for *their* sexual activities. I am ashamed of my curiosity about what they were doing at night; I am ashamed for my discoveries." (Ashamed and inhibited, that is, rather than watching, being excited, or aggressive [shame as complex affect].)

All this leads back to the following central conflict, the one side he expresses as follows: "I want to rebel against my overly intrusive, constantly pressuring mother, defy her angry and anxious invasion of me. But it is much too dangerous to defy her openly and compete with her power bluntly."

"On the other side I want to be loved. But all love, all respect is followed by coldness and disappointment, their admiration by indifference. My expectation of them always led to disillusionment. To show love or interest in closeness was, therefore, inevitably followed by a painful let-down and the sense of being unloved and unlovable. Shame is at core this conviction: I never can be loved. It's much too dangerous to love."

The basic damage to his development appears to have been done by the angry overintrusiveness and bossy dominance of his fear-ridden mother and grandmother, especially in regard to his bowel movements, their bossy dominance being perpetuated in the superego figure of the "drill sergeant within."

How does he then deal with this one basic conflict between hating an intrusive mother and feeling attraction for her?

Most of all by phobic avoidance: "If I am withdrawn and unloved I can remain safely at a distance from all those dangerous stimulations. True, I always expect shock and disappointment, instead of excitement and erection. But by such anticipated disillusionment I prevent all dangerous arousal and hence all overexcitement." Thus the fear of being intruded upon, and penetrated by man or woman, of being invaded emotionally and aroused sexually and intellectually, has frozen him into a state of general inhibition and nonperformance. His tremendous gifts have become almost completely blocked. He has turned to such generalized passivity as a protection against his active impulses and interests.

Along with such a phobic character go a host of phobic symptoms: "I deal with the fear of hatred and contempt by phobic projection: my fear of rats and cockroaches, my fear of social exposure and my generalized shame-proneness, my fear of all success or prominence or even of venturing away by traveling, and most of all my disgust about the female genital, all this leaves me withdrawn and inhibited." The intrusive and yet somehow enticing mother is thus safely devalued and dehumanized, then distanced and shunned.

Yet why this phobic solution eventuating in pervasive timidity and shame? I believe that at the core of his character neurosis stands an identification with the mother: "I identify with the despised and terror ridden mother. I am as bad, as worthless, as she is. I am just as fear-filled and incompetent, just as contemptible and castrated as I see her." Additionally, he identifies with her as with a victim of his own hostile wishes. How does one identify with someone else? Most of all by being with and looking at. "By looking at her I became her. Looking at her with hatred, defiance and scorn meant I myself turned into a hated, defied and scorned being. Hence I have to block my looking, my curiosity, my exploring, my attention. It is too dangerous to look and thus risk excitement. Both are part of shame: the fear to be seen, the fear to see. While thus I save myself from the dangers of all those activities and interests I end up with blinders on, my view and my exposure utterly restricted." There is probably far more to this need to block looking, but it has not yet become clearly recognized and integrated.

The result: his life has become unreal; his attitude of "Noli me tangere—don't touch me" is matched by the masochistic conviction: "Only if I am touched, especially if I am painfully touched, am I real." Put in the words of another, quite similar patient with a manifest masochistic perversion: "Tangor, ergo sum. I'm being touched, therefore I am." Masochism means: "My dangerous active impulses are more safely expended upon myself, in form of indirect revenge. I express my spite by proving that my parents and you all are failures. I fail in order to prove *you* to be impotent. What do you have to show for after more than 700 hours of effort? I am worse off, the chasm separating me from success is even wider than before I started. You are a pathetic fool, I prove you to be a fool by being a fool myself. It all ends in shame." That is his masochistic triumph, repeated in life and reiterated in the analysis as "negative therapeutic reaction."

Against this paralyzing identification with the terror-ridden mother stands one fantasy, one large and grandiose protection: "Against this identification with the victim of my contempt I have the homosexual fantasy: there my partner and I have both such a grand and nourishing penis, a monumental penis. We can assure each other: We do have a penis, penis, penis. It is: phallus, phallus über alles"

The fascinating consequence of this solution is a deep split in his personality. On the one side he is identified with the despised mother, hence pathetic and phobic. On the other side he looks to father, to the older brother, to me for an answer, the wished-for, idealized identity. When he feels unreal it means: "I don't want to be the one, and I cannot be the other." Since "being with" or "looking at" is equated with "becoming like" he avoids assuming the first form of identity by not being with a woman. Rather he tries to become strong, successful, and proudly defiant by being with the stronger man. "This explains," he says, "the idea of the unreality of my own being. I'm defined by the identity of the other."

The clue for his all-pervasive shame is thus the pernicious identification with the despised, castrated, terror-filled, and prohibition-ridden mother. His depersonalization is a way of denying that identity: "I am not this, I don't want to be this. But who am I? I cannot be whom I want and aspire to be. Why? Because excitement and spiteful self-assertion—hence success as a man—stand under absolute interdiction and would bring about intolerable guilt."

Thus he is caught between the Scylla of shame (in submission) and the Charybdis of guilt, of standing up "like a man." In short, his sense of self, his identity, had all along been violated by parental intrusion and disregard of his autonomy. In turn, withdrawal and defiance, now endlessly repeated in the transference (as silence or as negative therapeutic reaction) became his protecting cloak. Under a veneer of subservience this was the "obduracy of the spirit" described by Dickens.

We all are, of course, aware of the extent to which the description of shame gives specific content to the abstract and over-stretched concept of narcissism. That concept has become so broad that it covers almost everything and thus has lost most of its usefulness. All anxiety refers to self-esteem, all anxiety has, as Rangell recently stressed, the quality of "going to pieces, falling apart"—of fragmentation, in other words. There is not an anxiety specific to narcissism alone. Equally, all sexual or aggressive concerns go out from the self and reflect on the self—its valuation, its power, its defects. Every mental process has thus a narcissistic aspect, an implicit or explicit reference to self-valuation.

Even when we restrict that overextended concept to conflicts about self-esteem—expectations too high, estimations too low, over- or undervaluations of ourselves—we see how narcissism is simply one aspect of all conflicts and of all growth and development. To trust or not to trust, to be dependent or not, to love or not to love, to insist upon one's identity or not, to defy or not, to express sensual longings or not—all possess components of self-valuation. The more primitive those conflicts are, the stronger are their narcissistic components. Of course it is not true that the psychology of narcissism is somehow beyond conflict. The deeper the problems of self-valuation or exaggerated expectations of others, the more archaic are those conflicts—the conflicts about wanting to be and to get, to be admired and to admire, to be loved and recognized as special and as unique—and the more shocking the realization when these expectations are more or less cruelly thwarted.

Such narcissistic conflict is again beautifully described by Dickens in Mr. Dombey. Here are only a few sentences:

> "It is the curse of such a nature—it is a main part of the heavy retribution on itself it bears within itself—that while deference and concession swell its evil qualities, and are the food it grows upon, resistance and a questioning of its exacting claims, foster it too no less. The evil that is in it finds equally its means of growth and propagation in opposites. . . . It is of proof against conciliation, love, and confidence! against all gentle sympathy from without, all trust, all tenderness, all soft emotion; but to deep stabs in the selflove, it is as vulnerable as the bare breast to steel; and such tormenting festers rankle there as follow on no other wounds, no, though dealt with the mailed hand of Pride itself on weaker pride, disarmed and thrown down. Such wounds were his. He felt them sharply in the solitude of his old rooms, whither he now began often to retire again, and pass long solitary hours. It seemed his fate to be ever proud and powerful, ever humbled and powerless where he would be most strong." (pp. 581–582)

Who said that inner conflict was invented by psychoanalysis and then superseded by Jung's and Kohut's descriptions of the basic narcissistic configurations?

Narcissism is an aspect, a point of view, rather than a specific dynamic content—just as the centrality of conflict and the centrality of defect are two opposite philosophical vantage points allowing us to explain all mental and behavioral phenomena, but not all of them equally well all the time. (All neurotic symptoms are "defects" and were often treated as such by non-psychoanalysts; and in turn even the severest "Ego-defects" are related to conflicts and can be much reduced by the resolution of unconscious conflict.)

In contrast, shame is a fairly defined affect, conscious or unconscious, caused by a discrepancy between expectancy and realization; an inner or an outer discrepancy, an inner or an outer conflict. It is the polarity, the tension, between how I want to be seen and how I am. In its internalized version shame is thus the outcome of a very specific tension between the superego and the ego function of self-perception. The higher the self-expectation and the greater the demand for perfection, the likelier and the greater the discrepancy, and the harsher the need for self-chastizement by self-ridicule, self-scorn and by symbolic or real disappearance and self-effacement. Insofar as "narcissism" refers to the concept of "selfesteem" and "pathological narcissism" to that of "overvaluation" of oneself or of others (something "immoderate," "limitless," "exaggerated," "absolute"), any great discrepancy between self-expectation ("ideal self") and self-perception ("real self") is by definition a "narcissistic conflict," and it is *eo ipso* one that is *felt* as shame ("the complex affect of shame"). In other words, the more ambitious and peremptory (narcissistic) the ego ideal is, the more painful is the wound about failing and the more pervasive is the narcissistic anxiety about yet more mortifications of such nature—in other words, the more shame-prone is that person. At the same time radical narcissistic affects prevail, like envy, spite, and rage dealing with such shame, and, as in the case of Mr. and Mrs. Dombey, the need for a protective attitude may become overriding—that form of narcissism which is observed as withdrawal, unfeeling coldness, and haughty invulnerability as a prevention of shame. In Dickens's words: "the cold hard armor of pride in which he lived encased . . . the imperious asperity of his temper . . . his cold and lofty arrogance . . . he had kept his distant seat of state on the top of his throne, and she [his first wife] her humble station on its lowest step" (p. 581).

And similarly for Edith, his second wife: "Entrenched in her pride and power, and with all the obduracy of her spirit summoned about her" (p. 544); "immovable and proud and cold" (p. 522).

Yet so often such overweaning narcissistic claims are reflected not in one's outer demeanor, but in the demands placed on the self and in the ensuing self-chastisement from within. In the case of a very depressed woman who had endured a traumatic childhood:

> Hand on hip, foot on floor—always back to that omnipotent kid whom the mother told: "You drive me crazy—you will be the death of me yet." Yet I had this bad power. And on the other side was my sister, held up as a shining ideal. I was always the one who caused trouble, the biggest baddest kid around. For me to show anger would be disastrous. That blackest person, that horrible kid in me, had to be stepped on and squashed.

The result was that every sign of self-assertion and disagreement had to be hidden behind relentless goodness and the facade of a savior and protector of suffering children. This rescue attitude is compounded by contempt against the self: "Who in the world do you think you are? I'm going to take you by the scruff of your neck and shake you until you come to your senses." The patient said this with a sneering, snickering yell that made me shiver. She felt at times absolutely unlovable and, in spite of great accomplishments, she felt herself to be an unworthy failure.

This is expressed in the words of Selma Lagerlöf as follows: "Anden med isögonen, själv-iakttagelsens underliga ande, den bleka väktaren vid handlingarnas källa–självförhånandets gud . . ."—the spirit with icy eyes, the peculiar spirit of self-observation, the pale guard at the source of action, the god of self-contempt.

Another patient, 30-years old, with a massive masochistic perversion said: "I feel robbed of myself, of self-acceptance and self nurture. I have the image of a small child standing in black space, in silence, in an empty theater. It's a horrible feeling of not knowing what to do—of having no direction, of being without script, without director and without audience—only feeling very inadequate and unable to do the right thing. It numbs me and I feel very cold. The feeling of inadequacy to the task of living, of being excluded, that I'm somehow not worthy. When I had lunch by myself it seemed everybody was pointing at me: 'She doesn't have any friends; nobody wants her, she is such an outcast.' " In her case the origin was this: she was the oldest child of a hot and cold mother, an "emotionally stingy" woman, whose silent anger still expresses itself by icy withdrawal. Seeing at age 2 her newborn brother at the breast the patient was overcome by the sense of being excluded, a hungry deprived outcast, that she hurled a mug of milk at her mother in jealous rage. Now she is continually engaged in the triple process of eliminating all rivals, of punishing herself for such castrating, deprecating wishes by inviting real bodily harm, and by identifying with a mother who suddenly turns from being caring and warm to being faithless, treacherous, and cold. Not that shame is everything in this pattern of recollection and repetition but it is a very important part concentrated in the one feeling: "I am excluded because of all my failings and fundamental badness." Her superego repeats what her mother had begun, and its role as inner judge and executioner is vastly potentiated by her own wrath directed against that treacherous mother.

So far I have dealt with the shame about *what* is exposed, the content of what is shown. And whenever we trace it back in individual history we hit on a kind of basic triad of weakness, defectiveness, and dirtiness as the original content of shame: "I am unlovable because I am weak and failing; or because I'm defective and mutilated; or because my body, my wishes, my feelings are filthy." Those contents change greatly during development—to shame about sexual exposure, about social failings, about lack of control, about treachery, duplicity, falseness, about passivity.

So much about the *content* side of shame. But shame has another aspect to which we have noted a few allusions: the *movements* of self-exposure, the *acts* of perception themselves are also shame-laden. Instead of the contents, it is thus the *functions of showing oneself* and of *perceiving* that are being blocked.

In the words of another patient,

> If I look at you, I have the feeling of becoming more possessive, of giving freedom to my desires. I become one with

> people by looking, hearing, touching. By seeing I break the limits. I want the exposure of what is covered. I invade and transform and destroy everybody when I am in their presence. I want to touch and go inside. My eyes become like a penis entering you. Looking seems bad and makes me feel so ashamed, I have to hide my face.

Through looking she merges as might another merge in love and in physical union; but she also enters with power, and she rules and destroys: "When I look, I feel as if I had the power to control the other person, that I could create all that I imagine, but as soon as I am away from you, I see you dead. When I meet you again it is as if you had risen from the dead."

In turn, of course, the others would have equal power:

> If I did let them get close to me, they would devour and destroy me. I must create a space of nothingness between them and me. They are a puppet show without meaning. The puppets are dead, meaningless, unreal to me. I am alive, but isolated. Nobody I am separated from means anything to me.

For her, and many others like her, shame is the wall of separation that protects their fragile selves against the intrusive looks and words of others and guards them against any imprudent reaching out and self-uncovering. To express oneself in any form—by looks, by physiognomy, by words, by gesture—means self-surrender. To be seen means to be overwhelmed; to see means to exert horrendous power.

Hence union by perception, power by perception—both blocked by depersonalization: "Reality would lose all concreteness. Everything would flow and merge, and then become distant, scattered, and disconnected."

In another case—a girl with an acute catatonic break:

> I saw how my parents were killed by the shock of seeing me because I looked so dead. I saw things becoming disorganized all over the world because of me. I dreamed I was eating the eyes of the world. I was eating the eyes of Christ, blinding him by my eating and drinking. My eating created the darkness.

All her gestures and looks were felt to have that force of drawing out the energy of life from others. Seeing and being seen, speaking and listening; all had that magical power of draining the world. She was a monster of dependency and passivity. Only the most radical self-consciousness and withdrawal could protect world and self from the magical power of perception and expression.

I see an equally close correlation between shame—especially partly unconscious shame—and chronic severe depersonalization as exists between unconscious guilt and chronic severe depression. There is a particularly good description of this correlation given by Selma Lagerlöf (in *Gösta Berling's Saga*) in regard to Marianne Sinclaire, the girl completely made into a tool for her father's fantasy purposes and intentions. (That is, by the way, the deepest shame: Being treated as a means entails the complete disregard of oneself as a person in one's own right, a form of contempt: "Your feelings, your needs, and your decisions do not count at all, only *my* designs determine what you can do and will be." This contempt *must* evoke shame and rage when the human being is treated only as means, not as his or her own end.) Lagerlöf describes how the girl was split in half: on the one side the spirit of self observation—pale, watching, cold, contemptuous; and on the other side the empty spectacle of her actions—feelingless, unreal, a meaningless rolc. And the self-observation itself is watched, in endless perspective of watcher being watched (pp. 114–116)—the well-known endless sequence of shame about shame ("förlamande hjärtats rörelser och tankens kraft genom att hånle utan återvändo . . . Allt blev spel och overklighet under isögonen som vaktade henne under det att de återigen vaktades av ett par bakom dem, som vaktades av ett annat par i ett oändligt perspektiv"*).

Thus perception and expression become unreal, wholesale; their drive-qualities, their carrying the wishes for self-assertion or power, yearnings for trust, love and belonging—all being repressed.

If shame is a basic protection mechanism in the areas of perception and expression, a protection in the sense of pre-

*"Paralyzing the heart's feelings and the power of thought through incessant scorn . . . Everything became playacting and unreality under icy eyes watching her while these in turn were watched by a pair [of eyes] behind them, which were watched by another pair, in an endless perspective."

venting overstimulation in these two areas, as well as a "drive restraint" in the form of preventing dangerous impulses of curiosity and of self-exposure, then it is essential to study somewhat more closely the putative drive activity involved:

What are those drives?

They are: (1) the urges for active, magical exhibition—the wishes to fascinate; (2) their reverse: the fear to be passively exposed and stared at; (3) the urges for active curiosity; and (4) their reverse: the fear of being fascinated and overwhelmed by the spectacles offered by others.

Let me elaborate:

1. *Active, magic exhibition,* the wish to fascinate: This is often manifested in the form of the enigmatic, mystifying way of talking. It is as if every word should have a spellbinding, charming, overwhelming, and paralyzing quality. If this wish is blocked by shame anxiety, silence and a depersonalization of the voice ("my voice does not belong to me") occur.

2. *Passive exposure* is usually much more feared than wished. The patient feels dread when stared at, overcome and devoured by the looks of others and tries to fight back. Actually, the most typical defense, prompted by this fear of passive exposure, I found not in this area of exhibition and perception itself, but displaced onto orality: the gorging binge—bulimia—many of these patients experience. It serves to "counter-devour" the "devouring" looks of others. Such voracity is thus a weapon against shame, yet it becomes in turn a new source for shame—again the endless perspective.

3. *Active curiosity:* The patient wants, by knowing and looking, to conquer and to merge with the partner into an all powerful, autarchic union, and thus to incorporate the other person's strength and value. If therefore such attentivity and curiosity are blocked by shame, the patient is unable to learn, to explore, even to think by himself.

4. *Passive experience of the exhibition of others,* being fascinated: Since self-exposure may assume a fantastically overpowering and intruding effect, the exhibition by others, especially the bodily exhibition by family members, must be equally and extremely frightening. Like the looks of others, their self expression and exhibition is experienced as exerting a hyp-

notizing, paralyzing spell and again may be fought off with the help of the gorging binge.

Other versions of shame consequent to such bombardment by unbearable fascination may lie in the bland, dull attitude of the three monkeys: "I don't want to see anything, I don't want to hear anything, and I don't want to say anything." The blank stare and the masklike face express the global denial of traumatically intense active feelings (traumatic because they arouse anxiety, e.g. of castration or abandonment): "I don't want to respond to what I have witnessed by feeling." I believe it is such severely traumatogenic shame that underlies what is now often dubbed alexithymia (e.g., in drug addicts).

The condign punishment for exhibitionism (or as I prefer to call it *delophilia*), one then meted out by the superego, is: to freeze up, to become an inanimate object, like a statue or a picture, a puppet without life, to become rigid and expressionless. The commensurate penalty for scopophilia (or *theatophilia*) is: to be blinded, unable to perceive, to deny, and to be blocked in taking in what is happening and to turn into the horror, into the monster itself, to identify with what has been looked at illicitly. Yet these two forms of shame largely overlap.

Such punishment is anticipated and preventively employed against oneself by the defense of shame as a reaction formation: "I myself am the first to block all my attention and communication; I show myself but as a frozen, wooden, stiff mask in order not to suffer the fate of freezing, dehumanizing shame anxiety."

But there is far more to this. Perceptual-expressive interaction is the one area that is cardinally important for the development of the core of our identity. Only in seeing and being seen, in hearing and being heard, can the matching occur between our own self-concept and the concept others have of us. Tomkins (1982) stated:

> "The significance of the face in inter-personal relations cannot be exaggerated. It is not only a communication center for the sending and receiving of information of all kinds, but because it is the organ of affect expression and communication, it is necessarily brought under strict social control . . . the shared eye-to-eye interaction is the most intimate relationship possible between human beings." (p. 376)

The modes of *attentive*, curious grasping and of expressing oneself in nonverbal as well as verbal *communication* are the arena where in love and hatred, in mastery and defeat our self is forged and molded. If this interchange is blocked and warped, the core of the self-concept is severely disturbed and becomes permanently twisted and deformed.

Such interference may be due to the intensity of the inherited drives or drive restraints (an entirely hypothetical and probably unverifiable assumption) or it may be owing to the family environment, one that can be readily observed. It may consist of massive concealing and hiding or it may be imparted by constant intrusion and exposing. The consequence of such an interference is that expectations and reality never seem to fit: "The real (experienced) self of me never matches what 'they' expect, nor do 'they' ever match what I expect."

Perception and expression simply cannot be trusted. They have turned into mere vehicles for union, power, and destruction, not for accurate cognition and mastery of reality.

These studies of early childhood give us some clues about early shame: shame anxiety as a basic affect of warning in regard to such perceptual–expressive interaction; the attitude of shame as a precaution or correction of threats to such interaction; and the compound shame affect as an attempt to restore a safer level of it.

What has just been referred to in this multiple series of discrepancies has been summarized by Kohut in the disappointments about the "grandiose self" and the "omnipotent self object," largely due to inadequate empathy on the part of the parent.

Kohut stresses the archaic *images* of self and object. In contrast, I find it more useful to see these images on the one hand as expression of deep *desires*; on the other hand, at least potentially, as *defensive structures* against overwhelming anxiety (helplessness).

I see the "grandiose self" coordinated to the exhibitionistic (delophilic) drive, while the "idealized self-object" correlates with the scopophilic (theatophilic) drive. In the former the subject wants basically to overpower the object by the magic force of his expressions, of his or her looking, talking and thinking; the subject wants to fascinate, charm, spellbind, grip, mesmerize, magnetize, or subjugate the other and merge with him or her. In scopo- or theatophilia the magical force of the object is incorporated, identified with, and submitted to, with the help of looking, hearing, or being touched; one is filled with, gripped by the power of the awe-inspiring object and becomes enthusiastically enriched.

Turning now to the *development* of *both* branches of shame—the shame in regard to functions and the shame in regard to contents: It is obvious that there must be a strong inborn capacity to develop this affect, an "inherent program," as Nathanson calls it (Chapter 1, this volume) one that apparently does not *require* seeing for its development, since other forms of perception and expression suffice in persons born blind. It appears more and more persuasive that there is autochthonous *drive activity*, first of some original "curiosity" and then of "expression" reaching back to the very first weeks of life. The core of the self and object world is from its inception shaped by this double quest. Libido and aggression use this double drive for their own purposes of merger and conquest, and early damage in the interaction between baby and mother deleteriously affects the development of this double drive, leading to a separate developmental line of forms of anxiety as precursors of shame: "It is too dangerous to look or to hear, or to be perceived, I must withdraw."

Much of the early relationship between mother and child in humans does not rely on direct contact (clinging, cuddling), as in other mammals, and there is no following (as in imprinting in birds). Rather, the mother–child relationship relies heavily on the mutually attuned back-and-forth of the smiling response (Tomkins, 1982). For example, Beebe and Sloate (1982) describe a formerly psychotic mother who held her baby either too close or too distant. She "interfered with mutual gaze by frequently shifting her position, moving her body quite close to the infant, and then rapidly pulling back again ("swooping") so that not only was the distance inappropriate, but she also did not provide a steady 'target' on which the infant could focus." The central feature in the child within 3 months after birth was her extensive gaze aversion: "the pattern of extensive looking away was already being used by this infant to help modulate inappropriate stimulation" (pp. 605–606). In turn, such gaze aversion was taken by the mother as rejection; the stage had already been set for a power struggle around the infant's gaze patterns.

Such proto-defenses are precursors not only of the later range of shame affects and attitudes but also of that closely related protective mechanism that Dr. Nathanson (1986) has so well described: the "empathic wall," the protection against being overwhelmed by the moods and affects of others.

As to shame's *contents*: the basic forms are shame about a weak self unable to stand on its own two feet, shame about having dirty body contents, and shame about having only a minuscule and detachable penis, or none at all. It is striking in this light that the corresponding three fearsome and painful realizations—of a symbiotically bound self that tries to struggle free, of the necessity to submit to toilet training, and of the early castration anxiety and castration shame—all coincide developmentally with the first visible emergence of shame: during the rapprochement phase (15th to 20th month). Severe traumatization during this period might well lead to very strong shame-proneness.

Initially, I deferred the reply to an often asked question: "What is the difference between shame and guilt? Isn't the former simply condemnation experienced from without, and the latter condemnation internalized." I don't think this touches the basic difference between these two basically different affects. Both can be experienced as coming from without, both can be entirely coming from within. Yet which are the differentiating attributes of shame versus guilt? Clearly they often overlap: I cannot in this chapter undertake a detailed differentiation between these two so important affects which stand guard over all of our social life as well as our inner life and have such important functions both in normality and in pathology. A few comments should suffice:

Shame refers to some sort of failure, weakness or flaw of the *self*, while guilt refers to some violation or attack upon the *other*.

Both delimit the range of power in social interaction. Shame anxiety marks the boundary beyond which no one may intrude, while guilt anxiety signifies the limits beyond which the subject may not step. Shame guards the boundary of privacy and intimacy; guilt limits the expansion of power. Shame covers up weakness; guilt limits strength. Shame protects an integral image of the self; guilt protects the integrity of an object. Shame appears to have its original meaning as protector of the self's inmost privacy, hence as the safeguard of primary process thought, the language of the self. Guilt can be viewed as fulfilling the same purpose for object relations, hence for secondary process thought.

Many have commented that shame has a more global quality than guilt. The reason is not that it simply refers to an action or trait that affects the person as a whole. The pertinent global quality has to be sought at the other pole, the object pole, that is, the expectations that have not been met. In shame it is the ideal image against which we measure parts or all of ourselves. (And that ideal may itself be split and may even be in contradiction with itself.)

In guilt we use not an ideal image, but a complex system of ideal actions as a measure. This inner code is delimited and additive, not global. If it is appearance (in form of exposure) that is central in triggering shame, disappearance is the logical outcome of shame, and contempt is the form of aggression that aims to bring this about. If physical attack and violation of others' rights is central in guilt, punishment by hurt, mutilation, and murder is its retaliation.

There is a peculiar shame—guilt dialectic, a back and forth between the danger of appearing weak and failing, which is the position of shame; and the danger of exerting power and hurting another, which is the position of guilt. It is a dilemma typical for much of classical tragedy; but it also is the *tragic dilemma* so often faced in personal and national history.

A few words about defense against shame: one major way of defending against shame is by screen affects, by counterposed feelings to shut out the inner sense of shame. Most frequently this is performed by anger and rage. Then we have scorn: to show up others as contemptible and ridiculous instead of oneself. There is haughtiness: in cold arrogance or icy withdrawal one fights off the hurt of shame and engages in all those grandiose claims and fantasies now so often lumped together as narcissism. There may be *hybris*, the wanton disregard for the sensitivity of others. Spite, or defiance, is one of the most important affect defenses (and not just against shame) and one can engage in lying and other forms of trying to defeat authority within and without in order not to feel shame. Where there is envy, you find shame underneath. Numbness, the stony mask of alexithymia, may often be a defense against the most profound shame by the freezing of all feelings.

Besides those screen affects there are all the ways of externalizing this inner sense of shame, mostly by inviting degradation from the outside instead of suffering the nagging shame from within. Shame is particularly likely to be projected, as ideas of reference, delusions of being watched, spied upon, controlled; all eyes seem to express scorn and betrayal and to follow the individual's each step.

Not rarely have I been asked: "What about those people who appear to have no shame? Did they just not develop it?" In my observations shamelessness is rather a defense against shame than an absence of it. Instead of feeling shame about violation of ethical values and moral standards, such persons feel shame when they are caught in a vulnerable position. And what would catch them so? Kindness, friendship, love, and feeling committed in any way—being trapped or intruded upon, in their vocabulary. Their ruthlessness hides how shame-sensitive they really are. This, like so much else in personality development and especially in that of morality, is not due to any defect or lack, but to counter-identification and disidentification: "I'm not like her or him, and I never want to be!" This, by the way, is one example of a kind of double jeopardy shame: to be torn between two ideal images of oneself, and inevitably to fail one or the other, which is an unending source for inner shame.

Like guilt, shame is a protector of specific ideals and values as we saw covered with the Greek term *aidos*. It points beyond itself and beyond psychoanalysis to value philosophy and to the historical analysis of various cultures.* Shame in China or in

*Here I can only allude to this important topic. See chapters 2 and 3 of *The Mask of Shame*.

Jewish tradition is quite different from shame in modern America or Europe.

*Aidos* forms an important part of the attitude of nobility, a virtue far more important in the past and in cultures other than in ours. By nobility we mean the victory of form over passion, consistent self-restraint under the abiding guidance of an ideal.

Wherever, though, shame is, at its highest, the guardian that protects the core of integrity, and makes objection to the "compromise of integrity" described by Leo Rangell in *The Mind of Watergate*.

Very close to nobility is another virtue, much dishonored in its breach: loyalty to oneself, self-loyalty, remaining faithful to the best within oneself. I mentioned Goethe's reverence for oneself at the beginning. Ibsen wrote: "Do not try to change me! I want to be true to myself." Not to do so would be for him a source of deepest shame.

Socrates says in the *Apology*: "Wherever a man's place is . . . there he ought to remain in the hour of danger: he should not think of death or of anything but of disgrace. . . . I've always been the same in all my actions, public as well as private." To betray his identity would be utter shame.

And far way from him geographically, but close to him in time and spirit, Confucius said:

> Smooth words, flattering expression, exaggerated politeness—things like that Zuo Qiu Ming was ashamed of. I'm ashamed of them also. To hide one's anger and to be friendly with one's foe—things like that Dso Kiu Ming was ashamed of; I am ashamed of them also. . . . Only he is noble whose form and substance are in balance. . . . To have no income in a well ordered state, or to have income in a disordered state—that is shame. (Wilhelm, 1921)

Finally a few remarks about the implications of all these concerns for therapeutic technique. The essence of psychoanalysis lies not in revealing one side, but in studying all sides, moment by moment, of inner conflict—all sides without reproof and with utmost respect. Analytic neutrality should not be the often practiced attitude of rigid aloofness; rather what is meant by it is an impartiality vis-à-vis superego and drives, including such very important manifestations of the former as guilt and shame. As is well known the focus in psychoanalysis and to a considerable extent in exploratory psychotherapy as well has gradually shifted from the drives to the defenses. Careful defense analysis pays particular attention to superego analysis. "The superego . . . is in essence itself a defense structure" (Fenichel, 1941, p. 62).

Following some present writers, like Stone (1984) and Gray (1982), I would say that it is the *use of transference for suggestion* that marks psychotherapy. In other words, to be a good, giving authority, sometimes warning, even chiding, but always in the context of wanting to help the patient, that is of the essence in psychotherapy. The goal is to substitute a new, more tolerant superego figure for the original harsh, oppressive one.

In turn psychoanalysis at its essence is *teaching of self-observation*—in Martin Stein's phrasing: "we attempt to correct, by analysis, those distortions of self observation which become evident in the analytic situation" (1966, p. 276); in Paul Gray's expression: "that the patient can come to share the recognition with the analyst, that, unlike behavior, thinking has no limitations" (1973, p. 486). This means *to become able to think, to feel, and to say everything, without limitations, while ever more able not to do it.*

One finds elements of both in all psychoanalyses and most psychotherapies, but what is for hypnosis or psychotherapy strategically central may be tactically of value, but not of its essence in psychoanalysis proper, and vice versa. What is of the essence for the one, is peripheral for the other—a hallmark of all complementarity, here more of an *ego type of education in psychoanalysis* versus a *more superego type of teaching in psychotherapy.*

Thus in both analysis and psychotherapy the therapist has to be particularly attentive to hidden superego transference on the side of the patient and to the possible acting out of superego tendencies in subtle or not so subtle forms by himself. The more he allows himself to be placed into such a superego position the more he may directly effect an immediate behavioral change, but the more difficult will it be to bring about deeper long-term improvement. In other words, the more the therapist or analyst assumes the role of an approving or disapproving, an admiring or shaming, an exhorting or critical superego, the more he shifts from the psychoanalytic to the suggestive-hypnotic and educative paradigm. There is nothing wrong in and by itself with such a shift, but we need to be aware of what we do and of its often serious consequences, especially if such superego influence is exerted in *intensive* treatment, where, after all, overall regression in affect and perception is much encouraged. The residues of negative transference resulting from such real, and therefore unanalyzable, superego impositions can become unmanageable, both within and without the therapy.

I have come to the conviction that all through the fields of psychotherapy and psychoanalysis the role of such acting out of superego features in the countertransference is enormous, especially in the form of shaming and blaming. I believe it plays a central role in the spirit of blaming and attacking so prevalent in our groups, societies, and institutes. Much therapeutic stalemate and hence the much too liberal use of basically pejorative terms like borderline, narcissistic character, superego lacunae or defects, and ego weakness could perhaps be ascribed to such countertransferential acting out.

The careful analysis of shame requires great tact and patience. We have to respect the patient's need to hide behind layers of silence, of evasion, omission, intellectualization as dictated by such anxiety about exposure. We have to understand his need to assume a mask of hauteur and arrogance: "I don't care because I must avoid caring too much," as one of my patients expressed it. We have to respect it as rooted in anxiety, not in sinful self-indulgence. To attack these protective tactics as narcissism or just to accept them as a legitimate mode of self-expression, may often be a necessary expedient; but neither is part of an optimal psychoanalytic approach. With both eventually we may have to pay a heavy price in negative transference, in acting out, and in stagnation.

Most of all we thus violate our calling as authority in psychotherapy, for authority, *auctoritas*, means "warrant for (inner) growth," and *psyches therapeia*, "taking care of the soul in its identity."

## BIBLIOGRAPHY

Baron, J. L. (Ed). (1965) *A Treasury of Jewish Quotations*. South Brunswick: Yoseloff.

Beebe, B. & Sloate, P. (1982). Assessment and treatment of difficulties in mother–infant attunement in the first three years of life. *Psychoanalytic Inquiry, 1*:601–623.

Dickens, C. (1964). *Dombey and son*. New York: New American Library.

Euripides. (1959). *Tragedies*. tr. D. Greene & R. Lattimore. New York: Modern Library, Random House.

Fenichel, O. (1941). *Problems of psychoanalytic technique*. tr. D. Brunswick. New York: Psychoanalytic Quarterly.

Fenichel, O. (1945). *Psychoanalytic theory of neurosis*. New York: Norton.

Goethe, J. W. von (1969). *Wilhelm Meisters Wanderjahre*. (Vols. 17–18). Nördlingen: dtv Verlag. (Original work published 1829)

Gray, P. (1973). Psychoanalytic technique and the ego's capacity for viewing intra-psychic activity. *Journal of the American Psychoanalytic Association, 21*: 474–494.

Gray, P. (1982). "Developmental lag" in the evolution of technique for psychoanalysis of neurotic conflict. *Journal of the American Psychoanalytic Association, 30*:621–656.

Hesiod. (1959). *Works and days*. tr. R. Lattimore. Ann Arbor: University of Michigan Press.

Jaeger, W. (1965). *Paideia. The ideals of Greek culture*. Oxford: Blackwell. (Original work published 1933)

Kohut, H. (1971). *The analysis of the self*. New York: International Universities Press.

Lagerlöf, S. (1978). *Gösta Berlings saga*. Stockholm: Delfinserien, Bonniers. (Original work published 1891)

Lewis, H. B. (1971). *Shame and guilt in neurosis*. New York: International Universities Press.

Lynd, H. M. (1961). *On shame and the search for identity*, 2nd ed. New York: Science Edition.

Meyer, M. (1971). *Ibsen—a biography*. Garden City, NY: Doubleday.

Nathanson, D. L. (1986). The empathic wall and the ecology of affect. Psychoanalytic Study of the Child. 41:171–187.

Nietzsche, F. (1976). *Jenseits von Gut und Böse*. Stuttgart: A. Kröner. (Original work published 1885)

Nunberg, H. (1961). *Curiosity*. New York: International Universities Press.

Plato. (1952). *The dialogues*. tr. B. Jowett. Chicago: Great Books, Encyclopedia Britannica.

Rangell, L. (1980). *The mind of Watergate*. New York: Norton.

Rangell, L. (1982). The self in psychoanalytic theory. *Journal of the American Psychoanalytic Association, 30*:863–892.

Schneider, C. D. (1984). A mature sense of shame. Panel discussion, American Psychological Association, Los Angeles.

Simmel, G. (1901). Zur Psychologie der Scham. *Suhrkamp Taschenbuch der Wissenschaft, 434*:140–150.

Stein, M. H. (1966). Self observation, reality and the superego. In R. M. Loewenstein, L. M. Newman, M. Schur, & A. J. Solnit (Eds.), *Psychoanalysis—a general psychology* (pp. 275–297). New York: International Universities Press.

Sterba, R. (1934). The fate of the ego in analytic theory. *International Journal of Psychoanalysis, 15*:117–126.

Stone, L. (1984). *Transference and its context.* New York: Aronson.

Tomkins, S. S. (1978). Script theory: Differential magnification of affects. H. E. Howe, Jr. and R. A. Dienstbier, Eds., *Nebraska Symposium of Motivation* Vol 26:201–236. Lincoln, NE: University of Nebraska Press.

Tomkins, S. S. (1982). Affect theory. In P. Ekman (Ed.), *Emotion in the human face* (pp. 353–395). Cambridge, England: Cambridge University Press (2nd edition).

Wilhelm, R. (1921). *Kung Fu Tse: Gespräche. Lun Yü.* Jena: Diederichs.

Wurmser, L. (1981). *The mask of shame.* Baltimore: Johns Hopkins University Press.

Wurmser, L. (1984). More respect for the neurotic process. *Journal of Substance Abuse Treatment, 1*:37–45.

Wurmser, L. (1984). The role of superego conflicts in substance abuse and their treatment. *International Journal of Psychoanalysis and Psychotherapy, 10*:227–258.

# 3

# Shame and the Narcissistic Personality

HELEN BLOCK LEWIS

*Like many of those who have recognized the centrality of shame conflict in the lives of those who come to us for treatment, Lewis was drawn to her study of shame by the sober analysis of therapeutic failure. Patients who had terminated what was thought to be a successful analysis returned some years later with new complaints of even greater intensity. An experimental psychologist who had worked with Witkin (Witkin et al., 1954) to develop the concept of "field dependence," she came to recognize that proneness to shame or guilt was based on a host of developmental factors and would lead to predictable variations in neurotic symptomatology. This new viewpoint allowed her to set up the experimental protocol which led to the landmark book* Shame and Guilt in Neurosis *(1971).*

*Lewis was not the only psychoanalyst engaged in the study of therapeutic inefficacy. Contemporaneous with her focus on the importance of unanalyzed shame, Kohut (1971) and Kernberg (1975) were developing their major theoretical positions, both describing patients intractable to classical psychoanalytic technique. Broucek (1982) calls attention to the existence of distinct narcissistic subtypes—the craving, the paranoid, the manipulative, the egotistical, the dissociative, and the*

Helen Block Lewis. Late Professor Emerita (Adjunct) of Psychology, Yale University; Former Editor, *Psychoanalytic Psychology*.

*phallic-narcissistic, all of which are deeply involved with shame issues. He suggests that underlying the differences between Kohut's view of defects stemming from problems in narcissistic development, and Kernberg's delineation of the borderline personality, lies not the considerable difference in their theoretical orientations but the difference in the patient population each chose to analyze—the former deriving a theoretical system from what Broucek calls the egotistic type and the latter from the dissociative type.*

*In this contribution, Lewis approaches the literature on the narcissistic personality from the standpoint of her own research demonstrating shame as the key emotion. The reader will find rewarding her clear focus on the alterations in therapeutic technique necessitated by this understanding, especially the refinements in interpretation made possible by clear distinctions between shame and guilt.*

## INTRODUCTION

In this chapter, I shall develop the thesis that the phenomena of shame are at the root of the behavior and symptoms of many so-called "narcissistic" or "borderline" personalities. The clinical distinction between narcissistic personalities and classical transference neurotics (Kernberg, 1975; Kohut, 1971) has many parallels to the distinction between the phenomena of shame and guilt. The techniques of treatment emphasized by the "self-psychologists" (e.g., Stolorow & Lachmann, 1980), in particular, the use of empathetic mirroring to signify acceptance of the patient's self, can readily be understood as techniques that are needed to help patients cope with their shame experiences.

Attention to the psychoanalysis of shame and guilt has proven to be a therapeutic boon. My analytic focus on the sequelae of these states, especially the way in which unanalyzed humiliation fury leads back into shame and guilt can also help to prevent iatrogenic increases in symptoms during treatment. It seems possible that some of the unexpected flare-ups of pathology during classical treatment (Kohut, 1971) of neurotics may have been triggered by unanalyzed shame in the patient–therapist relationship (Lewis, 1980).

In recent years, there has been an upsurge of interest in the psychoanalysis of shame (Lewis, 1971; Lindsay-Hartz, 1984;

Miller, 1985; Wurmser, 1981). A number of recent publications have also recognized the overlap between shame and the phenomena of narcissism (Broucek, 1983; A. Morrison, 1983; N. Morrison, 1985). This volume itself is ample testimony that the development of the psychoanalysis of shame is well begun.

This chapter will be organized into five sections. Section 1 will describe in some detail the overlap between the phenomena of shame and of narcissism. It will also compare the treatment implications of a focus on shame and guilt with a focus on narcissistic phenomena. Section 2 will trace the development of my clinical interest in shame. Two influences can be traced: the first was the unexpected therapeutic failures that I was encountering in my work as an analyst. These failures seem to me to correspond to the difficulties Kohut (1971) described with his patients. Quite independently, however, I was pushed to hypothesize that what may have been operating was the neglect of shame, rather than a new kind of unrecognized neurotic disorder, namely, the "narcissistic personality." My attention to shame grew out of my research on the cognitive style now called "field dependence" (Witkin et al., 1954). In thinking about the clinical implications of field dependence I found it necessary to distinguish carefully between states of shame and guilt (Lewis, 1971). Section 2 will briefly describe field dependence and its clinical implications. Section 3 contains a condensed summary of the phenomenological distinctions between states of shame and guilt on which my treatment focus rests. In Section 4, I offer a variety of clinical vignettes that illustrate the way I work at the psychoanalysis of sequences from undischarged shame and guilt into symptom formation. Finally, in Section 5, I offer further clinical examples of the neglect of shame.

## *1. THE OVERLAP BETWEEN SHAME AND NARCISSISM*

The phenomena of shame and of narcissism are clearly related in being experiences in which the *self* is central. Shame is a negative experience of the self; it is an "implosion" or a momentary "destruction" of the self in acute self-denigration. Narcissism is a positive experience of the self; it is the state of loving or admiring oneself. Narcissism is recognized not only by psychoanalysts, but by folk-wisdom as a defense against the hatred of the self in shame. Moreover, it is recognized as a dangerous defense. Some 30 years ago, Grace Stuart (1956), in her book on narcissism, pointed out the ancient Greek belief that seeing one's own image was a forerunner of death. In a collection of writings on dreams (N. Lewis, 1976) we find that dreaming of looking at oneself in a mirror was considered a bad omen even in the Egyptian "dream book," which may date from as early as 2000 B.C.

Most observant people are aware that narcissists are warding off humiliation or shame by their conceited airs. What psychoanalysts since Freud have assumed from clinical observation is that being in a chronic state of guilt is a defense against forbidden grandiosity or narcissism. Reik's (1941) description of the forbidden narcissism in masochism remains a classic. Some patients unconsciously cultivate a sense of their own worthlessness because they cannot bear their own triumph over the beloved people in their lives (Bergler, 1952; Berliner, 1958; Bibring, 1953; Menaker, 1953; Reik, 1941).

Although all of these students of masochistic defenses were describing the way in which the self is experienced as defective or shameful in order to maintain loving connections to beloved "introjects," there was then no viable psychoanalytic concept of the self in which to embed these descriptions. Menaker (1953), for example, specifically described masochism as a defense reaction of the "ego," stressing the theoretical point that masochism is more than an instinctual reversal. These formulations about the ego were essentially derived from Freud's concept, put forward in *The Ego and the Id* (1923) that psychiatric disturbances rest on a malfunctioning or archaic superego. In this formulation, unconscious or archaic *guilt* was assumed to be operating against the ego. That shame of the *self* was also a component of masochism was always apparent in its clinical descriptions. No theoretical place had been found, however, for either the concept of the *self* or the affective-cognitive state of *shame*. In fact, the negative and positive forms of "narcissism" were often confused, so that narcissism came to be loosely applied to "grandiosity," to the self and to shame. This confusion is easy to understand, since both shame and "narcissism" so directly involve the self at the center of experience, either being scorned or admired.

Let us look now at the descriptions that Kohut and Kernberg give us of "narcissistic personalities," to see how the descriptions overlap the phenomena of shame and guilt. Kernberg (1975) tells us also that narcissistic personalities show an "unusual degree of self-reference in their interaction with other people, a great need to be admired by others and a curious apparent contradiction between a very inflated concept of themselves and an inordinate need of tribute from others" (pp. 17–18). Kernberg also describes narcissistic patients as having "deficiencies for experiencing guilt feelings and feelings of concern for objects. Over-idealized object-images and components of the ego-ideal . . . interfere with their superego integration" (p. 35). In the first quotation, Kernberg is pointing to the *self* as the *center* of experience, one of the chief characteristics of experience of shame. The contradiction between an "inflated" self-concept and a self that needs reassurance of its worth becomes less "curious" if we assume that what is being described is the operation of shame. In the second quotation, Kernberg is pointing to the fact that, in shame the "other" remains "over-idealized" or powerful if only because s/he is admired by the self. The apparent deficiency of (guilt) feelings of concern for the other as injured, or needing the self to be active, neatly parallel the distinction between the self as active in guilt and passive in shame. "Narcissistic personalities," however, need not be regarded as lacking in superego integration because they are so often caught up in coping with shame (see Lewis, 1971, for a fuller treatment of his point). Kohut (1971) tells us that narcissistic personalities are specifically unable to regulate self-esteem. "The specific (pathogenic) experiences . . . fall into a spectrum ranging from anxious grandiosity and excitement on the one hand to mild embarrassment and self-consciousness or severe shame, hypochondria and depression on the other" (p. 200). Narcissistic personalities are thus clearly suffering from shame. The connection Kohut makes between narcissism and depression also parallels the connection I have made between shame and depression (Lewis, 1971). There is now fairly strong evidence that shame ("low self-esteem") plays a central role in depression (Lewis, 1986).

Kohut contrasts the transference neuroses with the narcissistic personalities as follows: In the former, castration anxiety is the leading source of discomfort, with fear of loss of object coming second, while in the narcissistic personality disturbance, this order is reversed, that is, fear of loss of object comes first. As I have shown, following Piers and Singer (1953) and Erikson (1950), shame arises out of the fear of "loss of love" and rests primarily on anaclitic identifications, while guilt is the internalization of the castration threat and rests primarily on defensive identifications. I can thus easily translate Kohut's contrast between the transference neuroses and the narcissistic personality disturbance to say that the superego of narcissistic patients is shame-prone, while the superego of transference neurosis patients is guilt-prone. Both kinds of patients, however, have developed superegos that include both shame and guilt.

When we turn to a principal clinical example of narcissistic personality, Kohut's case of the research chemist, Mr. A, we find clear-cut indications that the patient was shame-prone. He had a tendency to feel vaguely depressed, lacking in zest and energy, and this mood was triggered by the vulnerability of his self-esteem, that is, by his sensitivity to criticism, to lack of interest in himself, or to the absence of praise from the people he experienced as his elders or superiors. Thus, although he was a man of considerable intelligence who performed his tasks with skill and creative ability (let me here interject that obviously Mr. A's ego was not defective), he was forever in search of guidance and approval. At slight signs of disapproval, however, or of loss of interest in him, he would feel drained and depressed, would tend to become enraged and then cold, haughty, and isolated, and his creativeness and work capacity deteriorated. Kohut tells us further that Mr. A was ashamed of his father's failures, that is, of father's inability to withstand the impact of defeat. Kohut describes the patient as also being unable to enjoy his own powers. As we read Kohut's account of Mr. A, it seems that the patient was far from being narcissistic in the ordinary usage of the term. Narcissists are people who are so overtly conceited, arrogant, and thick-skinned that it is virtually impossible to insult them; they are usually impervious to anything so mild as disapproval. If anything, Mr. A fits the description of a "moral masochist," with the masochist's familiar readiness to experience himself as inferior and to suffer under the resulting humiliation. For example, Mr. A's being ashamed of his father presumably involved him in some forbidden feelings of superiority over his father. Triumphant feelings and fantasies that denigrate beloved others evoke not only guilt for the implied injuries but shame (of the self) for the implied loss of the beloved.

Shame, however, is an acutely painful state, which adults regard as childish or inappropriate. Mr. A's mechanism for warding off the shame that he experienced both in the transference and in the patient–therapist relationship was to appear to be without transference feelings for the analyst. The process involved would most clearly fit the mechanism I have described as "by-passing" shame. As we shall see when we now consider Kohut's (1979) two analyses of Mr. Z, identifying both bypassed and overt, unacknowledged shame helps to illuminate the sequence from shame into humiliated ("narcissistic") fury and insoluble guilt.

Let us look first at how Mr. Z presented in his first analysis. Z complained of "mild, somatic symptoms—extra-systoles, sweaty palms . . . and of feeling socially isolated because he was unable to relate to girls" (p. 3). Mr. Z's formal statement of his shyness with girls is a statement (not necessarily accompanied by overt shame) in which he refers to the threat of overt shame. The anxiety symptoms he describes suggest the accompaniments of overt shame. In any case, his presenting complaints implicate shame experience. Kohut tells us, moreover, that "the revelation of Mr. Z's problems proceeded at first slowly and *against resistance motivated by shame*" (p. 5); (emphasis added). In the first analysis, however, shame was not explicitly identified except as a resistance motivation. As a result, the inevitable sequence that shame evokes shame-rage and thence into insoluble guilt was not recognized and therefore not analyzed. I have suggested elsewhere (Lewis, 1986b) that resistance might be considered a misnomer for shame and guilt.

The history of Mr. Z's relations with his family, although it inevitably underwent many revisions during two analyses, can also be understood as reflecting the shame of personal betrayal at the hands of the persons most important to him. First his father deserted the family, when the patient was 3, thus evoking the shame of abandonment. Then father returned, evoking the shame of betrayal on mother's part, now that Mr. Z was once again part of the oedipal triangle. Even more important, however, was the noxious event that occurred during Mr. Z's early adolescence. The adult, beloved male "friend," his camp counsellor, violated Mr. Z sexually, thus evoking the profound shame that this betrayal of trust always occasions. Humiliated fury has very little place to go except back down on the self, when one has been seduced, to become a component of one's humiliation. It is for this reason that the violation of the incest barrier between the powerful adult and the relatively powerless youngster is so damaging.

When we turn to the theoretical convictions that Kohut describes as informing his interpretations, we can see how Kohut's first "classical" theory ignores shame, while his self-psychology makes more room for it in the treatment process. Kohut tells us that the first analysis of Mr. Z proceeded "according to the convictions of a classical analyst who saw the material that the patient presented in terms of infantile drives and of conflicts about them, and of agencies of a mental apparatus either clashing or cooperating with each other" (p. 15).

Specifically, in the first analysis, Kohut states:

> the theme that was most conspicuous during the first year of the analysis was that of a regressive mother transference, particularly as it was associated with the patient's narcissism, that is, as we then saw it, with his unrealistic, deluded grandiosity and his demands that the psychoanalytic situation should reinstate the position of exclusive control, of being admired and catered to by a doting mother. . . . For a long time the patient opposed these interpretations with intense resistances. He blew up in rages at me, time after time. . . . The first year and a half of his analysis was dominated by his rage. These attacks arose in response to my interpretations concerning his narcissistic demands and his arrogant feelings of "entitlement." (p. 5)

Only after a year and a half did the patient's rage abate and then it abated in response to something Kohut had said, without consciously realizing its implications. What mitigated Z's rage was Kohut's saying: "of course it hurts when one is not given what one assumes to be one's due" (p. 5). Kohut was thus implying that Mr. Z was in some way entitled to his "narcissistic" rage, instead of just "arrogant." As I interpret what happened, Kohut was now treating Z's humiliated fury as an inevitable or at least an appropriate response to which he was entitled because he had experienced an injury to the self—he had not been given his "due." As I interpret the change, Kohut now understood and accepted that Z was processing shame-rage.

In the second analysis, Mr. Z's demandingness was met by Kohut with an underlying belief not in classical drive theory, but with the assumption that Mr. Z had actually suffered a serious deficiency in the quality of his self-objects. Kohut interpreted Mr. Z's rage not as an irrational response to Kohut's failure to be the doting mother, but as an unproductive "burdensome iatrogenic artifact" (p. 12).

One does not need to take sides in the controversy between classical analysis and self-psychology over the nature of neurotic developmental history to see that Kohut was confronting Mr. Z's shame-rage. In the first year and a half Kohut did not understand that Mr. Z was "entitled" to his shame-rage whenever he perceived that Kohut was shaming him by interpreting Mr. Z's behavior as "infantile," "deluded," "arrogant," or "grandiose." Wile (1984) has given us an excellent review of the interpretations made by Kohut and Kernberg as "accusatory." While I agree that they are accusatory, I would amend Wile's term to call the interpretations shaming. Patients are not being interpreted as having commited moral transgressions so much as they are implicitly being told that they are failing in their adulthood.

Whether or not Mr. Z's mother was doting or intrusive and so evoked his Oedipus complex, thus depriving him of a mirroring self-object for his healthy exhibitionism (Kohut, 1979), she was bound to have evoked Mr. Z's shame and humiliated fury by either her positive or negative excessive attention. The question of how to understand and how to further interpret Mr. Z's humiliated fury or shame-rage thus becomes the essential point of therapeutic technique. Humiliated fury needs to be understood and therefore interpreted as a "feeling trap." On the one hand, it is a "subjective" reaction; it is "only" about the self. It is thus being processed by the person as "inappropriate," or shameful. Shame breeds more shame of being "inappropriate." It is simultaneously evoking a rage reaction both at the self for being humiliated and at the other, who has been experienced as betraying, disapproving, or scornful. Humiliated fury is inevitably directed against the offending other, and retaliatory impulses are evoked to "turn the tables" on the other. (Freud described this dynamism beautifully in *A Child Is Being Beaten*, 1919). To the extent that the other is beloved, however, there is much risk in retaliatory fantasies and impulses. Not only is there the risk of further estrangement and loss, but of injury to the other, for which the self is immediately in a state of guilt. Humiliated fury is a state to which one does and does not feel *entitled*. Whether or not one feels entitled to it, it is a state one cannot help. The contrast between humiliated fury and righteous indignation to which one does feel unambiguosly entitled makes it easier to follow the course of humiliated fury. Horowitz (1981) has observed the humiliated fury in the state he calls "*self*-righteous rage." Kohut's realization that Mr. Z was somehow entitled to his rage seems to me to be a step toward the recognition of the inevitability of humiliated fury when one is shamed. The recognition of shame as a universal fact of the human attachment condition rather than ipso facto a pathologic remnant of primitive narcissism creates a more accepting atmosphere for states of shame. Kohut has thus come a long way from his 1971 formulation of shame as a result of the flooding of the ego with "unneutralized exhibitionism" (p. 181). What is flooded in shame is not the ego but the self. If the ego were not simultaneously registering an incongruity there would be no shame. In short, there is a mixed cognitive message in shame-rage: that one *is* and is *not* entitled to this rage. This ambiguity can be crazy-making. In any case, Kohut's acceptance of Mr. Z's rage as a "burdensome iatrogenic artifact" (p. 12) seems to coincide with my observation that failure to analyze the shame that is existential in the patient–therapist relationship is a frequent source of therapeutic impasse.

## 2. *SHAME AND FIELD DEPENDENCE*

My attention to the phenomena of shame developed only gradually over the first 15 years of my work as a practicing analyst.

The idea that shame is neglected in treatment became particularly salient as I tried to understand my own, unpredicted therapeutic failures. At the same time, I was actively collaborating with H. A. Witkin and others in the research on the cognitive style we came to call "field dependence" (Witkin et al., 1954).

Very briefly, field dependence/independence refers to performance on a series of standardized tests of a person's capacity to disembed a "figure" from its embedding context or ground. There are stable, consistent individual differences from early adolescence on in the extent of field dependence. One test requires a person to find a hidden geometric figure in a maze of embedding lines. Even when the position of the self is at issue, people differ in the extent to which they can "decontextualize." For example, forced to rely only on a luminous tilted frame (in an otherwise darkened room) some people perceive a luminous stick as "straight" when it is parallel to the tilted frame. These same people experience their bodies as "straight" when the chair in which they are sitting is tilted 35 degrees in the same direction as a tilted room. Other people experience the stick or the self as upright in space no matter what the degree of tilt in the framework.

Our hypothesis, since confirmed in more than 30 years of research, (Witkin, 1965) was that this cognitive style would have many clinical implications, one of which is a connection to shame and guilt.

Field dependence is a construct that we pursued partly because it was congenial to a psychodynamic view of perception. The idea that personality style might be reflected in characteristic modes of orienting oneself in space was developed as part of the "New Look" at cognition that characterized the psychology of perception in the late 1940s and early 1950s. Field dependence is a cognitive style that catches the self in relation not only to its physical surround but in relation to significant others. It should also be noted in passing, that the Gestalt psychologist, Wertheimer, whose work we were extending, had a working concept of the self as early as 1912. Similarly, Freudian revisionists during the 1940s and 1950s, principally Horney and H. S. Sullivan, were also developing a working concept of the self. It is thus somewhat ironic that self-psychology has only recently been rediscovered by Kohut and others as a necessary addition to classical psychoanalytic thinking.

During the 1960s, Witkin, Edmund Weil, and myself (Witkin, Lewis, & Weil, 1968) planned and executed a study in which we predicted that field-dependent patients would be more prone to shame than to guilt in their first therapeutic encounters, whereas field-independent patients would be more prone to guilt than to shame. The transcripts of the first two psychotherapy sessions of "pairs" of field-dependent and field-independent patients in treatment with the same therapist were assessed for their implied affective content by Gottschalk and Gleser's (1969) reliable and valid method. As predicted, field-dependent patients showed significantly more shame anxiety than guilt anxiety, whereas field-independent patients showed significantly more guilt than shame.

Our success in predicting the occurrence of shame and guilt in therapeutic sessions helped to persuade me that my focus on shame was grounded on some psychological realities. I was also encouraged to undertake my phenomenologic study of shame and guilt (Lewis, 1971).

Our study of field-dependent and field-independent patients also yielded evidence that, as one might expect on an introspective basis alone, shame and self-directed hostility occur in conjunction with each other. This finding was subsequently confirmed (Safer, 1975; Smith, 1972). Guilt, in contrast and surprisingly, occurred in our transcripts in conjunction with hostility directed outward and inward with about equal frequency.

Once the results on shame and field dependence and on guilt and field independence were in place, they joined a network of connections for predicting forms of psychopathology (Witkin, 1965), including sex differences in proneness to depression and paranoia (Lewis, 1976, 1985). Robust evidence now connects field dependence and depression. Field independence, as might be expected, is linked to paranoia. The well-established sex difference in field dependence neatly parallels the sex differences in proneness to depression and paranoia, especially between the ages of 15 and 35 (Lewis, 1976, 1985). This congruence between sex differences in cognitive style and in forms of pathology may be connected to shame and guilt as possible mediators of the differences. Smith (1972) predicted and confirmed a connection between shame and depression. Izard (1972) has amassed good evidence for the existence of shame in the emotion profiles of depressed patients. The projection of guilt in paranoia has been an accepted clinical observation since Freud's (1911) unraveling of Schreber's delusions. The empirical evidence, however, for the connection between guilt and paranoia is less well developed than the evidence for a connection between shame and depression.

It is worth noting, in passing, that the distinction between shame and guilt may be of use in differentiating varieties of depression. Blatt's (1974) contrast between anaclitic and introjective depression may overlap the categories of shame and guilt, respectively. Grinker, Werble, and Drye's (1968) description of the depression experience particularly characterized by "loneliness and emptiness" may parallel both Blatt's anaclitic depression and the shame-prone superego mode.

An empirical study of guilt and conscience in the major depressive disorders suggests that "negative self-esteem" rather than guilt "forms the cornerstone" in depressed patients of all types (Prosen, Clark, Harrow, & Fawcett, 1983). Shame may be understood as the affective-cognitive state that accompanies "low self-esteem."

Evidence from cognitive and behavioral approaches to depression strongly suggests the usefulness of considering shame as a major component of depression (Lewis, 1986a). In a reformulation of learned helplessness theory, for example, Abramson, Seligman, and Teasdale (1978) suggest that depression is the end product of a faulty attributional style in which people focus on their personal helplessness. Specifically, learned helplessness theory assumes that people who attribute the causes of "bad events" to "internal," "stable," and "global" personal traits (what have been called ISG attributions) are likely to be depressed.

In a further refinement of ISG style, Peterson, Schwartz, and Seligman (1981) have found that depressed women undergraduates were more likely to blame their *characters* for bad events than they were to blame specific *behaviors*. (If anything, blame for behaviors was negatively correlated with depression.) If we equate blame of the self for its character with shame and blame for behaviors with guilt, we may glimpse a convergence of evidence from behavioral and psychoanalytic sources suggesting the role of shame in depression. Indeed, the most hopeful sign of fruitful collaboration between behavior theorists and psychoanalysts is the evidence provided by Peterson, Luborsky, and Seligman (1983) that depressive mood can be predicted from ISG attributions.

Behavior theorists have described a cognitive paradox in depression: If depressed people are as helpless as they feel, logic dictates that they should not also feel self-reproaches (guilt) for what they are unable to do (Abramson & Sackeim, 1977; Peterson, 1977; Rizley, 1978). This paradox vanishes, however, if we assume that depressed people are helpless to change the vicarious experience of another's negative feeling about the self (i.e., to get out of a state of shame). Humiliated fury won't do it; expressing such fury is likely to get the self into even more trouble with the other, especially as humiliated fury is felt by the self to be inappropriate and blameworthy, leading to guilt as well as shame.

One small finding of a behavioral study (Lamont, 1973) seems to capture the essence of the connection between shame and depression. In this study, the following cognitive message was demonstrated to have a strong effect on dysphoric people. It read: "We don't have that much control over other people's feelings [no shame at loss] and we don't have to feel responsible for how other people feel [no guilt]" (p. 320; the brackets enclose my interpolations).

## 3. *THE PHENOMENOLOGY OF SHAME AND GUILT*

As already indicated, an important source for my study of the two states was the 180 transcripts of psychotherapy sessions collected in the course of our research into the connection between field dependence and shame and guilt (Witkin *et al.*, 1968). The phenomenology of shame and guilt involves an examination of the two affective states with respect to the position of the self in the field of experience. From the fact that it is necessary (often difficult) to identify states of shame and guilt and their sequelae, it is obvious that both states involve considerable gaps in awareness. In this respect, I follow Freud's description of the superego as partly unconscious. In particular, states of shame and guilt often exist without being correctly identified by the patient. In addition, shame is often unacknowledged because it is extremely painful and perceived as irrational. There is also a state I call "bypassed" shame, in which events that might evoke shame are registered or noted by a "wince" or "jolt" to the self. Ensuing ideation then takes the form of thinking about what negative (shaming) thoughts the therapist would have about the patient. The ideation following bypassed shame is often difficult to distinguish from guilty ideation. Acute, unidentified, or unacknowledged shame is often hard to distinguish from its rapid transformation into depressive ideation. Unidentified guilt is usually experienced in transformation as obsessive worry or fear (dread) of specific happenings, which are unconsciously assumed to be appropriate punishments.

There are three aspects of the concept of the self that are involved in a comparison of the states. These are: the self as an "identity," the self as a "boundary," and the self as a "localization" of experience "inside" or "outside" the self.

The self refers to a registration of experience as belonging to one's own *identity*. In this respect, shame and guilt are both registered as one's own experience. Shame, however, involves more self-consciousness and more self-imaging than guilt. The experience of shame is directly about the self, which is the focus of a negative evaluation. In guilt, it is the thing done or undone that is the direct focus of negative evaluation. We say, "I am ashamed of myself" and "I am guilty of having done (or not done) something." Because the self is the focus of awareness in shame, "identity" imagery is usually evoked. At the same time that this identity imagery is registering as one's own experience, there is also vivid imagery of the self in the other's eyes. This creates a "doubleness of experience," which is characteristic of shame. This double experience is a frequent basis for what Freud called "internal theater" of the self in its own and other's eyes that is so characteristic of hysterical patients.

A second aspect of the self is that it has boundaries that distinguish the self's experiences and the "other's" experiences. The boundaries are often routinely and safely crossed when one has a vicarious experience with someone emotionally close. Even when two people have not been previously close, the self may function vicariously. In experiments involving the Zeigarnik (1927) effect, it could be demonstrated that when two people were working cooperatively, there was no difference in recall between those tasks personally completed and those actually completed by the cooperating partner (Lewis, 1944; Lewis and Franklin, 1944). Shame is the vicarious experience of the other's negative evaluation. In order for shame to occur, there must be a relationship between the self and the other in which the self cares about the other's evaluation. This is a particularly important point because shame is often given the narrow meaning of either "fear of getting caught" or else a "narcissistic" reaction. The other is also an important figure in the shame experience, usually in the position of being admired. Fascination with the other and sensitivity to the other's treatment of the self renders the self more vulnerable to shame. Shame is actually close to the feeling of awe. It is also the feeling state in which one is susceptible to falling in love.

Guilt also involves the self in vicarious experience. But it is the experience of the other's harm, injury, or suffering. By implication, the self is able, has done, or has not done something. At the moment of shame, in contrast, the self is unable to avoid the vicarious experience of the other's negative evaluation of the self. In guilt, vicarious experience involves a self suffering the (admired or beloved) other's disapproval or scorn.

A third aspect of the self is that it is a perceptual product that localizes experiences as originating "out there" or "within the self." Both localizations, however, are registered as one's own experience. Shame, which involves more self-consciousness and more self-imaging than guilt, is likely to involve a greater increase in feedback from all perceptual modalities. Shame thus has a special affinity for stirring autonomic reactions, including blushing, sweating, and increased heart rate. Shame usually involves more bodily awareness than guilt, as well as visual and verbal imaging of the self from the other's point of view. Shame is thus a more acutely painful experience than guilt. Because the self is involved in imagery of itself in relation to others, it can appear as if shame originates "out there," whereas guilt appears to originate "within." This characteristic makes shame appear to be a more primitive or irrational reaction than guilt. Both states, however, involve the self in trying to maintain affectional ties to significant others. Shame is the experience of losing self-esteem in one's own and others' eyes. It is the experience of failure. Guilt is the experience of injuring others or things and requires that one make appropriate reparation.

There are intrinsic difficulties in the states of shame and guilt that can impede their resolution or discharge. These may be grouped under three headings. First, difficulties in recognizing one's own psychological state can arise from the fact that shame and guilt are often fused and therefore confused. Shame and guilt may both be evoked simultaneously by a moral transgression. The two states then tend to fuse as the experience of guilt. The dictionary confirms this observation by defining shame as an acute or "emotional" sense of guilt (Lewis, 1971). Shame of oneself is thus likely to be operating underneath guilt for transgression.

The self-reproaches that are likely to be formed as guilty ideation develops might run as follows: "How could I have *done that?* What an injurious *thing to do.* How I have *hurt* so-and-so. What a moral lapse that *act* was. What will *happen to* (or *become of*) him or her? How should I be *punished?* What must I *do* to *make amends? Mea culpa!*" Simultaneously, shame ideation says; "How could *I* have done that? What a *fool*—what a *bad person*—not like *so-and-so,* who does not do such things. *How worthless I am. For shame!*"

When shame and guilt are evoked simultaneously by transgression, the shame or personal failure component, although acute, can be buried in guilty ideation and remain active even after appropriate amends have been made. This is a frequent source of unresolved obsessive dilemmas.

A second difficulty in the resolution of states of shame and guilt arises from the fact that the stimulus to shame can be twofold: Either a moral transgression or a failure can evoke shame. Ausubel (1955) has drawn attention to the twofold stimulus evoking shame, distinguishing between moral and nonmoral shame. When nonmoral shame is evoked, it readily connects with moral shame. For example, under the press of shame for competitive defeat or sexual rebuff, one can begin an immediate search for the transgressions that make sense of the injury one has suffered. Thus, shame has a potential for a wide range of associative connections between failures of the self and its transgressions.

There are many varieties of shame phenomena that need to be identified accurately. Mortification, humiliation, embarrassment, feeling ridiculous, chagrin, shyness, and modesty are all different psychological states, but with the common property of being directly about the self and overtly involving the other as referent in the experience. As a beginning to the study of these states, I treat them as variants of the shame family, but with different admixtures of pride and of self-directed hostility. Humiliation, for example, is experienced either in one's own or in the other's eyes and can involve rapid shifts of position of the self from one stance to the other. Embarrassment, to take another example, involves the self in a feeling of temporary paralysis or loss of powers in relation to the other. Mortification, in contrast, has a clear element of conscious, wounded pride and involves the self in a more distant relationship to the other.

Most important for the appropriate discharge of the shame state is the awareness that shame can be discharged in good-humored laughter at the self and its relation to the other. After all, shame is "only about the self." This is an observation that Freud (1905) first made in his remarkable study of the way jokes dissolve humiliation (for a fuller treatment, see Lewis, 1983). Because shame responses are so florid and so painful, however, there has been a tendency to regard them as pathologic regressions, a view that coincides with the patient's shameful imagery of himself or herself. One is ashamed of being ashamed, thus compounding the difficulty of finding a rational solution in some gentle ridicule. Retzinger (1985), using videotapes of people experiencing resentment has demonstrated experimentally that laughter reduces both shame and hostility.

Guilt, in contrast, is about things. It therefore has an "objective" quality (Heider, 1958). It is this objective quality that has led theoreticians to regard guilt as a higher order response than shame. It is often difficult, however, to assess the degree of one's responsibility or to assess the degree of punishment that is appropriate. When guilt is evoked, it can thus merge into a "problem" of the rational assignment of motivation, responsibility, and consequences. As the person becomes involved in these problems, it can happen that guilty affect subsides, whereas ideation about how to make amends continues. Guilt thus has an affinity for "insoluble dilemmas" in which the self is active, self-contained, but unable to stop thinking about what to do. (The Rat Man is a classic example of the profound connection between unresolved guilt, bypassed shame, and insoluble obsessive dilemmas; see Lewis, 1971.) In addition, the unconscious gratification of being in a morally elevated state of guilt sometimes keeps the state active beyond the time of restitution or expiation.

A third difficulty intrinsic in both shame and guilt is encountered in discharging the hostility that is naturally evoked in both states. In shame, hostility against the self is experienced in the passive mode, as emanating from the other. (Indeed, in many instances, this perception is accurate.) When shame is evoked by personal betrayal or by unrequited love, the self feels crushed by the rejection. The self feels not in control but overwhelmed and paralyzed by the hostility directed against it. One could "crawl through a hole," "sink through the floor," or "die" with shame. The self feels small, helpless, and childish. So long as shame is to the fore in consciousness, it is the other who is experienced as the source of hostility. Hostility against the rejecting or betraying other is almost simultaneously evoked. But it is humiliated fury, or shame-rage, which is simultaneously being processed as "inappropriate" or "unjust" fury. To be furious and enraged with someone because one is unloved by him (or her) renders one easily and simultaneously guilty for being unjustly enraged. Evoked hostility is readily redirected back on the vulnerable self in the form of more shame and guilt. Evoked shame-rage, moreover, inevitably produces retaliatory feelings that "turn the tables" on the other. But so long as the other continues to be loved or valued, the awareness of one's humiliated fury is muted, and it is "turned back upon the self" transformed into depression.

When hostility is evoked in connection with guilt, what is experienced is righteous indignation, which is considered an "appropriate" reaction. The consciousness of guilt and its appropriateness may actually be a quiet source of gratification in being morally elevated. Righteous indignation requires the correct assessment of blame, and the ideation that develops is busy determining responsibility both of the self and of others. The position of the self as the initiator of guilt puts the self "in charge" of the allocation of blame and of the assessment of happenings in the field. The active role of the self in guilt opens the possibility that hostility may be directed not only against the self but against the other and against forces in the field, thus creating an affinity between guilt and the projection of hostility. The affinity between guilt and the necessity to do something to make amends creates a readiness to transform guilt into obsessive ideation. The projection of hostility outward creates the familiar transformation of guilt into paranoia.

Table 3-1 summarizes the phenomenologic description of shame and guilt and the working concepts that emerge.

## *4. TECHNIQUES OF ANALYZING SHAME AND GUILT*

My technique of conducting psychoanalysis has changed radically since my first case under "classical" Freudian supervision in 1945. The kernel of my present technique is a focus on the sequelae of unresolved states of shame and guilt into symptom formulation. Freud's original discovery was that neurotic symptoms develop out of forbidden sexual longings. My focus on shame and guilt picks up on the "forbidden" aspects of experience. It relies heavily on Freud's description of primary process transformations—symptoms and dream content—that are created under the press of forbidden longings. In its microscopic analysis of patients' streams of consciousness, my technique is thus very classical, but in other respects, it is quite unorthodox.

Elsewhere (Lewis, 1981, 1983) I have detailed the changes in Freud's theoretical formulations that I now consider necessary. I list these here only very briefly.

1. I have abandoned Freud's metapsychology because it rests on a mistaken concept of primary human narcissism. This is contrary to our newer information about infants' extraordinary sociability.
2. I have replaced Freud's narrow theoretical framework with a broader theory that assumes the cultural or social nature of human beings. This is more consonant with anthropological

**Table 3-1.** Summary of Phenomenology of Shame and Guilt

| | Shame | Guilt |
|---|---|---|
| Stimulus | Disappointment, defeat, or moral transgression | Moral transgression |
| | Deficiency of *self* | Event; *thing* for which self is responsible |
| | Involuntary; self *unable*, as in unrequited love | Voluntary; self able |
| | Encounter with "other" or within the self | Within the self |
| Conscious content | Painful emotion | Affect may or may not be present |
| | Autonomic responses: rage, blushing, tears | Autonomic responses less pronounced |
| | Global characteristics of self | Specific activities of self |
| | Identity thoughts; "internal theater" | No identity thoughts |
| Position of self in field | Self passive | Self active |
| | Self focal in awareness | Self absorbed in action or thought |
| | Self-imaging and consciousness; multiple functions of self | Self intact, functioning silently |
| | Vicarious experience of other's negative view of self | Pity; concern for welfare |
| Nature and discharge of hostility | Humiliated fury | Righteous indignation |
| | Discharge blocked by guilt and/or love of "other" | Discharge on self and other |
| Characteristic symptoms | Depression; hysteria "affect disorder" | Obsessional; paranoid "thought disorder" |

Shame variants: humiliation, mortification, embarrassment, chagrin, shyness
Guilt variants: responsibility, obligation, fault, blame

evidence that human beings are everywhere organized into societies governed by moral law.

3. I have adopted the hypothesis that human culture is our species' evolutionary adaptation to life. Moral law is thus immanent in human life.
4. In this new framework, the self, however narcissistic or egotistical it appears, is a quintessentially social phenomenon.
5. Sex differences in the organization of the self are inevitable as a result of differences.
6. I assume that shame and guilt are the affective-cognitive signals to the self that its basic affectional ties are threatened.
7. Symptoms arise when both shame and guilt are evoked and cannot be appropriately discharged.
8. Differences in symptom formation depend on whether shame or guilt is to the fore in the person's experience (see Table 3-1).

This focus on evoked, undischarged states of shame and guilt and their sequelae is very different from my earlier mode of listening for echoes of the past in the context of the "timeless unconscious." The focus sharply distinguishes between the transference and the patient–therapist relationship. Not all the events that occur in the patient–therapist relationship are transferential, because shame and guilt are part of every session. The focus thus intensifies the "existensial" analysis of the patient–therapist relationship. This vigilance in pursuing the patient–therapist relationship makes it easier to retrieve and rework illuminating transferences from the past. Even more important, it helps prevent symptom formation as a side effect of treatment itself.

It has been my experience that patients benefit from this guided tour through their own "superego" upheavals. A particular therapeutic boon is that the focus makes it easier for the patient to see that it is s/he who is being judgmental, not the therapist. The therapeutic situation becomes less painful because the therapist is experienced as more accepting and supportive of the self than is the patient. The inevitable shame evoked by this contrast is itself a fruitful source of insight into the sequence from shame into humiliated fury and thence into guilt for "unjustified" hostility. It has been my experience that patients who do not have the prior expectation that treatment should last several years have been able to terminate in a relatively short time. I now routinely practice a form of dynamic focused psychotherapy that often, although not always, turns out to be short term. Professional therapists in training with me are one exception to this description. The endless demand on one's shame and guilt that being a therapist entails requires a more rigorous code of self-understanding than most non-therapists need. For the rest, although I am not in a hurry to terminate, I am much more receptive to patients' suggestions that they are ready than I used to be when a 2-year stretch seemed the irreducible minimum that could be useful.

There are a number of specific ways in which a focus on the sequences from undischarged shame into humiliated fury and guilt improves therapeutic efficiency. I have often been asked whether there are not other emotional states that are of equal interest to the analyst.

My answer is that of course there are many other important emotions, but we who deal with mental illness are mainly dealing with people's forbidden longing—their unresolved moral dilemmas about how to manage the risks of attachment. In any case, there is now fairly strong empirical evidence that neurotics differ from their normal counterparts not so much in the deficiency of their moral judgments and behavior (i.e., in their moral transgressions) as in the pervasiveness of their low self-esteem (Wylie, 1979).

### *Achieving Benign Neutrality*

The first advantage of a focus on sequences from undischarged shame and guilt is that the analyst can more readily achieve the stance of benign neutrality that is so essential to the therapeutic enterprise. Because the analyst is listening for the affective state, s/he is less likely to become caught up in the cognitive content or "reality" of the patient's guilty or shameful ideation.

The reality or correctness of a patient's self-description is always difficult to assess. What the analyst (and the patient) can be sure of is the immediate feeling state out of which the self-description emerges, and the negative or positive feeling state that this self-description thus reflects. Freud (1917), it will be remembered, had difficulty assessing the "reality" of the depressive patient's self-reproaches. On the one hand, he wondered "why a man has to be ill before he can be accessible to a truth [namely, that he is] . . . petty, egoistic, dishonest, lacking in independence, one whose sole aim is to hide the weakness of his own nature" (p. 246). On the other hand (and on the next page), Freud takes the view that there is "no correspondence, so far as we can judge between the degree of self-abasement and its real justification. A good, capable, conscientious woman will speak no better of herself after she develops melancholia than one who is in fact worthless" (p. 247). The analyst is clearly on firmer ground if s/he does not take a position on the content of the patient's self-reproaches, but rather calls the patient's attention to his or her affective state of shame or guilt. My technique thus minimizes the danger that the therapist will get caught up in analyzing the *content* of the patient's (often rational) self-reproaches, without first calling the patient's attention to his or her implicit state of shame or guilt.

Here is a vignette that illustrates the problem. In his first consultation hour with me, Patient Y, a 25-year-old man, a successful intellectual, stated the reason for seeking treatment as follows:

> I am totally self-destructive. That's what Q says [the wife of one of his closest friends, who had urged him to undertake treatment], and she's right. I used to be a leader. Now I'm withdrawn in a corner, not myself, brooding, depressed [shame]. I know what the trouble is: [guilt] I'm jealous. I need a job that gives me more scope. If I thought that getting a better job would make me happy, I wouldn't go into treatment. But I know better.

In this account by the patient of his difficulties, we find a sweeping, global negative generalization about himself. The patient feels he is so self-destructive that even if he *did something*, that is, get a better job, he wouldn't be happy and would still need treatment. The patient is somewhat aware of his guilt over jealousy but much less aware of shame.

It is tempting for the therapist to get caught up in the cognitive content of the patient's shameful and guilty ideation. For example, one could set the analytic task as finding the childhood reasons why Y is so jealous and so self-destructive. Instead, it is important to point out to the patient that he is in an acute state of being ashamed of himself and guilty, as well, for jealousy.

The patient is dissatisfied with himself for "jealousy"; his idea about it is that jealousy has transformed him into a brooding, depressed person. Although he is quite aware of the feeling of jealousy and is guilty about it, he is not aware that he is ashamed of this feeling and, moreover, that being in a state of jealousy (more accurately, envy) is a feeling of being somehow inferior to the other (i.e., ashamed). That rage accompanies this feeling, and that humiliated fury finds the self as its principal target, is what needs to be unraveled so that the sequence between feeling "jealous" (shame) and feeling depressed does not automatically occur.

In this first consultation session, the problem was set as "finding the sequence" that leads to depression. It was also possible to convey to the patient that he felt as guilty about his jealousy as if it were a "voluntary" reaction instead of a "natural" or inescapable reaction. The sweeping generalization implied in his remarks about himself was thus made more specific. That he was processing shame was also called to his attention.

### *Distinguishing Between Shame and Guilt Improves the Accuracy of Interpretation*

A brief reinterpretation of an acknowledged "mistake" by a distinguished psychoanalyst can be used to illustrate the difficulty that arises from inaccuracy. Malan (1976) describes an incident early in his work with brief dynamic psychotherapy in which an ill-chosen interpretation may have contributed to a worsening of the patient's condition. Here is the incident:

> A man walked into a hospital where I was casualty officer, complaining of the fear that he might kill his wife. Questioning revealed that while he was serving abroad in the Army during the war his wife had an affair with another man and had had a child. Being inexperienced and full of enthusiasm for the power of interpretation, I said to him: "So you have good reason to want to kill your wife." He made no clear response to this and went off. Two days later he came back in an exalted state, demanding of everybody: "Do you believe in the Lord?" He was clearly psychotic and had to be admitted as an emergency patient.

Malan's interpretation had sympathized with and probably increased the patient's humiliated fury. It did not pick up on the patient's more proximal complaint: that he was afraid he would kill his wife. The patient was, without being aware of it, in a state of guilt for what he wanted to do to his wife. Translating "I am afraid I will kill her" into "You must be in a state of guilt for wanting to kill her" is not only accurate, but it reminds the patient of his own good judgment. Although the patient's guilt state is unrecognized by him, its existence is nevertheless the source of his fear of what he might compulsively do: commit a crime and an injustice in the name of bringing justice to his wife. Guilt clearly rests on the humiliated fury or shame-rage that the patient has been harboring and simultaneously recognizing as unjust. His psychotic symptom can be understood as a condensation of his scorn or ridicule of the therapist who tacitly gives him permission to kill as if he (and the therapist) were the Lord.

*Identifying Rational-Sounding Obsessive Ideation.*

Attention to the sequence from shame into guilt helps to identify obsessive ideation that is rational in content (egosyntonic) but nevertheless represents a primary process transformation.

Here is a brief vignette from the analysis of a 26-year-old man—attractive, successful, intellectual—who entered analysis with me for sexual impotence of 4 years duration. Some 4 years previously, at the moment when he had overcome severe conscientious scruples (guilt) against intercourse (without lasting commitment to his fiancee) and had had first intercourse with her, she remarked that she was "worried" about his potency because he had been so tardy in taking her to bed. The patient was unaware of a shame reaction to his fiancee's unconsciously cruel (shaming) remark. He remembered vividly, however her saying "I was worried about you" at the same time that he noticed "the semen running down her thighs." He remembered being nagged by the thought, later that night, that there was "something wrong with his capacity to love" since he had not been so joyous as he expected to be after their first intercourse. A few months later, he and his fiancee broke up, and she shortly married someone else. The next time he had intercourse with another woman, and then for the subsequent 4 years with different women, he lost his erection.

It was possible to show the patient the sequence from bypassed shame at his lover's interpretation of his scruples into humiliated fury and thence into obsessive ideation. It should be noted that the initial absence of fury left the image of his beloved intact—it was her shaming view of him that he somehow internalized. The ensuing obsessive ideation about his potency was not "crazy," since he was regularly losing his erection. The patient was himself aware that it would be better if he were not so "anxious." But he could not shake his anxiety. Once he connected his bypassed shame with his inevitable shame-rage at his beloved, he could see the sequence from this state into unbidden, intrusive, persistent thoughts (obsessive ideation) about the potency she had devalued. It should be noted that I use the term primary-process to describe the sequence and the transformation of thought under the press of undischarged shame and guilt, without assuming that we understand the processes involved, only that we can describe a relatively predictable sequence.

## *5. SOME CLINICAL EXAMPLES OF THE NEGLECT OF SHAME*

### *The Case of Dora*

Perhaps the clearest way to illustrate the clinical implications of recognizing the role of shame in depression is to review a much studied case, that of Dora (Freud, 1905). The difficulty Freud experienced in treating his young depressed-hysterical woman patient, Dora, is a classic example of the neglect of shame, and a classic example, as well, of sexism in psychiatry (still apparent today). As we read the case today, we can see that even though Dora had experienced personal betrayal at the hands of the people she loved most dearly—her father, Herr K, and Frau K—both Freud and Dora missed her most powerful feeling: the shame of personal betrayal, that is, of lost trust or broken attachment. Even when they explicitly named her feeling "mortification" (a shame variant), neither Freud nor Dora permitted themselves to take it "seriously." Because they were both unable to deal with Dora's shame, except to deprecate the rage it evoked as "exaggerated," Dora unexpectedly left treatment in what Freud felt, quite accurately, was a burst of revenge. But Freud had no idea of what he had done to deserve it. And Dora must have come away from the experience with the feeling that she could not find vindication anywhere, while still being ashamed of wanting it. Twenty-five years later, when Felix Deutsch was called into psychiatric consultation for her, Dora was still struggling with feelings of mortification.

Dora's actual situation at the time of her suicide note was this: Her father was having an affair with Frau K. Because of this affair with his friend's wife, it was convenient for Dora's father to look away from the sexual advances Herr K was making toward his adolescent daughter. When Dora told her father about being molested, her father said he did not believe her, although she knew quite well that he actually *did* believe her. His disbelief was dishonest, and thus a double personal betrayal. Frau K, whom Dora loved and for whose children she had often been a devoted "sitter," also disbelieved her. And Herr K, in whose affection for her she had once trusted, had become a sexual molester, not an indulgent father-figure. It is fascinating to realize the profound influence of the patriarchal system in which these events took place. Freud himself was of the opinion that the normal "female" response to Herr K's advances should have been pleasure, and that Dora's disgust was a measure of her unconscious guilt for oedipal fantasies. That her inevitable response to personal betrayal would be shame-rage was simply not recognized by either Freud or Dora, although Dora was clearly in the grip of humiliated fury. Freud puts it this way: "When she was feeling embittered she used to be overcome by the idea that she had been handed over to Herr K as the price of his tolerating the relations between her father and his wife; and the rage at her father for making such use of her was visible behind her affection for him. At other times she was quite well aware that she had been guilty of exaggerating in talk like this. The two men had, of course, *never made a formal agreement in which she was the object of barter;* her father in particular would have been horrified at any such suggestion" (p. 50, my emphasis). There was clearly no place in Freud's cognitive system for the shame-rage that broken attachment evokes. Dora was also all too ready to repair her attachment bond with her father by exculpating him and blaming herself, a state that generated her depression as well as her hysterical symptoms. Although Freud intuitively connected her symptoms to the molestation she had suffered, it was his neglect of shame in both the sexual abuse and the personal betrayal that made the analysis a failure.

*A Field-Dependent Young Woman Depressive*

Some excerpts from the transcripts of dynamic psychotherapy sessions with a 21-year-old woman, a college senior, extremely field-dependent, who participated in our study of field-dependent and field-independent patients (Witkin *et al.*, 1968) illustrate with great clarity the neglect of shame. The excerpts also illustrate that pejorative attitudes toward attachment and shame are still current in psychoanalytic psychotherapy nearly a hundred years after Freud treated Dora.

This patient, FD2, had applied for treatment for depression and, also with the hope that treatment might alleviate the facial tics with which she had been afflicted since childhood. The first excerpt illustrates how acutely painful a shame reaction can be. Although the patient is describing acute shame in a metaphor of death, the therapist's response is not an empathetic one; he counters by questioning her metaphor. The patient dutifully retreats to a literal meaning, but continues to express her shame in another metaphor. She also indicates quite clearly that her tics are increased when she is in a shame state, but the therapist does not pursue the connection. Throughout the lengthy transcript from which this excerpt is derived neither the patient nor the therapist actually labelled her state as "shame."

P: When I find somebody looking at me [at her tics] I could die.

T: Could die?

P: Well, not literally (*slight laugh*) that's when I sort of have the feeling that I could crawl through a hole. That's when I do these habits the most.

The second excerpt illustrates the way in which laughter

tends to relieve shame. Once again, however, the therapist takes a questioning rather than an empathetic stance toward the patient's laughter. Once again, the patient dutifully agrees that "it's not funny," but continues to describe how laughter relieves shame. The patient makes very clear also how shame dissipates when she is reassured that an important affectional tie—to her boyfriend—is no longer in jeopardy. The therapist, however, interprets her shame about her tics as if it were an irrational "way of keeping other people from knowing about it" rather than as a natural phenomenon, in which concealment of defects seems urgent in order to maintain affectional bonds. The patient had been describing how "her own mother" used to shame her about the tics. "I was told that I was very stupid and if I only knew how I looked, I wouldn't do it (*slight laugh*). So I mean if my own mother told me that it looks horrible, I believed her (*laugh*)."

P: I was always very self-conscious in a—with people around, and always imagining that I looked horrible. And as I said, I don't really know how I look. It's just, well you know—and it disturbs me a lot. And I feel very—like when people kept looking at me (*slight laugh*).

T: Feel like everybody's looking at you?

P: Yeah. I feel like I'm such an oddity that everybody's looking. "What is that girl doing?" (*laugh*)

T: But you smile and laugh as you say that—

P: Well . . . (*slight laugh*) not that I think it's funny, but it's a curious feeling that I have, I perhaps can laugh. I can laugh about it now, more than I could even last year. I mean up until last year I couldn't even talk about it, much less laugh about it. You know it was a very, very sensitive sore spot, and the reason I can more or less laugh at it—if you want to call it that—it's not really funny, but I started talking about it with my boyfriend . . . he was the first one I ever discussed it with; and it was so hard for me I couldn't even look him straight in the face. It was just really a horrible experience, but after I spoke about it, I felt much better.

T: Do you think it made any difference to the twitches?

P: No, it didn't (*slight laugh*). It didn't disappear. It didn't subside or anything. The only difference it made was in how I felt about having them myself, and the fact that I didn't have to worry about my boyfriend. He knew about it and he didn't care.

T: It sounds as if you're not talking about it, is just some kind way of keeping other people from knowing about it.

The next excerpt illustrates the way in which the patient's depression is evoked in direct response to her mother's shaming of her boyfriend. She is describing her mother's disapproving reaction to the patient's engagement to be married. The sequence from humiliated fury into depression is discernible.

P: As a child . . . I—we were very affectionate, we were very close. We were just about inseparable. But as I got older and I started dating . . . well, suddenly so much dissension and disagreement and not getting along. . . . She doesn't let me feel optimistic in any way. . . . She has no faith in me, and she has no faith in my boyfriend. And she doesn't know how I feel . . . about constantly ridiculing and criticizing him. Even if she feels that it's true and that she's justified, I don't feel she should do it. Because if I love him, I feel she should take it into consideration and try to give me more confidence in myself and him. She doesn't. No confidence. Constantly criticizing and doom doom doom . . . and I start to believe it because I hear it all the time. And then, if my boyfriend happens to go down in the dumps—I go right with him. I need him; he's my morale . . . he's gotta be there to tell me that things will be all right and that we will have money and that we will be happy. . . . Because when I'm with my family—I might just lay down and die.

T: You take on your mother's opinion?

P: Yeah, I can't help it. I try to fight against—when I'm with them I'll fight down to the end, and yet when I leave I get so depressed, I'm so down in the dumps. And I feel inside of me, a kind of sickness comes over me, and they always do this to me.

The next excerpt illustrates clearly the sequence from shame into humiliated fury and thence into guilt for unjust rage. The patient is describing her reaction to the therapist's failure to keep an appointment without notifying her.

P: But just waiting for the bus—oh (*laugh*) You know I was

really upset (*slight laugh*) because I was upset at the time; I was on the verge of tears . . . because I had this test. I hate just wasting time. I generally am a great time-waster anyway, but I can blame no one but myself. But here I have no control over the situation. You know, I hate that feeling. I hate the feeling of being helpless, and not being able to do anything about. I guess everyone hates that feeling. But it just wore off—given a few days it generally wears off. But the point is . . . I knew that you couldn't be here . . . I am just angry at the situation in general, that you weren't here and I had wasted the day . . . things like this often happen and I just hate the feeling of not being able to do anything . . . it's a sort of like the whole world's against me (*slight laugh*).

T: The whole world instead of me?

P: Yeah, just things in general . . . and there's no one really you can blame . . . rationally, you know, and really feel right about blaming the person. In fact, if I had blamed you I would have felt downright guilty, because I feel I had no grounds. I would have no grounds to be angry at you because you couldn't help it. . . . But it still doesn't take away the feeling of anger, or . . . the frustration.

The final excerpt illustrates the patient's natural tendency to "turn the tables" on the therapist and the therapist's neglect of this aspect of the shame-rage sequence. As we shall see, the consequence is an increase in the patient's symptoms. In this instance, shame in the patient–therapist relationship is probably compounded of the (mutual) assumption of the "doctor's superior wisdom" and the fact that the therapist is a much older (superior) man. We come on the therapy session at a point where the patient is telling the therapist about how easily her mother makes her feel guilty and how "silly" she knows it is for her to feel this way, but she can't help it. As an example, the patient had offered the therapist the prediction that her mother would make her feel guilty about having Thanksgiving dinner with her boyfriend, away from home. The therapist, responding in the spirit of minimizing the mother's power, had suggested that the patient was "worrying too much in advance." The patient's opening comments in the next session, although phrased as a trivial point, were to the effect that the therapist was "wrong." The patient was "right"; her mother did make her feel guilty. The therapist caught that he was being disputed. The patient was signaling to him by her embarrassed laughter that she was making a trivial point—one that he would "hardly later remember." She was already ashamed (guilty) of her need to put him down, but this aspect of the shame-rage sequence went by him. He interpreted her need to show him wrong as a neurotic defense (of which he obviously disapproved). In the next moment, the patient was apparently having some tics. And she was terribly disconcerted by the therapist's calling them to her attention. She actually thought that he might be out to trick her, but for benign therapeutic reasons! She then lost her train of thought, and within moments was off on a depressed train of thought about her many failings: lapses of memory, inability to keep things organized, and excessive anxiety. These failings even include her inability to keep her appointments straight—the very lapse the therapist had made when he had failed to keep their appointment without notifying her. In other words, under the press of unanalyzed shame *vis-à-vis* the trusted male therapist, the patient experienced a temporary increase in her neurotic symptoms.

T: What's on your mind? (*Opening the session*)

P: I just wanted to tell you that . . . the last time when we were talking about . . . I said my mother would have a certain reaction . . . and you sort of thought—at least you sounded like you thought—I didn't have much basis for, you know, thinking that. But sure enough I got the reaction I expected, I mean, frankly, I would have been surprised if . . . maybe even disappointed if I didn't get it. And I got it.

T: You were right.

P: Yeah, when I told her that—you probably have forgotten this thing about my eating over [at] my boyfriend's house Thanksgiving and—I was afraid to tell her because I knew there was gonna be a big uproar and at first just like last year the same pattern. (*A description follows of her quarrel with her mother.*) I mean, I knew she was going to get me upset and that she would make me feel bad—and I was right. And so there you are (*slight laugh*). I wasn't, you know, just making it up. I do have grounds for it because it happens so often.

T: And?

P: I just wanted to tell you, you know, that was the outcome. It did happen.

T: You wanted to tell me you were right.

P: Hm? Because I—you seemed to think that I was showing some sort of pattern there about—I forgot what it was now, but you didn't seem to think that . . . you thought that it was sort silly of me to say that because . . . you know to predict something like that because it might not come true at all. Or something like that. I can't remember exactly. But it did. I didn't [sic!] wanna show you my mother is a rat (*laugh*). (The patient herself had actually called her problem about guilt and Thanksgiving a "silly" one.)

T: But it looks like you want to show me how wrong I was too.

The patient here responds, haltingly, that she was only trying to be helpful. In the next moment, the therapist calls her attention to tics.

T: I got the impression that just there for a moment you were doing some of this nervous twitching.

P: No (*pause*) I . . .

T: No?

P: Not now. Right before you . . .

T: (*Pause*) No?

P: If I was then (*slight laugh*) don't say that!

T: Maybe it's what?

P: If I was and I don't realize it, that's bad (*slight laugh*) Well, if I was (*inaudible*) then I certainly wasn't aware of it and I've never had anyone tell me I was doing it, when I wasn't aware of it. But I really didn't . . . not at that instant.

T: So I must be wrong.

P: Hm?

T: I must be wrong.

P: (*Laugh*) No (*laugh*). What is it a mistaken perception or something like that?

T: I'm seeing things.

P: Yeah (*laugh*) You're not wrong, you're just seeing things (*pause*). Well, you could, you know, just, I, I don't think you can say right or wrong in this situation . . . Did you just say that?

T: What do you mean?

P: (*Laugh*) Are you trying to trick me?

The patient continues to doubt that the therapist actually saw a tic and the he actually said what he did say. The therapist responds by saying, somewhat sarcastically, "You have the feeling that I'm sitting here trying very hard to think up ways of trapping you." He also implies that she ought not to assume that he would "play tricks" on her.

P: No, not really play tricks. You know, I just thought you were trying to bring out a point that I'm trying to disagree with you. Or trying to say that you know "I'm right and you're wrong." I mean I thought you were just trying to illustrate a point. Not really trick me.

T: Go on.

P: (*Pause*) Well what do you want—I forgot (*slight laugh*) where I was.

T: Well, where were you?

P: I, I finished my thought, and then you said "go on."

T: Maybe there's another one.

P: You know, you're making me angry (*slight laugh*).

T: I (*pause*)—is that what the smile says?

There follows a sequence in which the therapist asks her to introspect how her anger "feels." She says it makes her feel sort of "bad and put down." She tries to explain that she got angry because she thought he was "annoyed" at her for challenging him. The therapist responds by interpreting her anger as inappropriate because she didn't "wonder very much whether" he was annoyed or not, so that her anger was not really "justified."

A few minutes later in the session we find the patient talking about her many failings.

P: Another thing that you know I find—like when I happen to have a lot of things to do, not even in school, but just in gen . . . not tests, but making appointments to see people, and to see more than one person, and doing little things . . . unless I make a long list of things that I have to do, I'm constantly rehashing it in my mind. And I go crazy . . . I get so nervous, and I do it over and over and over again, and I leave one out and then I have to go back and do it all over. And I say there is supposed to be ten and I can only count nine. You know I really can't take it. I really get very upset when I have a lot of things to think about. I just can't handle it (*pause*). And that's what I have now . . . that's what happens to me . . . all sorts of things pile up . . . papers to do and tests and all sorts of things that I've stuck—and I'm always afraid that I'm gonna forget to do them. Even *forget to go to an appointment* (*emphasis added*).

T: You have to keep telling yourself over and over again about the appointments.

P: Yeah. Because I'll forget. I mean if I don't keep on reminding myself I'm gonna forget completely. I have a terrible memory. I know it . . . ever since this therapy has been going on."

The sequence from shame in the patient–therapist relationship, into humiliated fury, with its natural impulse to "turn the tables," thence into guilt for "unjustified anger" is thus apparent. The patient is now back down into her familiar state of low self-esteem. And neither the therapist nor the patient is aware that in what is a rational-sounding "primary process transformation," the patient is failing in the ability to keep appointments, not the therapist.

And so we are reminded of Freud's (1917) original, brilliant clinical observations that, in depression, the self-reproaches are unconsciously meant for "someone whom the patient loves or has loved or should love. Every time one examines the facts this conjecture is confirmed" (p. 248). Including the superego experience of shame and of shame-rage in the dynamics of depression helps to illuminate the process by which this substitution takes place. It helps us also to understand that many "narcissistic" reactions reflect our deepest affectional ties.

## References

Abramson L., & Sackeim, H. (1977). A paradox in depression: Uncontrollability and self blame. *Psychological Bulletin, 84*, 838–857.

Abramson, L., Seligman, M., & Teasdale, J. (1978). Learned helpness in humans: Critique and reformulation. *Journal of Abnormal Psychology, 87*, 49–74.

Ausubel, D. (1955). Relationships between shame and guilt in the socializing process. *Psychological Review, 62*; 378–390.

Bergler, E. (1952). *The superego: Unconscious conscience.* New York: Grune & Stratton.

Berliner, B. (1958). The role of object relations in moral masochism. *Psychoanalytic Quarterly, 27*, 38–56.

Bibring, E. (1953). The mechanism of depression. In P. Greenacre (Ed.), *Affective disorders.* New York: International Universities Press.

Blatt, S. (1974). Levels of object representation in anaclitic and introjective depression. *Psychoanalytic Study of the Child, 29*, 107–157.

Broucek, F. (1982). Shame and its relationship to early narcissistic development. *International Journal of Psychoanalysis, 65*, 369–378.

Erikson, E. (1950). *Childhood and society.* New York: Norton.

Freud, S. (1905). Jokes and their relation to the unconscious. *Standard Edition, 8.* London: Hogarth Press.

Freud, S. (1905). Fragments of an analysis of a case of hysteria. *Standard Edition, 2.* London: Hogarth Press.

Freud, S. (1911). Psychoanalytic notes on an autobiographical case of paranoia; (dementia paranoidea). *Standard Edition, 12.* London: Hogarth Press.

Freud, S. (1913). Totem and taboo. *Standard Edition, 13.* London: Hogarth Press.

Freud, S. (1917). Mourning and melancholia. *Standard Edition, 14.* London: Hogarth Press.

Freud, S. (1919). A child is being beaten. *Standard Edition, 17.* London: Hogarth Press.

Freud, S. (1923). The ego and the id. *Standard Edition, 19.* London: Hogarth Press.

Gottschalk, L., & Gleser, G. (1969). *The measurement of psychological states through verbal content.* Berkeley: University of California Press.

Grinker, R., Werble, B., & Drye, R.; (1968) *The borderline syndrome.* New York: Basic Books.

Heider, F. (1958). *The psychology of interpersonal relationships.* New York: Wiley.

Herman, J. L. (1981). *Father–daughter incest*; Cambridge, MA: Harvard University Press.

Herman, J. L. (1986). Histories of violence in an outpatient population. *American Journal of Orthopsychiatry, 56*, 137–141.

Horowitz, M. (1981). Self-righteous rage and the attribution of blame. *Archives of General Psychology, 38*, 133–138.

Izard, C. (1972). *Patterns of emotion: A new analysis of anxiety and depression.* New York: Academic.

Izard, C. (1977). *Human emotions.* New York: Plenum.

Kernberg, O. (1975). *Borderline conditions and pathological narcissism.* New York: Jason Aronson.

Kohut, H. (1971). *The analysis of the self.* New York: International Universities Press.

Kohut, H. (1979). The two analyses of Mr. Z. *International Journal of Psychoanalysis, 60*, 3–27.

Lamont, J. (1973). Depressed mood and power over other people's feelings. *Journal of Clinical Psychology, 29*, 319–321.

Lewis, H. B. (1944). An experimental study of the role of the ego in work. The role of the ego in cooperative work. *Journal of Experimental Psychology, 34*, 113–126.

Lewis, H. B. (1958). Overdifferentiation and underindividuation of the self. *Psychoanalysis and the Psychoanalytic Review, 45*, 3–24.

Lewis, H. B. (1971). *Shame and guilt in neurosis.* New York: International Universities Press.

Lewis, H. B. (1976). *Psychic war in men and women.* New York: New York University Press. (*Revised Edition: Sex and the superego.* Hillsdale, NJ: Analytic Press.)

Lewis, H. B. (1980). "Narcissistic personality," or "Shame-prone" superego mode. *Comprehensive Psychotherapy, 1*, 59–80.

Lewis, H. B. (1981). *Freud and modern psychology.* II. *The role of emotions in human behavior.* New York: Plenum.

Lewis, H.B. (1983). *Freud and modern psychology:* I. *The emotional basis of mental illness.* New York: Plenum.

Lewis, H. B. (1985). Depression versus paranoia: Why are there sex differences in mental illness? *Journal of Personality, 53*, 150–178.

Lewis, H. B. (1986a). The role of shame in depression. In M. Rutter, C. Izard, & P. Read (Eds.), *Depression in young people: Developmental and clinical perspectives.* New York: Guilford.

Lewis, H. B. (1986b). Resistance: A misnomer for shame and guilt. In D. S. Milman & G. D. Goldman (Eds.), *Techniques of working with resistance.* New York: Aronson.

Lewis, H. B., & Franklin M. (1944). An experimental study of the role of the ego in work. II. The significance of task-orientation in work. *Journal of Experimental Psychology, 34*, 195–215.

Lewis, N. (1976). *The interpretation of dreams and portents.* Toronto: Samuel, Stevens, Hakkert.

Lindsay-Hartz, J. (1984). Contrasting experiences of shame and guilt. *American Behavioral Scientist, 27*, 689–704.

Malan, D. (1976). *The frontier of brief psychotherapy.* New York: Plenum.

Masson, J. (1985). *The complete letters of Sigmund Freud to Wilhelm Fliess.* Cambridge, MA: Harvard University Press.

Menaker, E. (1953). Masochism: A defense reaction of the ego. *Psychoanalytic Quarterly, 22*, 205–220.

Miller, S. (1985). *The shame experience.* Hillsdale, NJ: Analytic Press.

Morrison, A. F. (1983). Shame, the ideal self, and narcissism. *Comtemporary Psychoanalysis, 19*, 295–318.

Morrison, N. (1985). Shame in the treatment of schizophrenia: Theoretical considerations with clinical illustration. *Yale Journal of Biology and Medicine, 58.*

Peterson, C. (1979). Uncontrollability and self-blame in depression: Investigations of the paradox in a college population. *Journal of Abnormal Psychology, 88*, 620–624.

Peterson, C., Luborsky, L., & Seligman, M. (1983). Attribution and depressed mood shifts: A case study using the symptom context method. *Journal of Abnormal Psychology, 92*, 96–104.

Peterson, C., Schwartz, S., & Seligman, M. (1981). Self-blame and depressive symptoms. *Journal of Personality and Social Psychology, 41*, 253–260.

Piers, G., & Singer, M. (1953). *Shame and guilt.* Springfield, IL: Thomas.

Prosen, M., Clark, D., Harrow, M., & Fawcett, J. (1983). Guilt and conscience in major depressive disorders. *American Journal of Psychiatry, 140*, 839–844.

Reik, T. (1941). *Masochism in modern man.* New York: Grove Press.

Retzinger, S. (1985). The resentment process: Videotape studies. *Psychoanalytic Psychology, 2*, 129–152.

Rizley, R. (1978). Depression and distortion in the attribution of causality. *Journal of Abnormal Psychology, 87*, 32–48.

Safer, J. (1975). *The effects of sex and psychological differentiation on response to a stressful group situation.* Unpublished doctoral dissertation, The New School for Social Research, New York.

Smith, R. (1972). The relative proneness to shame and guilt as an indicator of defensive style. Unpublished doctoral dissertation, Northwestern University.

Stuart, G. (1956). *Narcissus.* London: Allen and Unwin.

Stolorow, R., & Lachmann, F. (1980). *Psychoanalysis of developmental arrests.* New York: International Universities Press.

Wile, D. (1984). Kohut, Kernberg and accusatory interpretation. *Psychotherapy, 21*, 353–364.

Witkin, H. (1965). Psychological differentiation and forms of pathology. *Journal of Abnormal Psychology, 70*, 317–336.

Witkin, H., Lewis, H., Hertzman, M., Machover, K., Meissner, P., & Wapner, S. (1954). *Personality through perception.* New York: Wiley

Witkin, H., Lewis, H., & Weil, E. (1968). Affective reaction and patient–therapist interactions among more or less differentiated patients, early in therapy. *Journal of Nervous and Mental Disease, 146*, 193–208.

Wurmser, L. (1981). *The mask of shame*. Baltimore: Johns Hopkins University Press.

Wylie, R. (1979). *The self–concept: Theory and research on selected topics* (rev. ed.). Lincoln: University of Nebraska Press.

Zeigarnik, B. (1927). Ueber das behalten von erledigten und unerledigten handlungen. *Psychologische Forschungen, 9*, 231–238.

# 4

# Shame

SILVAN S. TOMKINS

*It is rare that one scientist working alone creates an entire field of study. Yet this is the importance of Silvan Tomkins and his life work. The theory of emotion he published a quarter century ago as* Affect Imagery/Consciousness *(1962, 1963) and known today simply as "affect theory," has been the basis of all contemporary research on the nature of emotion. Recent landmark books such as Stern's (1985)* The Interpersonal World of the Infant *and Lichtenberg's (1983)* Psychoanalysis and Infant Research, *focussed as they are on the critical importance of affect in the development of the infant and as the major communication system between infant and caregiver, owe much to Tomkins. Most surprising is that his work has been so basic, so immanent to the study of emotion, that many of those involved in emotion research quite literally forget to cite Tomkins even when they utilize and take for granted ideas originally his. So much of affect theory has crept into the literature of psychology as its solid base of knowledge that one forgets how recent it really is.*

*The actual relationship of affect to facial display, although apparently suggested by Darwin, must be credited to Tomkins. Darwin saw the face as a passive and quite secondary vehicle for the display of emotion, which he believed to be a central experience appearing only later on the face. Tomkins recognized that the innate affects were man-*

Silvan S. Tomkins. Department of Social Systems Sciences, University of Pennsylvania, Philadelphia, Pennsylvania.

*ifested on the face with such rapidity, and were capable of such quick shifts, that they could not be explained as secondary phenomena; further, he noted that affects were visible on the face of the newborn, and therefore appeared too early in development to be related to accumulated experience. He postulated that what we see (and feel) as facial display is the actual source of what we call emotion, an "inward feed" of information from the face to conscious awareness. Finally, he provided a logical definition of drive which made it impossible to maintain Freud's notion that the emotions were derivative of the drives.*

*It is my impression that the therapeutic efficacy of the tricyclic and monoamine axidase antidepressants in the treatment of depressive illness, and of lithium salts in the management of bipolar affective disorder have made many psychiatrists and psychoanalysts ask about the nature of these conditions that we have so blithely called "affective illnesses," and beyond that, what is affect? Psychoanalysis has forever been announcing that it does not have a workable theory of affect, apparently unaware that a powerful new theory existed in its sister science of psychology. Tomkins had presented ideas only recently confirmed by the legion of infant observers, and which draw our attention back to his theories as originally stated, rather than the highly derivative and sometimes questionable ways they have been restated by others. Because of the general unavailability of* Affect/Imagery/Consciousness, *in which he introduced his general theory of affect and the specific theory for shame, I asked Professor Tomkins if he would review his position in terms of our current interest in the superego and the emotions called shame and quilt.*

I regard shame as an affect auxiliary, and as a theoretical construct, rather than an entity unambiguously defined by the word "shame." Our languages of communication are rough-hewn devices, sometimes coarse and sometimes marvellously subtle, reflecting insights and purposes of past cultures, which in part continue to be vital to the present, but in part to be alien and irrelevant.

If one were to trace the varying meanings of the word "shame" over the past few thousand years, one would illuminate the rich textures of the varieties of cultural *mentalité* rather than find this primary human feeling to be a fundamental invariant. A word in ordinary language may or may not confer the precision necessary for a scientific language. Thus, to write "salt" is not the same as to write "NaCl" or "sodium chloride," especially since both sodium and chloride may be combined with other elements to make compounds for which the word "salt" might be as useful a name. Nonetheless "salt" may "do" as a rough equivalent of sodium chloride so long as one does not insist that potassium chloride *is* "salt" or is *entirely different* from table salt.

Similarly, the common word "shame" will be adequate for my needs as a rough equivalent of the theoretical entity referring to a specific affect auxiliary. It is important for one to understand that the *word* shame (today) refers more to feelings of inferiority than feelings of guilt, and therefore more to responses of proving oneself good" (in the sense of being superior) than to responses of proving oneself "good" in the moral sense. As for the *theoretical construct* shame, however, I will argue that these are *not* differences in shame, but rather differences in objects and sources, and differences in responses to both sources and affect. Therefore, strictly speaking one can be "ashamed" of *either* being inferior or being immoral and of striving either to overcome inferiority or immorality.

The reader at this point will have serious reservations that it does not "feel" the same to have failed and to have hurt someone, nor therefore to try to succeed or to make restitution. Nonetheless, I will argue that though the *total* complex of affect, source, and response may feel quite different in these two cases (and indeed prompting the invention of the word "guilt" to distinguish shame from guilt) that the component affect is nonetheless identical in both cases, could one abstract the elements from each of these complexes.

A comparison with other affects may be helpful. Consider Freud's distinction between fear and anxiety. In fear one "knows" what one is afraid of. In anxiety one does not. A phobia will prompt one to avoid a quite specific object. An anxiety attack will not. There is a nontrivial sense in which these "feel" to be very different experiences. Nonetheless I argue that the affect (whether one calls it fear, terror, or anxiety) is identical. It is extremely improbable that such a fundamental motivating mechanism could be split and differentiated into several mechanisms every time its trigger varied in source. Similarly, when the response to fear varies, the "feel" is also quite different, but no less misleading about the underlying affect mechanism. Thus in anorexia one starves for fear of eating, whereas in bulimia one eats compulsively for fear of starvation or emptiness. Different as these complexes are, I believe the affect of fear is identical in these otherwise opposed complexes of responses.

The differences in complexes of source, affect and response and the identity of affects must be preserved because the varieties of such differences are without limit and the difference between shame and guilt is but *one* of *many* possible variants of shame which we will examine later.

In order to understand the nature of shame as affect auxiliary, let us first examine the nature of the affect mechanism. The affect mechanism is *not* identical with our concepts of motivation, which latter refers to a much more unitary, compact, and reasonable phenomenon than does the construct of affect. Consider the relation between a phobia and free-floating terror. In the fear of dogs and in our avoidance of dogs, or in our escape from them, we are clear in our use of the concept of a motive. Dogs are the "cause" of our aversion *and therefore* of our attempts at avoidance or escape, and when we succeed in avoiding or escaping dogs we have *attained our goal* and are therefore no longer afraid. To have a motive (as we commonly use this word) is to have a *correlated* set of responses, of drives and of affects to a source, which are evoked by that source and which are in turn responsible for our *further* responses of approach or avoidance.

Freud radically complicated this assumption when he demonstrated the existence of unconscious motives, by which he appeared to mean that we sometimes acted *as if* we had motives other than we knew, but which an analyst *did* know. I wish to complicate further our understanding of the nature of motivation by stressing that the relations between the affect mechanism and its sources as triggers, and its further evoked responses, are at once amplifying, abstract, general, modular, correlating, and partial.

It is in many ways similar to the set of complex relationships between an alphabet, words, grammar, and semantic rules. An alphabet is *not* a word, but words require an alphabet. Grammar is not semantics, but semantics require a grammar. Any system requires the property of modularity, or varying combinatorial capacity, to generate complexity. The affect mechanism is one mechanism among many that together enable us to feel and act as "motivated." It is, in my view, the single most important component in motivation, but nonetheless partial and incomplete as a "motive" in the ordinary use of that term.

It is my view that affects are sets of muscular, glandular, and skin receptor responses located in the face (and also widely distributed throughout the body) that generate sensory feedback to a system that finds them either inherently "acceptable" or "unacceptable." These organized sets of responses are triggered at subcortical centers where specific "programs" for each distinct affect are stored, programs that are innately endowed and have been genetically inherited. They are capable, when activated, of simultaneously capturing such widely distributed structures as the face, the heart, and the endocrine glands and imposing on them a specific pattern of correlated responses. One does not learn to be afraid or to cry or to startle, any more than one learns to feel pain or to gasp for air.

Contrary to Freud, I do not view human beings as the battleground for their imperious drives, which urge them on blindly to pleasure and violence, to be contained only by a repressive society and its representations within—the ego and the superego. Rather, I see affect or feeling as *the primary innate biological motivating mechanism*, more urgent than drive deprivation and pleasure, and more urgent even than physical pain. Without its amplification, nothing else matters, and with its amplification anything can matter. It thus combines urgency, abstractness, and generality. It lends its power to memory, to perception, to thought, and to action no less than to the drives.

That this is so is not obvious, but it is readily demonstrated. Consider that almost any interference with breathing will immediately arouse the most desperate gasping for breath. Consider the drivenness of the tumescent, erect male. Consider the urgency of desperate hunger. These are the intractable driven states that prompted the answer "The human animal is driven to breathe, to have sex, to drink, and to eat." to the question "What do human beings really want?"

And yet this apparent urgency proves to be an illusion. It is *not* an illusion that one must have air, water, and food to maintain oneself, and sex to reproduce oneself. What is illusory is the biological and psychological source of the apparent *urgency* of the desperate quality of the hunger, air, and sex drives. Consider these drive states more closely. When someone puts his or her hand over my mouth and nose, I become terrified. But this panic, this terror, is in no way a part of the drive mechanism. I can be terrified at the possibility of losing my job, or of developing cancer, or at the possibility of the loss of my beloved. Fear (or terror) is an innate affect that can be triggered by a wide variety of circumstances. Not having enough air to breathe is one of many such circumstances. But if the rate of anoxic deprivation becomes slower, as, for example, in the case of wartime pilots who refused to wear oxygen masks at 30,000 feet, then there develops not a panic, but a euphoric state—some of these men met their deaths with smiles on their lips. The smile is the affect of enjoyment, in no way specific to slow anoxic deprivation.

Consider more closely the tumescent male with an erection. He is sexually excited, we say. He is indeed excited, but no one has ever observed an excited penis. It is a man who is excited and who breathes hard, not in the penis, but in the chest, the face, and the nose and nostrils. But such excitement is in no way peculiarly sexual. The same excitement can be experienced, without the benefit of an erection, to mathematics—beauty bare—to poetry, and to a rise in the stock market. Instead of viewing these as representing sublimations of sexuality, it is rather that sexuality, in order to become possible, must borrow its potency from the affect of excitement. The drive must be assisted by affect as an *amplifier* if it is to work at all. Freud knew, better than anyone else, that the blind, pushy, imperious id was the most fragile of impulses, readily disrupted by fear, by shame, by rage, by boredom. At the first sign of affect *other* than excitement, there is impotence and frigidity. The penis proves to be a paper tiger in the absence of appropriate affective amplification.

In short, I propose that affect is primarily facial behavior. When we become aware of these facial and/or visceral responses, we are aware of our affects. We may respond with these affects, however, without becoming aware of the feedback from them. Finally, we learn to generate, from memory, images of these same responses, images of which we can become aware with or without repetition of facial, skeletal, or visceral responses.

The affect system provides the primary blueprints for cognition, decision, and action. Humans are responsive to whatever circumstances activate positive and negative affects. Some of these circumstance innately activate the affects. At the same time, the affect system is also capable of being instigated by learned stimuli and responses. The human being is thus urged by nature and by nurture to explore, and to attempt to control, the circumstances which evoke his positive and negative affective responses. It is the freedom of the affect system that makes it possible for the human being to begin to implement and to progress toward what he regards as an ideal state—one that, however else s/he may describe it, implicitly or explicitly entails the maximizing of positive affect and the minimizing of negative affect.

What are the major affects, these primarily facial responses? I have distinguished nine innate affects, and separated them into two groups, positive affects and negative affects.

The positive affects are as follows: first, *interest* or *excitement*, in which we observe that the eyebrows are down and the stare tracking an object or fixed on it; second, *enjoyment* or *joy*, the smiling response; third, *surprise* or *startle*, with eyebrows raised and eyes blinking.

The negative affects are the following: first, *distress* or *anguish*, the crying response; second, *fear* or *terror*, in which the eyes may be frozen open in a fixed stare or moving away from the dreaded object to the side, the skin pale, cold, sweating, and trembling, and the hair erect; third, *shame* or *humiliation*, with eyes and head lowered; fourth, *dissmell*, with the upper lip raised; fifth, *disgust*, with the lower lip lowered and protruded; sixth, *anger* or *rage*, with a frown, clenched jaw, and red face.

If these are innately patterned responses, are there also innate activators of each affect? Consider the nature of the problem. Such a hypothesis must include the drives as innate but not exclusive activators. The neonate, for example, must respond with innate fear to any difficulty in breathing but must also be capable of being afraid of other objects. Each affect has to be capable of being activated by a *variety* of unlearned stimuli.

The child must be able to cry at hunger or loud sounds as well as at a diaper pin stuck in his or her flesh.

It must therefore be intrinsic to this system that each affect be activated by some general characteristic of neural stimulation, a characteristic common to both internal and external stimuli, and not too stimulus-specific (like a releaser). Next, the activator has to be correlated with biologically useful information. The young child must fear what is dangerous and smile at what is safe. The activator has to "know the address" of the subcortical center at which the appropriate affect program is stored—not unlike the problem of how the ear responds correctly to each tone.

Next, some of the activators must be capable of habituation, and others not; else a painful stimulus might too soon cease to be distressing and an exciting stimulus never be let go—such as a deer caught by a bright light. These are some of the characteristics to be built into the activation sensitivity of the affect mechanism. It would seem most economical to search for commonalities among the innate activators of each affect. This I have done, and I believe it is possible to account for the major phenomena with a few relatively simple assumptions about the general characteristics of the stimuli that innately activate affect.

I would account for the differences in affect activation by three general variants of a single principle—the density of neural firing or stimulation. By density, I mean the number of neural firings per unit of time. My theory posits three discrete classes of activators of affect, each of which further amplifies the sources that activate them. These are *stimulation increase*, *stimulation level*, and *stimulation decrease*. Thus, there is a provision for three distinct classes of motives; affects about stimulation that is on the increase, about stimulation that is level, and about stimulation that is on the decrease.

With respect to density of neural firing or stimulation, then, the human being is equipped for affective arousal for every major contingency. If internal or external sources of neural firing suddenly increase, s/he will startle or become afraid, or become interested, depending on the suddenness of the increase in stimulation. If internal or external sources of neural firing reach and maintain a high, constant level of stimulation, which deviates in excess of an optimal level of neural firing, s/he will respond with anger or distress, depending on the level of stimulation. If internal or external sources of neural firing suddenly decrease, s/he will laugh or smile with enjoyment, depending on the suddenness of the decrease in stimulation.

The general advantage of a system that allows affective arousal to such a broad spectrum of levels (and changes of level) of neural firing is to make the individual care about quite different states of affairs in different ways.

Such a neural theory must be able to account for how "meaning" in such neural messages operates without the benefit of a homunculus who "appraises" every message before instructing the individual to become interested or afraid. (It is clear that any theory of affect activation must be capable of accounting for affect that is triggered in either an unlearned or a learned fashion.) Certainly the infant who emits his or her birth cry on exit from the birth canal had not "appraised" the new environment as a vale of tears before s/he cries. It is equally certain that s/he will later learn to cry on receiving communications telling of the death of a beloved person; this does depend on meaning and its appraisal. I would argue that learned information *can* activate affects only through the general neural profiles I have postulated.

Thus, for a joke to "work," the novelty of information adequate to trigger interest, and the final laughter depend on the *rate of acceleration of information* in the first case and in the *rate of deceleration* in the second case. If we hear the same information a second time, there is a sense in which it may be appraised as essentially a repetition, but, because we now "see it coming," there is neither interest nor enjoyment because the gradients of neural firing are now much flatter (because compressed) than when the information was first received.

Similarly, with the startle response, a pistol shot is adequate as an unlearned activator, but so is the sudden appearance of a man with two heads. In such a case I would suggest that the rate of neural firing from the conjoint muscular responses of the double-take and the very rapid recruitment of information from memory to check the nature of the apparent message also have the requisite square wave profile of neural firing called for in my model. In short, "meaning" operates through the very general profiles of acceleration, deceleration, or level of neural firing as these are produced by either cognitive, memorial, perceptual, or motor responses. Any such responses singly or in concert can, through their correlation between meaning and the profiles of neural firing, "innately" fire innate affect programs by stimuli or responses that are themselves learned.

The conjoint characteristics of urgency, abstractness, generality and modularity together produce both match and (in varying degrees) mismatch between affect and other mechanisms, making it seem sometimes blind and inert, other times intuitive and flexible: sometimes brief and transient, other times enduring and committing; sometimes primarily biological, other times largely psychological, social, cultural or historical; sometimes aesthetic, other times instrumental; sometimes private and solipsistic, other times communicative and expressive; sometimes explosive, other times overcontrolled and backed up.

If the objects of affects are abstract and depend for their particularity on supplementary information from perception, memory, and cognition then clearly the "same" affect is rarely *experienced* in entirely the same way. My experiences of excitement at sexuality, poetry, mathematics, or at another's face can never be described as entirely identical "feelings," despite the identity of the triggered affects. Further, any impediment to such excitement evokes unequal varieties of "shame," with respect to experience, despite identity of the affect of shame.

This is complicated by the fact that shame is not a primary affect as I conceive it, but rather an affect auxiliary. In our consideration of the nature of auxiliary mechanisms, let us first study drive auxiliaries.

Dissmell and disgust are innate defensive responses, which are auxiliary to the hunger, thirst and oxygen drives. Their function is clear. If the food about to be ingested activates dissmell, the upper lip and nose are raised and the head is drawn away from the apparent source of the offending odor. If the food has been taken into the mouth, it may, if disgusting, be spit out. If it has been swallowed and is toxic, it may produce nausea and be vomited out, either through the mouth or nostrils. The early warning response via the nose is dissmell; the next level of response, from mouth or stomach, is disgust.

If dissmell and disgust were limited to these functions, we should not define them as affects but rather as auxiliary drive mechanisms. However, their status is somewhat unique in that dissmell, disgust, and nausea also function as signals and motives to others, as well as to the self, of feelings of rejection. They readily accompany a wide spectrum of entities that need not be tasted, smelled, or ingested. Dissmell and disgust appear to be evolving from the status of drive-reducing acts to those that have as well a more general motivating and signal function, both to the individual who emits this signal and to the one who receives it.

Just as dissmell and disgust are drive auxiliary acts, I posit shame as an innate affect auxiliary response and a specific inhibitor of continuing interest and enjoyment. As disgust operates only after something has been taken in, shame operates only after interest or enjoyment has been activated; it inhibits one, or the other, or both.

The innate activator of shame is the incomplete reduction of interest or joy. Such a barrier might arise because one is suddenly looked at by another who is strange; or because one wishes to look at, or commune with, another person but suddenly cannot because s/he is strange; or one expected him to be familiar but he suddenly appears unfamiliar; or one started to smile but found one was smiling at a stranger. It might also arise as a consequence of discouragement after having tried and failed, and then lowered one's head in apparent "defeat." The response of shame includes lowering the eyelid, decreasing the tonus of all facial muscles, lowering the head via a reduction in tonus of the neck muscles, or a tilting of the head in one direction.

Discouragement, shyness, shame, and guilt are identical as affects, though not so experienced because of differential coassembly of perceived causes and consequences. Shyness is about strangeness of the other; guilt is about moral transgression; shame is about inferiority; discouragement is about temporary defeat; but the core affect in all four is identical, although the coassembled perceptions, cognitions, and intentions may be vastly different.

Biologically, disgust and dissmell are drive auxiliary responses that have evolved to protect the human being from coming too close to noxious-smelling objects and to regurgitate these if they have been ingested. Through learning, these responses have come to be emitted to biologically neutral stimuli, including, for example, disgusting and dirty thoughts. Shame, in contrast, is an affect auxiliary to the affects of interest-excitement.

Any perceived barrier to positive affect with the other will evoke lowering of the eyelids and loss of tonus in the face and neck muscles, producing a head hung in shame. The child who is burning with excitement to explore the face of the stranger is nonetheless vulnerable to shame just because the other is perceived as strange. Characteristically, however, intimacy with the good and exciting other is eventually consummated. In contrast, the disgusting other is to be kept at a safe distance permanently.

If shame is activated by the incomplete reduction of interest or joy, then the varieties of these circumstances depend first on what are either the innate or the learned sources of positive affect, and second on what are either the innate or learned sources of the incomplete reduction of positive affect. Such circumstances go far beyond the questions of inferiority and guilt which have dominated the discussion of shame versus guilt. In effect this implicates all the positive values of human beings *and* all the problems that interfere with these values, but not to the extent of *complete* and *enduring* interference.

In shame the individual wishes to resume his or her commerce with the exciting state of affairs, to reconnect with the other, to recapture the relationship that existed before the situation turned problematic. In this respect shame is radically different from the drive auxiliary responses of disgust and dissmell. In disgust the bad other is spit out, or vomited forth. In dissmell the bad other is kept at a distance because of an offensive smell. No one wishes to eat again the food that disgusts, or to come closer to the smell that repels. The food is both rejected now and rejected for all time to come, as are the symbolic objects of dissmell and disgust, as are untouchables in a caste society. Disgust and dissmell are responses appropriate to a hierarchically ordered society.

These are not appropriate in a more egalitarian, democratic society where, hopefully, the offending other is only partially or temporarily less than completely exciting or enjoyable. The distinction between the distancing by shame and distancing by disgust and dissmell may be seen also in the difference between disgust and dissmell. Consider that in disgust one permitted the offending object into the closeness of taste and *then* rejected it, whereas in dissmell one keeps the offensive other at a safe distance.

I have determined that if one poses this option of varying distance toward symbolic objects, those who respond with shame rather than with disgust or dissmell will opt for disgust rather than dissmell if asked to choose, as for example, between the opinions "life sometimes leaves a bad taste in the mouth" or "life sometimes smells bad." This finding was part of a more general investigation into the differential magnification of all affects and its relationship to ideology.

I have been concerned for some time with a field I have called the "psychology of knowledge," an analog of the sociology of knowledge. It is a concern with the varieties of cognitive style, with the types of evidence that an individual finds persuasive and, most particularly, with his or her ideology. (I have defined ideology as any organized, set ideas about which humans are at once most articulate, ideas that produce enduring controversy over long periods of time, that evoke passionate partisanship, and about which humans are least certain because there is insufficent evidence.) Ideology therefore abounds at the frontier of any science. Today's ideology may (tomorrow) be confirmed or disconfirmed and so cease to be ideology. In a review of 2,000 years of ideological controversy in Western civilization, I have detected a sustained recurrent polarity between the *humanistic* and the *normative* orientations appearing in such diverse domains as the foundations of mathematics, the theory of aesthetics, political theory, epistemology, theory of perception, theory of value, theory of child rearing, theory of psychotherapy, and personality testing.

The issues are simple enough. Is man the measure, and end in himself, active, creative, thinking, desiring, loving force in nature? Or must man realize himself, attain his full stature, only through struggle toward, participation in, and conformity to a norm, a measure, an ideal essence basically prior to and independent of man? This polarity appeared first in Greek philosophy between the work of Protagoras and the work of Plato. Western thought has been an elaborate series of footnotes to the conflict between the conception of man as the measure of reality and value, versus that of man and nature as alike unreal and valueless in comparison to the realm of essence that exists independently of space and time. More simply, this polarity represents an idealization of man—a positive idealization in the humanistic ideology and a negative idealization in the normative ideology. Human beings, in Western civilization, have tended toward self-celebration, positive or negative. In Oriental thought another alternative is represented, that of harmony between man and nature.

I have further assumed that the individual resonates to any organized ideology because of an underlying ideo-affective posture, which is a set of feelings that is more loosely organized than any highly organized ideology.

Some insight into these ideological concepts held by an individual may be obtained through use of my polarity scale. The polarity scale assesses the individual's normative or humanistic position on a broad spectrum of ideological issues in mathematics, science, art, education, politics, child rearing, and theory of personality. Following are a few sample items from the scale. The normative position will be A, the humanistic B. The individual is permitted four choices: A, B, A and B, and neither A nor B.

*1.*

A. Numbers were discovered.

B. Numbers were invented.

*2.*

A. Play is childish.

B. Nobody is too old to play.

*3.*

A. The mind is like a mirror.

B. The mind is like a lamp.

*4.*

A. If you have had a bad experience with someone, the way to characterize this is that it leaves a bad smell.

B. If you have had a bad experience with someone, the way to characterize this is that it leaves a bad taste in the mouth.

5.

A. To see an adult cry is disgusting.

B. To see an adult cry is pathetic.

I have assumed that the ideo-affective posture is the result of systematic differences in the socialization of affects. For example, the attitudes toward distress in the items above could be a consequence of the following differences in distress socialization: When the infant or child cries, the parent, following his or her own ideo-affective posture and more articulate ideology, may elect to convert the distress of the child into a rewarding scene by putting his arms around the child and comforting him. The parent may, however, amplify the punishment inherent in the distress response by putting him- or herself into opposition to the child and the child's distress. S/he will require that the child stop crying, insisting that the child's crying results from some norm violation, and threaten to increase the child's suffering if s/he does not suppress the response. "If you don't stop crying, I will really give you something to cry about."

If the child internalizes his or her parent's ideo-affective posture and his or her ideology, the child has learned a very basic posture toward suffering, which will have important consequences for resonance to ideological beliefs quite remote from the nursery and the home. This is exemplified by the following items from the polarity scale: "The maintenance of law and order is the most important duty of any government" versus "Promotion of the welfare of the people is the most important function of a government."

The significance of the socialization of distress is amplified by the differential socialization of all the affects, including surprise, enjoyment, excitement, anger, fear, shame, dissmell, and disgust. I have outlined elsewhere (Tomkins, 1979) a systematic program of differential socialization of each of these affects, which together produce an ideo-affective posture that inclines the individual to resonate differentially to ideology. In the preceding example, excitement and enjoyment are implicated along with distress, anger, shame, fear, dissmell, and disgust, as is the relative importance of the reward of positive affects versus the importance of the punishment of negative affects that is involved in law and order versus welfare.

What is less obvious is that similar differences in ideo-affective posture influence such remote ideological options as the following items from the polarity scale: "Numbers were invented" versus "Numbers were discovered"; "The mind is like a lamp which illuminates whatever it shines on" versus "The mind is like a mirror which reflects whatever strikes it"; "Reason is the chief means by which human beings make great discoveries" versus "Reason has to be continually disciplined and corrected by reality and hard facts"; "Human beings are basically good" versus "Human beings are basically evil." The structure of ideology and the relationships among the socialization of affects, the ideoaffective postures, and ideology are more complex than can be discussed here. I wish to present just enough of this theory to enable the reader to understand the relationship of the theory to the face.

I have assumed that the humanistic position is one that attempts to maximize positive affect for individuals and for all their interpersonal relationships. In contrast, the normative position is that norm compliance is the primary value and that positive affect is a consequence of norm compliance, not to be directly sought as a goal. Indeed, the suffering of negative affect is assumed to be a frequent experience and an inevitable consequence of the human condition. Therefore, in any interpersonal transaction, the humanist self-consciously strives to maximize positive affect insofar as it is possible.

The first hypothesis concerning the face is that humanists would smile more frequently than the normatively oriented, both because they experienced the smile of enjoyment more frequently during their socialization and because they internalized the ideo-affective posture that one should attempt to increase positive affect for the other as well as the self. The learned smile does not always imply that the individual feels happy. As often as not, it is a consequence of a wish to communicate to the other that one wishes him to feel smiled upon and to evoke the smile from the other. This smile is often the oil spread over troubled human waters to extinguish the fires of distress, hate, and shame.

It was known from previous investigations with the stereoscope (Tomkins 1965, 1975), that when one presented humanists and normatives with two pictures of the same face (one of which was smiling and one of which was not), the humanists tended to suppress the nonsmiling face significantly more often than did the normatives. Vasquez (1975) confirmed that humanist subjects actually smile more frequently while talking with an experimenter than do normative subjects. There is, however, no such difference when subjects are alone, displaying affect spontaneously.

The second hypothesis is that humanists would respond more frequently with distress, and normatives would respond more frequently with anger. The rationale for this is that when an interpersonal relationship is troubled, the humanist will try to absorb as much punishment as possible and so display distress rather than anger; anger, being more likely to escalate into conflict, is a more blaming extrapunitive response than distress. It was assumed that the normative subjects would more frequently respond with anger because they are more extrapunitive, more pious and blaming, and less concerned with sparing the feelings of others, as their internalized models did not spare their own feelings. This hypothesis was not confirmed, but neither was it reversed. This failure may have arisen because the differences in polarity scale scores were not as great as I would have wished. In part, this was a consequence of a strong humanistic bias among college students at the time of testing and because of the reluctance of known normatives to volunteer for testing. This is consistent with prior research, including my own, which indicates that volunteers in general are more sociophilic and friendly.

The third hypothesis is that humanists would more frequently respond with shame and that normatives would respond less frequently with shame but more frequently with disgust and dissmell. The rationale is that shame represents an impunitive response to what is interpreted as an interruption to communion (as, e.g., in shyness) and that it will ultimately be replaced by full communication.

In contrast, dissmell and disgust are responses to a bad other and the termination of intimacy with such a one is assumed to be permanent unless the other one changes significantly. These hypotheses were confirmed for shame and disgust but not for dissmell. Humanistic subjects, although displaying affect spontaneously, did respond more frequently with shame responses than did normative subjects, whereas normative subjects displayed significantly more disgust responses than did humanistic subjects.

In conclusion, it was predicted and confirmed that humanistic subjects respond more frequently with smiling to the good other and with shame if there is any perceived barrier to intimacy. Normative subjects smile less frequently to the other and emit disgust more frequently to the other who is tested and found wanting. The differences represent a correlation between cognition and affect, as affect is displayed on the faces of those who differ significantly in what they believe about the world in which they live.

If shame is an affect attenuation of excitement and enjoyment it is essentially *impunitive* rather than extrapunitive or intropunitive compared with disgust and dissmell. This is not to say that it does not hurt and sting, but rather that it is *less* malignant than are the drive auxiliaries of disgust and dissmell.

I have stressed the partial and temporary nature of shame. The reader may wonder about those who experience frequent and enduring mortification by shame. Can this be anything but malignant? I would distinguish in this case between shame as affect amplification and shame as affect magnification. Any affect may be radically increased in toxicity by undue magnification. Even excitement, rewarding as it may be, can become malignant if its density is unduly magnified in frequency, duration, and intensity.

Similarly, shame, if magnified in frequency, duration, and intensity such that the head is in a permanent posture of depression, can become malignant in the extreme. But this is a consequence of the magnification of affect, rather than of its nature as an amplifier. Analogous would be the lesser inherent toxicity of distress compared with terror. Nonetheless a continuing intense distress would be toxic in the extreme as would any negative affect if it became greatly magnified. Yet chronic distress over a period of months, as in infant "colic," can be tolerated both biologically and psychologically better than could a chronic intense state of terror. Even a chronic state of intense shame nurtures the hope and wish to resume the state of full excitement or enjoyment partially reduced in shame and by shame. This is why even intense shame or shame as guilt is not only compatible with continuing sexual excitement but may by contrast heighten such conflicted sexual excitement.

Further, the experience of shame may be made malignant by excessive recruitment of other affect with which it is then combined, as in that severe combination of shame, and distress or fear, and reduction in the nonspecific reticular amplification, that together constitute "depression."

The experience of shame itself characteristically recruits secondary and tertiary positive or negative affects toward shame. Thus one may develop secondary excitement at the sequence excitement-shame, as in awaiting the response of an audience to a play one has written, or in which one acts, or in awaiting the beginning of an adversarial contest as player or as audience, or in awaiting a sexual encounter. Thus some fighters, speakers, or lovers who cannot generate secondary excitement at the excitement-shame sequence report that they are in such cases incapable of adequate performance because the *absence* of shame or fear attenuates both primary and anticipatory excitement.

Similarly one may have fear of such anticipated sequences of excitement-shame as stage fright, which typically is dissipated by pure excitement or joy after the play (dramatic or adversarial) begins. Fear may also be generated prior to an uncertain sexual encounter which promises not only excitement but also possible shame as distancing, or as guilt.

Next one may recruit anger at the excitement-shame sequence, either afterward or as anticipatory anger. The increased amplification of the conjunction of excitement followed by shame may deeply anger the self at its victimization, or direct such anger at the other, or at the dyad for being equally "inhibited" either in the expression of excitement or of shame or of sexuality, as incompetence or as guilt, or as shyness, or as discouragement. Thus one may become furious at one's victimization by guilt, which is experienced as ego-alien.

Such victimization by shame or by shame as guilt may also recruit dense distress, in which one celebrates one's impotence to free a self that wishes to liberate itself but does not know how.

Excitement-shame may, as we have noted before, also recruit secondary shame at this sequence, so that the individual becomes ashamed of shame itself. I may, however, recruit disgust or dissmell rather than shame. In such a case we have the paradox of one part of the self performing psychic surgery on another part of itself, so that the self which feels ashamed is totally and permanently split off and rejected by a judging self that has no tolerance for its more humble and hesitant self. If disgust is recruited, there is a lingering acknowledgement that the offending self was once better, but is now offensive. If it is dissmell, the other part of the self is represented as completely and enduringly offensive. Such disapprobation may be united with anger against both the fear and shame of death, as in the poet's protest not to go "gently" into the night but to rage and rage.

Magnification of shame occurs not only by combining multiple affects about the same scene, as when a rape victim may experience not only shame, but disgust, dissmell, anger, and distress as well as terror, but also by combining multiple sources of *shame* about the same scene. Thus an impotent failure of sexuality may generate multiple feelings of deep shame such that the individual not only feels the shame of sexual inferiority, but of a totally inferior self, along with shyness, along with discouragement, guilt, defeat, and alienation. These are *all* the same affect of shame but to different aspects of the same scene.

Consider a classic shame scene such as toilet training by a mother who taunts her child as "baby" on the occasion of loss of control of anal or urethral function. Such a child may feel multiple sources of shame as well as multiple other negative affects. S/he has lost love, and lost respect from the mother, evoked too much attention and control from her, and also too much turning away in disgust and dissmell. The child has not only done something "wrong" as immoral but also wrong as incompetent. S/he not only failed in this act, but the competence of the self may have also been called into question. The distance now between the child and his mother is experienced as shyness. The difficulty of controlling himself or herself and maintaining the mother's love and respect is experienced as discouragement as well as defeat and indignity. Added to multiple sources of shame may be anger at the impatient mother, disgust at her disgust, dissmell at her dissmell, terror at his own affects as well as at her, and distress at the loss of what was once mutually enjoyed. Such a scene's magnification implicates all varieties of violations of values: moral—"soiling is wrong"; aesthetic—"soiling is ugly"; truth—"you promised to control yourself"; instrumental—"you have no skill"; and they are all "shameful."

Let us now examine more closely some of the varieties of shame, those sources of positive affect that may suffer partial and temporary attenuation which it is *hoped* will not become either permanent or complete.

First of all shame is in no way limited to the self, to the other, or to society. A once beautiful place, where one lived, and which is now ugly, for whatever reason, may cause the head to bow in regret and shame on being revisited in hope of recapturing idealized memories. But, as is characteristic of shame, one may also bow one's head in awe and shame at the unexpected grandeur and beauty of a sudden view of an ocean or mountain, never before encountered, that overwhelms by its beauty rather than by its ugliness. In such cases there is often an invidious contrast with the self as unequal to such beauty and grandeur, as in the confrontation with parents or parent surrogates who make the self feel small and unworthy by comparison.

Again, shame may be felt at the vicissitudes of fate, particularly in the face of death, when the self reluctantly acknowledges the fragility of cherished relationships. The head is bowed at a cemetery because one does not wish to give up the beloved but is required to do so. Shame is also experienced as a less permanent defeat in discouragement, following great effort that has so far come to naught. One bows one's head in acknowledgement of defeat for the time being but with the hope that it may one day be raised in pride.

Shame is experienced as shyness when one wishes to be intimate with the other but also feels some impediment to *immediate* intimacy. That impediment may be located either in the self, the other, or in the dyad, or in a third party who intrudes.

Shame is experienced as inferiority when discouragement is located in the self as an inability of the self to do what the self wishes to do. This is experienced differently than is the same phenomenon as discouragement, which stresses the failure of great effort, rather than the incapacity of the self.

Shame is experienced as guilt when positive affect is attenuated by virtue of moral normative sanctions experienced as conflicting with what is exciting or enjoyable. As in the case of any shame, such guilt requires a continuing interest or enjoyment which is only partially or temporarily attenuated. This is in contrast to moral outrage, moral disgust, or moral dissmell. In the extreme case immorality may be judged "beneath contempt," "inhuman," or "animalistic." All such feelings and evaluations differ from shame as "guilt" in totally and forever condemning what is judged immoral, whether by the self against another, or by the self against the self, as in "I can never forgive myself for what I did." In this case the self splits itself into two, a good self and totally bad self.

Feelings of shame or of shame as guilt may be experienced either as coming from without or from within. The common distinction between shame and guilt as resting on the locus of evaluation is in error since I may feel inferior or guilty because someone so regards me, *or* because I so regard myself. Further, I may feel ashamed because *you* should feel ashamed or guilty but do not. I may feel ashamed or guilty because you feel ashamed or guilty but *should not*, as in the case of my sanctioning slavery reluctantly.

To the extent to which I have conflicting values or wishes I may feel ashamed or guilty for opposite reasons at the same time. Thus I may feel ashamed of my wish to exhibit myself and of my wish not to exhibit myself, and of my wish that you exhibit yourself and of my wish that you not exhibit yourself.

To the extent that any primary affect is conflicted I may be shamed equally by feeling it and by not feeling it. Thus I may feel shame at being distressed at the plight of the self or the other, as well as shame at *not* feeling distress at the plight of self or other. I may feel shame at my own fear and also at my own fearlessness to the extent that I have been socialized by one parent to be fearless and by another parent to be cautious.

In contrast to conflict and ambivalence as a source of shame, is a *narrow optimal bandwidth* for excitement or enjoyment and therefore for freedom from shame at partial reduction of the sources of positive affect. Thus, I may define acceptable intimacy by a restricted zone of optimal closeness. In such a case, if the other is too close s/he is experienced as shaming by intrusion, but if the other is too distant s/he is also experienced as shaming by not being close enough.

The experience of shame itself may become a further source of shame whenever there is a narrow optimal zone of shame as acceptable. Thus if I am *too* shamed or too shameless I may experience *either* as shaming.

The same dynamic may be experienced at the experience of *any* affect that violates a narrow optimal bandwidth. I may wish to be less excitable than I am, less prone to become angry or distressed or disgusted or dissmelling, or fearful. This is to be distinguished from shame at affect *conflict*, as described above. In this case there is no conflict about specific affects, but rather a strict set of criteria for the variety, frequency of sources of affect, or for the affect's intensity, duration, or density, or about its translation into action.

Shame may be evoked by a *complete* rejection of *any* affect (including shame). It is not that there is a narrow bandwidth of acceptable sources, affect density, or responses to affect but rather a total intolerance of specific affects, their sources and action in response. The affect is simply condemned, so that whenever it appears it is capable of shaming the individual who wishes it had not appeared. Any affect may be condemned for one of a variety of reasons other than conflict. It may be condemned as unaesthetic and ugly, as engulfing the individual, as immoral, as typical of a lower class, as offensive to a beloved, as exaggerating and illusory, as too costly to one's commitments. These varieties may in turn generate varieties of shame.

The experience of shame is inevitable for any human being insofar as desire outruns fulfillment sufficiently to attenuate interest without destroying it. "I want, but . . ." is the essential condition for the activation of shame. Clearly not any barrier will evoke shame since many barriers either completely reduce interest so that the object is renounced, or heighten excitement so that the barrier is removed or overcome. If shame is dependent on barriers to excitement and enjoyment then the pluralism of desires must be matched by a pluralism of shame. One person's source of shame can always be another person's fulfillment, satiety, or indifference.

Insofar as human beings are excited by or enjoy their work, other human beings, their bodies, selves, and the surrounding inanimate world, they are vulnerable to a variety of vicissitudes in the form of barriers, lacks, losses, accidents, imperfections, conflicts, and ambiguities that will impoverish, attenuate, impair, or otherwise prevent total pursuit and enjoyment of work, of others, of sexuality and other drive satisfactions, and of the surrounding physical and social world.

The history of shame is also a history of civilizations. We will close this essay by an examination of some of the history of a perennial source of shame (and of shame as guilt): sexuality.

Sexuality has from the beginning of time engaged shame. Such shame was in no way a modern invention, appearing in recorded history at least as early as *Genesis* in the Old Testament. This shame was linked to the unholy thirst for knowledge of all kinds, with carnal knowledge only a special case, and was judged shameful because of its adversarial pretension to godliness, and its violation of God's wishes and prohibitions.

In Plato and in classical Greek ethics there were two, related, but partly independent sources of sexual shame: carnal knowledge was of two kinds, essential, eternal and illusory, transitory. So just as all knowledge might be essential or illusory, so too platonic love was invidiously contrasted with transitory imperfect sexual desire as shameful and degrading. This is an essentially *cognitive* interpretation of the shamefulness of sexuality. The second source of shame reflects the primacy of an active political life in an honor-dominated democracy. Here the critical question became: Was it right for a young man to take pleasure in a passive homosexual position? The issue was not of homosexuality versus heterosexuality inasmuch as it was judged acceptable for a man to be a husband, father, and head of household and at the same time the lover and protector of a young boy. But the Greek polis was not only a democracy, but a warrior nation based on slavery. Therefore the critical question became whether a young man could be *penetrated* (as a woman or slave might be) and not jeopardize his future virile role of future father, head of household, and of citizen. The active role was assigned only to the male. The passive role was an essentially dishonorable and therefore shameful one.

With the Romans, the ideal of love turned heterosexual and was located within marriage as the privileged and natural state of sexual relations. Monogamy and procreation were magnified as "natural" because both promoted reproduction. Plutarch did not distinguish platonic from physical love, but considered the sexual a unified impulse with two forms, the homosexual and the heterosexual. To some extent the privatization of the sexual life was part of the growing decadence of Roman public life and the reduction in vigor of its political institutions, compared with the Greek polis. The reverse trend against romantic love and sex and the family may be observed in the Soviet Union in the 1920s after the Russian revolution, when a self-conscious attempt was made to ridicule and control any idealization of sexuality and love within the bourgeois family lest it attenuate the virtue of Marxist citizens.

In addition to the Roman privatization of marital love and sexuality, there was also another magnification of individualism that had fateful consequences for the theme of shame in sexuality. Although the Greeks had distinguished temperate sexuality from intemperate sexuality, the Roman Stoics shifted Socrates' maxim "the unexamined life is not worth living" away from cognition to will, action, and ataraxia, the indifference to desire itself. Thus Epictetus substituted austere programs of self-mastery for the Socratic self-understanding. It is will, not knowing, that becomes the critical virtue and it is desire whose imperfect control becomes a major source of shame. It is *not*, as it was for the Greeks, an invidious contrast between platonic, knowing love and mere physical desire, but between *all* desire and the strong individual *will*.

As any society limits excessively the freedom of its citizens, one classical alternative to shame and the unrenounced quest for satisfaction is to renounce not only those desires limited by the society, but to renounce all affect and desire, and to value only a self that is capable of such renunciation. In my view, for such renunciation to occur, the intolerability of shame and suspended desire must be radically magnified, at the same time that the self *cannot* accept its own impotence and shame. Under these conjoint conditions a new self may be invented which preemptively strikes out at destiny and so frees itself from both shame and intolerable longing. It makes a virtue of necessity. Such asceticism may be general, including sexuality as a special case, or it *may* be able to coexist with an aestheticism of sexuality free equally of shame and of shame as guilt.

Thus in India it proved possible to combine the conception of Nirvana with an aesthetic of sexuality, in the detailed and explicit cultivation of the art of love which implicated a renunciation of desire, neither Greek in its cognitive mode, nor Roman in its mode of renunciation. If one *understood* the nature of reality, the cessation of desire toward *illusion* was an easy consequence. One did not have to become a stoic gymnast of will. Sexuality and shame are necessarily influenced by the differential relative magnification of truth, by aesthetic or by moral values, as well as by other values. The further consequence of the differential magnification of truth, aesthetic, and moral values is in the differential magnification of those human functions believed to underly these values. Thus when truth is valued, cognition is valued; when morality is valued, will, cognition, and behavior contest for supremacy; when the aesthetic is valued, the perceptual, drive, and affect functions are valued above will, action, and cognition.

When we move to the Christian conception of sexuality and shame we move to a pluralism of ideologies and sectarian controversies, as in most religions. It is, however, clear that sexuality and shame become primarily moral and religious matters. Sexuality became one among many marks of the human being's fall from innocence and from love of and by God, for which s/he lived in the shadow of eternal damnation. Not only has sexuality turned from shame to guilt, but a massive burden of terror has been added to the sexual act. Sexuality is no longer aesthetic or unaesthetic, platonic or illusory, a threat to the active, honorable political life, a threat to the reproduction of the species and to the monogamous family, nor a threat to the will of the individual; it is now above all else a sign of disobedience to the will of God, demanding that the individual risk a variety of punishments, including an eternity in Hell. Shame and terror are now tightly fused. When such a Christian was confronted with sexuality s/he was not only tempted by a shameful and shame-evocative Satan, but by the wrath of a dangerous and wrathful, albeit loving God. The varieties of differential amplification of love, hate, terror, distress, and shame in the history of Christianity are beyond the scope of this Chapter, crucial though they may be to an understanding of our sexuality and of our sense of shame. We will, however, review one part of this history as it has recently been described by the philosopher Edward Leites (1985).

Leites has shown that the mainstream of seventeenth and

eighteenth century English Puritanism made moral constancy a core virtue. In marriage, public life, commerce, child raising, and religious behavior the Puritans demanded emotional steadiness and self-control. Puritan ministers exhorted spouses to maintain steady emotional tonicity *and* emotional warmth and erotic delight—spouses were asked to couple spontaneity and sobriety. The pleasures of marriage should be both sensuous and spiritual, a style of feeling and action that was at once self-controlled *and* free.

According to Leites, self-control or constancy had the following distinctive features: First, it was opposed to the oscillating temperament. Second, it called for a reduction in self-involvement and for paying increased attention to others, but without excessive emotion. Third, it demanded the separation of selves and thus prompted the creation of the modern individual with a private, interior life. Thus Addison and Steele, in *The Spectator* (1965) had urged that in the interest of maintaining "good humor" when one feels unpleasant emotions one must absent oneself until one has recovered an even temperament. For the Puritans such a private realm was primarily for the benefit of others, not for the self. Fourth, self-control or constancy entailed a new notion of *capacity* for constancy in both morals and emotions that can be achieved by the proper socialization of children. This is of course in the starkest contrast to that other Christian conception of the Roman Catholic Church—that of sin and guilt, repentance and forgiveness via the confession. Five, the Puritans held up the ideal of integration and harmony within the self, rather than that of repressive asceticism. The Puritans, according to Leites, and against Max Weber (1958) rejected the monastic life, and opposed the idea that the voluntary celibate life was in any way spiritually superior to the life of the married person. Within the confines of the marriage bed, sexuality and sexual pleasure were not only permitted but seen as good things. In Leites' view they thought of this delight as a moderate feeling which did not ordinarily lead to extremes of passion.

As a consequence of these moral dictates, new sources of shame in marriage and in sexuality were generated. If one were too intense in love and sex, too oscillating and labile in affect, too *split* in libido between marital and extramarital sex, too self-involved in one's sexuality and excitement, too ascetic or chaste to satisfy oneself and one's mate, one should properly feel ashamed (and or guilty).

Leites suggests that the difficulty of maintaining sexual excitement in marriage, which was examined at length in Restoration drama, was in part a consequence of the demandingness of this Puritan ideal of the integration of erotic and spiritual satisfaction in marriage. He traces another sequel to this ideal in an analysis of Richardson's *Pamela.* Here there was a partitioning of masculine adversarial sexuality and feminine sexual purity, each superior in its special way. Integration was replaced by the opposition of *purity versus sexuality* in the eighteenth century culture of England. This paradoxically splits shame in many ways into the masculine shame of excessive (immoral) excited lust invidiously compared with feminine modest shame, but also a shame of the effeminate, insufficiently bold sexual adventurer who fails to excite his mistress. For the female it splits shame into a furtive wish to be the object of masculine lust (against her pure and modest resistance) but also a shame of being the overly weak captive of the dominating male on the one hand, and the excessively prudish and shy female on the other who ambivalently cannot respond to the excitement of the bold lusty male.

The complexities of the varieties of sexual shame, which depend on the varieties of sexual excitement and sexual enjoyment, is but a special but poignant case of the more general ways in which human beings learn to lower their eyes and bow their head to the impediments to their deepest wishes.

## REFERENCES

Addison, J., Steele, R. (1965). *The spectator,* 5 Vol. D F. Bond (Ed.). Oxford: Clarendon Press.

Leites, E. (1985). *The Puritan Conscience and Modern Sexuality.* New Haven: Yale University Press.

Lichtenberg, J. D. (1983). *Psychoanalysis and Infant Research.* Hillsdale, NJ: Analytic Press.

Stern, D. N. (1985). *The Interpersonal World of the Infant.* New York: Basic Books.

Tomkins, S. S. (1962). *Affect/Imagery/Consciousness: I. The positive affects.* New York: Springer.

Tomkins, S. S. (1963). *Affect/Imagery/Consciousness: II. The negative affects.* New York: Springer.

Tomkins, S. S. (1965). Affect and the psychology of knowledge. In S. S. Tomkins and C. Izard (Eds.), *Affect, cognition and personality.* New York: Springer.

Tomkins, S. S. (1975). The phantasy behind the face. *Journal of Personality Assessment, 39:* 551–562.

Tomkins, S. S. (1979) Script theory: Differential magnification of affects. In H. E. Howe & R. H. Dienstbier (Eds.), *Nebraska Symposium of Motivation,* Vol. 26. Lincoln: University of Nebraska Press.

Vasquez, J. (1975). *The face and ideology.* Unpublished doctoral dissertation, Rutgers University.

Weber, M. (1958). *The protestant ethic and the spirit of capitalism* (T. Parsons, Trans.). New York: Charles Scribner's Sons.

# 5

# Shame and the Other: Reflections on the Theme of Shame in French Psychoanalysis*

EMMETT WILSON, JR.

*On a flight home from London, seated next to the Cambridge University Professor who directed the British Arctic and Antarctic Expeditions, I learned of his experiences as the only Westerner accompanying the recent Russian polar expedition. Describing his attempt to savor a small glass of sherry from the one bottle he had brought for the extended trip, he warned me, "Never open a bottle around Russians. Any open bottle must be finished. Its a matter of national pride." I suspect that most of us know the Russian character only from fiction or film, for political differences and unconscious prejudice foster the transmutation of propaganda into staunchly held beliefs. This polarization of views is compounded by the fact that we rarely get an opportunity to study the normal workings of the Soviet system. I was fascinated by this explorer's description of Russian communal life in the unbelievably cold realm of the polar ice cap, and their concept of the shared responsibility necessary to survival.*

*I wish to thank René Major, Léon Wurmser, Victor Smirnoff, Donald Nathanson, and Margaret Wilson for their very helpful discussions and suggestions which have aided me in the preparation of this chapter.

Emmett Wilson, Jr. Private Practice, Princeton, New Jersey.

*"One day" he continued, "one of the Russians was found smoking a cigarette in the commons room. A colleague asked him to stop, but the smoker compromised only to the extent of opening a window—not a good compromise when you realize that the loss of valuable heat (in this sixty-below climate) was not worth the exchange of clean for smoky air." A row ensued, and the group leader called a meeting to discuss the issue. The dozen or so members of the expedition sat around the room, each in turn giving his reasons that smoking was bad for the group. Last spoke the smoker, who stated flatly that he liked to smoke, wanted to smoke, felt he was within his rights to smoke, and intended to smoke. Once again, each in turn, the members of the group stated their opposition to smoking; once again the smoker defended his position. Patiently, the leader encouraged still a third round of statements, the meeting well into its fourth hour. "This time, however, the smoker recognized the error of his ways, and thanked the group for teaching him true communal responsibility." Is not this equally an example of the balance between shame (as exposure) and conformity as a defense against shame, as of the workings of the communal system?*

*We only hear about the failures of the communist system, not its successes. Western psychiatrists react reflexively to the Soviet equation of dissidence and protest with mental illness; yet the example given above suggests that the conformity achieved through a process of group discussion aimed toward concensus may represent a* normal *facet of the Russian personality. Of course I am aware that a view of normality that* demands *concensus is easily capable of perversion into a totalitarian system; but the ease with which such a system can be accepted in Russia may be a clue that the affect shame is socialized differently in that culture. We are used to the concept of "face" in the psychology and philsophy of Japan and China—the face is the locus of affect display and the seat of shame—and Eastern psychology is shame psychology. I suspect that the Russian character is far closer to the Oriental than most have thought—skin color does not define personality structure.*

*If, in drawing together so disparate a group of scholars to discuss these many faces of shame I have convinced the reader that ours, too, is a shame society, this volume will have been quite successful. Learning that Emmett Wilson was bilingual, had studied in Paris, and was well versed in the French psychoanalytic literature, I asked him to review the concept of shame in French culture. It was my feeling, considering the can-can and the bikini as against the French sense of tact and privacy, that the national character of France involved a quite partic-*

*ular balance of exhibitionism and prudery. The historical concern with the concept of self and other, with shame as a powerful force making us aware of the difference, illuminates his study. Wilson's meticulous survey of basic writings from the time of Descartes to the present allows us to peek into that national character, to contrast ours against it, and to learn more about shame itself.*

At first blush it would seem that French psychoanalysis has ignored shame and its cognate concepts. Few writings focus directly and self-consciously on the topic of shame. Those that are available are often not easy to find, for in France it seems almost bad form to use a title that would immediately betray the contents of an article or book. Shame has certainly not become a catchword in French psychoanalytic circles. This is surprising in view of what may seem at times a virtual preoccupation with themes of *gloire, honneur,* and *amour propre* in French literature and in French culture. The language even has several terms for shame: *honte, vergogne, pudeur*. One would have thought that, of all concepts, shame would be thoroughly dealt with in the French analytic literature. In view of this relative neglect by French analysts, how is it that the current Anglo-American interest in shame seems so immediately within the French psychoanalytic tradition?

To explain this phenomenon, some background is necessary. Anglo-American psychoanalysis tends to turn to philosophy only when it gets into a quandary, as a way out of some problem or other. In contrast, French psychoanalysis has participated in the general intellectual life of that country in a way that is not found in the United States. Analysts in France have been very much influenced by philosophical concerns; they have never strayed very far from their philosophical heritage. These shared intellectual interests show up clearly in the French psychoanalytic literature. It is in the history of these pursuits that we may find the background necessary to place the concept of shame in perspective and thus clarify its influence on French psychoanalysis.

## PHILOSOPHICAL DISCUSSIONS OF SHAME AND THE GAZE (*LE REGARD*)

### *Descartes and the* Cogito

Most readers will be familiar at least in outline with the famous *cogito* of René Descartes: "I think, therefore I am." This was Descartes's attempt to find an indubitable starting point for philosophy, one unassailable by skepticism. With this move, Descartes attempted to found the true principle of philsophical certainty in the existing, thinking self, as the metaphysical point of departure for all philosophical knowledge. In the *cogito* and in the study of its implications Descartes sought an intuitive, indubitable, and self-evident basis for metaphysical truths.

We need not go into all the details of the subsequent history of the *cogito* here, for the unpacking of its implications accounts for much of the history of modern philosophy. The problems have been many, however. Most readers will know something of so-called Cartesian dualism, the view that there are two distinct realms: one of thinking substance, or mind, and the other of unthinking matter, or body. This position is often held responsible for the "mind/body problem." Various theories of interactionism, occasionalism, or parallelism, as well as more sophisticated contemporary proposals have been put forward as explanations for the manner in which the two realms are related. A stark dichotomization of mind and matter, of inner and outer reality, seemed to be the corollary of Descartes's move, and is certainly found in some philosophers inspired by Descartes.

Real or imagined difficulties with Cartesianism, of course, are not new to American psychoanalytic theorists. Many of them have criticized Descartes for fostering a "false" dichotomy of mind and body, as well as other "false" dichotomies such as that between objective science and subjective experience. Few, however, appreciate the difficult epistemological and metaphysical problems Descartes was trying to deal with in the *cogito*. Nor is there much appreciation of the intriguing complexities of Descartes's position, the issues Descartes himself raised about the mind/body problem, or his disavowal of the simplistic interpretation of the mind or soul as the "man in the machine." Few know his statement: "I am not . . . lodged in my body as a pilot in a vessel" (Descartes, 1955, Vol. 1, pp. 118, 192). Nor is there much recognition of his very modern view of the importance of language as the distinguishing characteristic of that which is human. Instead, his approach is schematically designated the Cartesian position, or Cartesianism, and Descartes is blamed for the scientific model supposedly derived from Cartesianism, and according to some critics, imposed on psychoanalysis.

## *THE PHENOMENOLOGISTS' CRITIQUE OF THE COGITO**

On the Continent, philosophers have often been concerned with the equally troublesome danger that this so-called reflective stream in philosophy might collapse into idealism or solipsism, whether of the Berkeleian or Hegelian variety. Solipsism refers to the philosophical position in which the self can know only itself as the only existent thing. Continental philosophers have often worried about this supposed commitment to solipsism in the *cogito*, with the thinking subject isolated, alone, certain only of his own certainty, while the rest of experience is reduced to possibly deceptive images and sensations. The *cogito* seemed to lead back to the skepticism it had meant to resolve. Though clearly a starting point for philosophy, the *cogito* became a most problematic one. For some, too, the Cartesian position represented the triumph of a sterile rationalistic approach, and many felt it would have been better to start from something like: "I feel, therefore I am."

The phenomenologists (and later, the existentialists) thought there was both more and less in the *cogito* than Descartes realized. These philosophers propounded alterative analyses of the *cogito* that are important for our purposes here. One of the central philosophical issues has been what is often called "alterity" on the Continent, or what Anglo-American philosophers refer to as the problem of other minds. These philosophical concerns about the other have led to the discovery of impli-

*See Spiegelberg (1960) and Schroeder (1984).

cations of the *cogito* that are perhaps different from or at odds with conclusions some Cartesians have drawn from it. In particular, continental philosophers have sought a way out of the apparent solipsistic collapse of the *cogito* by emphasizing an intuitive knowledge of another's presence in the "gaze of the other," and in the shame one feels under this gaze.

The theme of shame was dealt with somewhat perfunctorily by Descartes, in his *Passions of the Soul* (1953, p. 791f.). This work, published toward the end of Descartes's life, contains his fanciful theory of the pineal gland as the locus of the interaction between mind and body. It contains discussions of other issues as well, for he considers speculative psychological problems, the emotions, and morals—what would now be called philosophical psychology. Shame is a form of sadness founded on self-love, which comes from the belief or the fear that one is going to be blamed by others. Descartes concluded that we need the opinion of others even though they judge badly at times.

This is rather bland, coming from the man whose *cogito* initiated modern philosophy. The intersubjective element, however, is clearly present. It was to be seen even more clearly by Baruch Spinoza. Jerome Neu, in his description of the philosophical background for the psychoanalytic theory of the emotions, mentions Spinoza's discussion of "social emotions." Neu (1977) writes:

> The *capacity* to be ashamed depends on a prior understanding of blame (the pain with which a person turns away from another person's action, the purpose of which is to harm him). Without this concept, one could have no reason for thinking one was ashamed rather than merely repentant (which does not require awareness of our bad intention by another, the bad effects repented of might not even involve another). Even if we use "shame" in its looser more modern sense, where it is assimilated to Spinoza's use of "repentance," one could not feel shame (as opposed to, say, embarrassment, discomfort, or unease) unless one had concepts like "guilt" and "responsibility" and was able to apply them (even if misapplied on a particular occasion). One cannot feel shame *simpliciter*. (p. 94)

Some of the notions we are considering are to be found in the work of G. F. Hegel, in his discussion of self-consciousness.

For Hegel, self-consciousness exists by the fact that it exists for another consciousness. It is only by being recognized or acknowledged by others—as the result of *intersubjective* relationships—that consciousness of the self comes into being. There are also various other important Hegelian notions concerning the relationship of one consciousness to another: the master–slave dialectic, the theme of lordship and bondage, and the themes of mastery, control, and submission to the other. These will recur in our discussion of the various psychoanalytic aspects of shame. Unfortunately Hegel's insights tended to be obscured by the complexities of the philosophical system he developed, and by the prose in which he expounded it.

It was not until the work of the phenomenologists that the full implications of the theme of intersubjectivity were developed. We will first consider the German-speaking philosophers Brentano, Husserl, and Scheler, before moving on to the particularly French version of phenomenology that developed with Sartre and Merleau-Ponty.

Franz Brentano (1874/1973) stressed the intentionality of mental acts as a key element in his psychological theory. Mental acts are always directed *toward* something: a fear is a fear *of* something, love is love *for* something, and so forth. This notion has been important for the phenomenological position. Some have even thought that it may have influenced Freud in his recognition of the meaningfulness of unconsciously motivated behavior, for it is known that Freud attended Brentano's lectures at the University of Vienna. Edmund Husserl, who was very much influenced by Brentano, made the *cogito* one of the central themes in his work. In his *Cartesian Meditations* (1931/1960), Husserl set out to examine the *cogito* anew and in so doing to find what he called the "structures of consciousness" and how the ego apprehended them. He developed the notion of the intentionality of consciousness further.

The philosopher Max Scheler (1913/1970) extended this theme of intersubjectivity with his view of the direct perception of other selves. He maintained that there was an intuitive perception, not an inference of the other person. One does not perceive a body, but a person; one does not see someone's eyes, but rather his gaze. There is at first a neutral primordial stream of consciousness, which is then differentiated into consciousness of the self and the other—a view now familiar to analysts influenced by studies of infant development and early object relations.

We need not be concerned with the intricacies of the phenomenological doctrine, but the psychology that developed from it has had a great influence on French philosophy and on French psychoanalysis. Though much influenced by Husserl and Scheler, a peculiarly French version of phenomenology developed. The theme of otherness, however, continued to be a preoccupation. As Vincent Descombes (1980) remarks in his history of French philosophy, "The 'problem of the other' . . . furnished the writings of French phenomenology with their principal subject matter" (p. 22). Both Jean-Paul Sartre (1943/1956) and Maurice Merleau-Ponty (1968) refused to follow Descartes into either the dualism or solipsism to which classical Cartesianism was thought to lead, and both sought other meanings in the *cogito.* The theme of intersubjectivity occupies Sartre's attention in his major philosophical work, *Being and Nothingness* (1943/1956). In this treatise Sartre takes shame as the emotion to examine most fully in discussing the existence of others. In the feeling of shame—as we saw even in Descartes's discussion of the emotions—there is an immediate intersubjective field. Sartre places his emphasis on shame *before somebody*. Shame is not reached by reflection, as the *cogito* is. Instead, "I am ashamed of myself as I *appear* to the Other. . . . Shame is shame *of oneself before the Other*; these two structures are inseparable" (p. 222). Sartre thus understands shame as epistemologically and metaphysically an indication of a basic relatedness to others.

In summary, we might characterize the phenomenologists' critique of Descartes by modifying the cogito to read: *pudeo ergo sumus,* "I am ashamed, therefore we exist." Even more apt, since the verbal form for shame is usually impersonal in Latin: *pudet, ergo sumus,* "It shames, therefore we exist." In this aphoristic way we might summarize the role of shame in leading from an undifferentiated experiential matrix to the development of two self-conscious subjects. Their intersubjective existence for each other is discovered in the experience of shame. Because of shame, because of my concern with how I appear to the other, I become aware that others exist together with me in an intersubjective field.

## PSYCHOANALYTIC DISCUSSIONS OF SHAME

In France, the tendency for philosophical ideas to be taken up in other areas of intellectual endeavor, and to be reflected in the general intellectual life of the country, means that we encounter these same themes in psychoanalytic discussions. One of the main issues in French psychoanalysis, from its beginnings through Lacan to the present day, has involved a revolt against the solipsistic implications of Cartesianism similar to that in philosophical circles. Alterity has thus been a central theme in French psychoanalysis. Though there are parallels to the Anglo-American concept of object relations, including a parallel in the emphasis on object relatedness, there are major differences in approach.

Furthermore, French psychoanalytic writing contains many discussions that in a sense presuppose or derive from issues about shame. When seen from this perspective, much of French psychoanalysis falls into place as a series of discussions with a continuing and central focus on the development of early object relations and the development of the sense of self. Jacques Lacan's work on the mirror stage (1949/1977), for example, can be understood in this sense. The sympathetic hearing so often found in France for Kleinian formulations is also a manifestation of this interest in early object relations. Lacan's work, too, has stimulated the discussion of narcissism in France, as have the discussions of narcissism that emphasize its centrifugal or object-seeking aspects (Grunberger, 1958/1979a; Pasche, 1965/1980). The French have taken eagerly to contemporary research on infant psychiatry, whether it be by American "nursery neo-Kleinians" such as Eleanor Galenson and Herman Roiphe, or by French researchers such as Colette Chiland and Serge Lebovici. This, too, can be seen as part of the intense interest in early object relations. All these themes can be correlated as attempts to delineate the development of an intersubjective world and the nature of intersubjective experience.

### *JACQUES LACAN*

One of the chapters in Lacan's *The Four Fundamental Concepts of Psychoanalysis* (1978) deals with the gaze (*le regard*). Lacan calls

Sartre's comments on the gaze "one of the most brilliant passages of *Being and Nothingness*," and proceeds to discuss the gaze at length, exploring and developing its implications for psychology and philosophy. As Lacan states in his inimitably grandiloquent manner:

> Sartre . . . brings [the gaze] into function in the dimension of the existence of others. Others would remain suspended in the same, partially de-realizing conditions that are, in Sartre's definition, those of objectivity, were it not for the gaze. The gaze, as conceived by Sartre, is the gaze by which I am surprised—surprised in so far as it changes all the perspectives, the lines of force, of my world, orders it, from the point of nothingness where I am, in a sort of radiated reticulation of the organisms. (p. 84)

This passage, which certainly demonstrates some of the density and obscurity of Lacanian prose, means roughly that the other person's gaze functions as an organizer for our experience, structuring the psychological field as an intersubjective one, with all its attendant tensions and forces.

Lacan has two notions of otherness. There is the Other (*Autre*) with a capital letter. This Lacanian notion of the Other assigns considerable importance to language. For Lacan, the self-consciousness that thinks is a speaking self-consciousness—it has the use of language. This exercise of language is the foundation of subjectivity and of intersubjectivity. The speaking subject is sustained by language, by discourse, that is, by the "chain of signifiers." There is an "order of signifiers"—an "arrangement of relationships"—that has enough stability and firmness to be called a "law", or "the Law". This is, for Lacan, the "Law of the Father", the universal discourse into which one is integrated. Lacan designates this "order of signifiers in all its complexity" as "the Other," that is, "as pure Alterity as such".

There is another other in Lacan: *objet petit a*, the other with a small letter (i.e., *autre*). Lacan is also interested in bringing the gaze into relation with this other, which seems to be a composite of the Freudian concept of object relation and phenomenological alterity. He is not wholly in agreement with Sartre's view of the gaze and its role in the development of intersubjectivity, and he introduces another current into the discussion, the Hegelian notion of Desire, the peculiarly human and unfulfillable need and demand for love. For Lacan, Sartre's analysis of the gaze is not a correct phenomenological analysis. Sartre speaks of being caught spying. It is not merely a gaze that he sees, but, according to Lacan, "a gaze which surprises him in the function of voyeur, disturbs him, overwhelms him and reduces him to a feeling of shame. . . . [It is] a gaze imagined . . . in the field of the Other" (1978, p. 84). If one does not stress the dialectic of Desire, according to Lacan, it is not possible to understand why the gaze of others should so disorganize the field of perception.

There is a strong Hegelian influence in French philosophy. In the Anglo-American intellectual tradition, a combination of good sense and analytic philosophy, perhaps in that order, has more or less minimized Hegel's influence. Not so in France. An interpreter of Hegel, Alexandre Kojève (1969)— whose Hegel was more Kojève than Hegel—influenced a generation of French intellectuals, Lacan and Merleau-Ponty among them, through lectures at the École des Hautes Études in the 1930's. In addition to the theme of Desire, the Hegelian theme of master and slave afforded a focus for French intellectual discussion among philosophers and novelists, and among analysts as well, as we shall see later when some of these Hegelian themes recur in our consideration of masochism, exhibitionism, and narcissism.

## TOWARD A PSYCHOANALYTIC THEORY OF SHAME

We have reviewed the emphasis on intersubjectivity with its roots in Sartre's discussion of the gaze, and in Lacan's further development of this theme around the topic of alterity. The theme of shame has not, to my knowledge, been taken up again as an overarching or central concept since these early writings. I am in complete agreement, however, with the view expressed by Octave Mannoni (1982, p. 78), who feels that shame has not received its due place in psychoanalytic theory.

Mannoni makes these comments in the course of a study of countertransference contributions to interpretation. Unfortunately he accords only a few brief but important pages to the topic of shame. He suggests that the neglect may be due to Freud's difficulties about shame. Early in the development of psychoanalysis, Freud broached the topic when, in the course of his analysis of his dream of Count Thun, he mentions a scene from his childhood that had been described to him. At age 2, after a reproach from his father for bed-wetting, he was said to have consoled his father by promising to buy a new bed for him. Freud "short-circuits" the development of a theory of shame by referring immediately to the "intimate connection between bed-wetting and the character trait of ambition" (Freud, 1900, p. 216). Mannoni suggests that we can read similar themes into Freud's analysis of his Uncle Josef dream, a dream that was motivated by ambitions concerning an academic appointment. This dream suggests a further development of the themes of ambition, narcissism, and shame. Freud, according to Mannoni, eventually came to provide a theory of shame without ever mentioning it by name, at the beginning of the Postscript to his discussion of group psychology (1921, p. 134). Here Freud discusses Schiller's play *Wallensteins Lager*, and the ridicule that befell a sergeant who tried to identify himself with the general-in-chief, Wallenstein himself. Instead of shame, however, Freud focuses on ridicule. He uses the theme of ridicule to develop further the contrast between an identification at the level of the ego ideal and one at the level of the ego. An identification at the level of ego ideal has organizing and goal-setting characteristics for an individual. Had the sergeant made Wallenstein his ego ideal, he would have been the most devoted of junior officers. However, an identification at the level of the ego leads merely to mimicry and counterfeit imitation, and subjects the sergeant to ridicule. Mannoni thinks this is Freud's unenunciated theory of shame, and perhaps the only theory of shame that has been developed in psychoanalysis.

Mannoni indicates, however, that it is merely a false first impression that there is not much in the psychoanalytic literature on shame. I cannot therefore agree with him that Freud's sketch of a theory is our only theory of shame. The current interest in shame in Anglo-American psychoanalysis has shown how a great many apparently disparate themes are interconnected around the theme of shame—as derivative from or related to it in various ways. Léon Wurmser (1981), for example, links many themes from the study of the perversions (such as scoptophilia, exhibitionism, and masochism) with the notion of humiliation, subjugation, and control. He places such topics as narcissism and the self in relation to the theme of shame. In France these issues have been the subject of lively interest and have been treated with a typically French sensitivity to nuance and detail. Excellent clinical and theoretical discussions are interwoven with the theme of shame. As I hope to show in a brief, and admittedly incomplete survey of the writings of some contemporary French psychoanalytic theorists, a psychoanalytic theory of shame is in the process of developing and coalescing, however inchoate and unformed it may be as yet.

## *PSYCHOANALYTIC LITERARY CRITICISM*

In literary studies the influence of the phenomenological discussions of the gaze and shame is widespread. In Charles Badouin's (1943/1972) study of Victor Hugo, which is for the most part a brilliant but standard oedipal intepretation, there is a section called "Eye and Mystery," in which Badouin discusses what he calls the *complex spectaculaire*. There Badouin introduces the problems of seeing, being seen, showing and hiding—relating all these to oedipal conflict.

The critic Jean Starobinski, who is important to us because of his psychoanalytic sophistication, also takes up the theme. In his *L'Oeil vivant* (1961), he discusses the gaze and its relationship to objects. From this critique he develops the concept of "the hidden," defined as the other side of a presence. In his consideration of the gaze Starobinski touches on the other and on narcissistic regression. He discusses looking as an action that aims to place the other under guard or control. The act of looking is not over with immediately, for it brings along with it a persevering conquest or the desire of conquest. Starobinski in effect engages in a psychoanalysis of scoptophilia, and finds that seeing is unconsciously a dangerous act. Mythology and legend are unanimous on this, as he shows in the myths of Orpheus, Narcissus, Oedipus, Psyche, and Medusa. These myths are elaborations on the theme that the attempt to extend the scope of one's gaze leads the soul to blindness and death. He expands the theme in a study of Corneille, Racine, Stendhal, and especially Rousseau, to whom he later devoted a monograph (1971; see Clancier, 1973).

## *CLINICAL STUDIES*

### *The Perversions in General*

Clinical psychoanalytic studies present a rich exploration of areas subsidiary and adjacent to the topic of shame. The subject of perversion in particular has been extensively considered in the French psychoanalytic literature. If we take the notion of shame to be a central concept in narcissism, these studies of the perversions and of the role of humiliation, shame, and narcissism may lead eventually to the development of a coherent theory of shame.

Of the perversions, fetishism and sadomasochism have been perhaps the most thoroughly researched. All this work stresses the role of narcissism. Victor Smirnoff (1970/1980), in a major work on fetishism, brings out the importance of the component instincts, and includes cruelty, scoptophilia, and narcissism as central features of the fetishistic perversion. In a more recent study of fetishism, André Lussier (1983) comments:

> The voyeur, the exhibitionist, the sadist all have a very specific problem to resolve, a specific anxiety to reduce to silence, a proof to establish, a trauma to master. The fetishist also has this specific problem, but he goes much farther in his ambitious regression, in an attempt to refind the lost epoch, to find the lost object of the past, and, in a manner quite different from the psychotic, he is successful. . . . The fetishist, infinitely more than any other pervert, lives in the inextinguishable nostalgia of a maternal paradise. (pp. 23–24)

Masochism has also been related to this theme of narcissism. In one of the most interesting studies on masochism M. de M'Uzan (1972/1973) reports a case that is exceptional in the intensity of the sadomasochism and horror. He suggests that pain in this case, and perhaps in many cases of masochism, is the means rather than the aim of the perversion; masochism, then, is to be construed not so much from the point of view of castration anxiety, but as outside the oedipal conflict and more in the context of an attempt to heal the primordial narcissistic wound.

*Scoptophilia*

The visual perversions have been to some extent slighted in this context, but a recent extensive study of exhibitionism and voyeurism by Gérard Bonnet (1981) corrects this relative neglect. Bonnet's study is especially relevent in that he continues the theme of the gaze and the other, so important in the earlier works we have examined. Bonnet deals with the clinical as well as the metapsychological aspects of the pair of opposites: seeing and being seen. He provides extensive clinical studies of the various manifestations of exhibitionism and voyeurism, including such usually ignored phenomena as streaking, or group exhibitionism. He also presents a detailed case of female exhibitionism.

Lacan stressed that the true partner of a voyeur is another voyeur, someone who takes the place of the voyeur at the moment that the voyeur, surprised in the act, becomes the person seen. Lacan made this criticism of Sartre's discussion of the gaze, we may recall, when he pointed out that Sartre does not actually speak of seeing another's gaze, but of being himself surprised in the act of looking through a keyhole. Bonnet suggests that a similiar process is involved in exhibitionism, for the exhibitionist has the secret desire that his or her "victim" exhibit himself or herself also. When looking is forced on the "victim," the victim responds. He or she is provoked to institute punishment, for example, in the type of exhibitionism that Bonnet calls "penal exhibitionism," in which the exhibitionist seems to set himself up to be caught and punished. In "anonymous exhibitionism," on the other hand, the exhibitionist is not caught, but the "victim" exhibits his or her responses. The victim is provoked to fear, shock, and to telling about the encounter. For Bonnet, the victim's exhibitionism lies in the reports he or she gives of the incident, and he examines these reports at length to corroborate his thesis. This emphasis on the response of the victim is extremely important for our topic, for it shows how the victim becomes an integral part of the dyad depicted by the theorists of shame we discussed earlier.

Bonnet discusses the themes of opposites, reversal, and turning round upon the self. However, he tries to avoid the structuralism that has led many French psychoanalytic writers to emphasize the grammatical or syntactical aspects of such mechanisms as turning around and reversal. He considers various efforts to clarify these themes, including Lacan's *Four Fundamental Concepts* (1978) and Laplanche's *Life and Death in Psychoanalysis* (1970/1976).

Rather than involve the reader in these rather abstract, difficult, but important issues of psychoanalytic theory, perhaps I could characterize Bonnet's discussion by reference to a familiar joke. "Beat me!" pleads the masochist. "No, I won't!" taunts the sadist. This simple, classic joke suggests that the sadist does not take a masochist for his partner and it is likely such a relationship would be insupportable. Bonnet feels that Freud missed this in the metapsychological papers, a lapse he is trying to rectify.

Bonnet thus argues that there is no direct relationship between the various pairs of perversions. It cannot be assumed that there is a simple pair of opposites, for example, to see and to be seen, to hurt and to be hurt. There is not a simple dualism. There are, Bonnet points out, referential pairs, functional pairs, positional pairs, theoretical pairs, differential pairs, constitutive pairs, symmetrical pairs, asymmetrical pairs, and so on. All dogmatism becomes ludicrous and untenable in view of this complexity. If there is a pair of opposites, a coupled or linked set of impulses with complementarity, it is not to be sought on the same terrain as the manifest content of the perversion. In the manifest content, the unconscious currents are separate in spite of appearances which suggest a set of mirror opposites. The complementarity is to be sought, rather, at the level of unconscious components.

Bonnet directs us back to Freud's early discussions, beginning even with Freud's own exhibitionism in revealing his dreams to Fliess, and he makes some interesting generalizations on the exhibitionistic element in analytic practice. He focuses especially on the discussion of dreams of nudity in *The Interpretation of Dreams* (1900). The dream of exhibition manifests, under the cover of anal eroticism, the infantile desire to give birth to a child by one's own means, to be recognized as a creator, the discoverer—possible only if the other intervenes as a spectator, as the public. Bonnet follows the theme of the "eye of the other" through Freud's works and case studies, discussing relevant passages in the article on hysterical blindness and in the study of jokes. In the Dora case, Freud traced the hysteric's conflicts about seeing, while the Rat Man's masturbation before a mirror provided Freud the opportunity to analyze these conflicts in an obsessional subject.

Bonnet's extensive study continues the themes we have been sketching concerning intersubjectivity. Ambivalence about "the eye of the other" plays an indispensable role in the organization of these conflicts about seeing and being seen.

## PSYCHOANALYTIC THEORIES OF SHAME

### *NARCISSISM AND SHAME*

We have noted the centrality of the theme of narcissism in the studies reviewed so far. We shall now move on to work that links narcissism and shame. In France there has been an intense interest in the problems of narcissism, stimulated of course by Lacan, in part by the research of such other French analysts as Béla Grunberger, Guy Rosolato, and Francis Pasche, and by the contributions of Heinz Kohut. The rather total rejection of American analytic contributions influenced by Hartmann, which has characterized French psychoanalysis up to now, has ironically given way to an intense interest in the contributions of Kohut, as if these in some way redeemed American analysis. Indeed, the French have watched with interest the tilting of lances between Kohut and Kernberg. An issue of the *Nouvelle Revue de Psychanalyse* in 1976 was devoted to the topic, with articles by Guy Rosolato, André Green, Colette Chiland, Joyce McDougall, and with translations of Otto Kernberg, Hans Lichtenstein, and Herbert Rosenfeld.

For our purposes, we can limit our observations to Béla Grunberger and André Green. Grunberger has traced the path of narcissism through all the psychosexual stages and shown its use of different modes in these successive phases. One of his articles (1960/1979b) discusses the anal object relationship in the language of shame, humiliation, and control of the other. The anal character seeks a particular form of object relationship in which the object is acquired or conquered, and its uniqueness and autonomy are obliterated through this subjugation and control. The object is held captive and persecuted. The objects whom the anal narcissist attempts to master are interchangeable and indifferent to him. What matters is, rather, the *energic relationship* between subject and object. The establishment of this relation alone is sufficient to ensure his instinctual gratification. The anal character considers the individuality of his object as an obstacle standing in his way, thwarting his mastery of the object. This obstacle evokes the anal character's aggression, and he feels forced to fight and to obliterate the individuality of the other. The anal character's aim is "to reduce the object to its original form, which is that of excrement" (p. 149). This permits the anal narcissist to free himself totally from his own oral dependency and to base his autonomy on his power to make his object totally dependent on him.

Grunberger feels that such phenomena as discrimination, value scales, social and organizational hierarchies, and social stratification are derivatives of the anal object relationship. The anal subject-object couple is, for Grunberger, an extreme form of the Hegelian theme of master and slave: "You are my object, I will do with you what I want, and you will have no way of opposing me" (ibid.). The anal narcissist does not try to love and be loved but instead to dominate a captive and persecuted object. Grunberger is clearly aware that anality, when integrated into the personality, makes a contribution to the normal evolution of the individual, for "all constructive forms of human activity depend on it. The most highly evolved psychic functions (consciousness, perception, the sense of reality, judgment, abstraction, etc.) have their roots in it" (p. 156). In the normal subject it is subsumed under genital primacy. Grunberger has, however, provided us with a study of some of the typical consequences of pathologic fixation at the anal narcissistic stage.

More directly focused on the topic of shame is an important discussion by André Green (1983). He considers shame in the course of exploring what he calls moral narcissism. Green distinguishes: (1) a corporeal narcissism, which concerns body feelings and body representations pertaining to the body experienced as an object of the gaze of the other; (2) an intellectual narcissism, with a cathexis of and an abusive confidence in intellectual mastery—a sort of secondary form of the omnipotence of thought; and (3) a moral narcissism, which involves a cathexis of the infantile narcissistic state of wholeness or completeness, with ascetic sacrifices and a preoccupation with honor.

Green believes that it is important to distinguish between this concept of moral *narcissism* and the better-known moral *masochism* that Freud described. Even though there are parallels, and the death instinct and instinctual renunciation are involved in both, in moral narcissism we are not dealing with the masochist's punitive, severe superego. The two entities are distinct in the type of unconscious fantasy material present. The masochist desires to be beaten, humiliated, sullied, reduced to passivity, but it is a passivity requiring the presence of the other. The masochist was described by Lacan as needing "the anxiety of the other." It is different for the narcissist, who wants to be pure, to be alone, to renounce *both* the pleasures and pains of the world. He situates himself beyond pleasure and unpleasure—he is not looking for pain. Rather, he makes godlike vows of poverty, nakedness, endurance, solitude. His aim is the effacement of any trace of the other in the Desire for the One, the return to the maternal bosom, the "degree zero." This is an intense asceticism such as that described in some adolescents, but in pathologic form. Suffering is not sought, nor is it avoided. Instead of wanting to be treated as a small child—as Freud described the masochist—the narcissist wants to be treated as the opposite. He is a child who wants to resemble the parents who he fantasizes have no problem in dominating their impulses. He wants to be a grownup, which he equates with being godlike.

Green contrasts shame and guilt through a consideration of two plays by Sophocles: *Oedipus Rex* and *Ajax*. The theme of shame is a keyword textually in the *Ajax*, as it is psychologically for the narcissist. Utilizing the discussions by E. R. Dodds (1951) and M. Piers and G. Singer (1953), Green explores the distinction between shame and guilt in these two plays and in the clinical situations they suggest. Individual psychopathology, according to Green, corroborates the themes developed by Dodds and by Piers and Singer. By linking shame to pregenital phases of development, we are able to explain not only its narcissistic element but also its intransigent, cruel character, which makes no reparation possible. Shame is global, primary, and absolute.

Though Ajax sought self-punishment, we must distinguish this from the self-punishment of the masochist. The masochist masks an unpunished fault under his masochism—he has sinned and feels blamable. Ajax, however, does not look for punishment but inflicts it on himself to save his honor—the other keyword of narcissism. The moral narcissist has not committed a sin or crime, but has remained fixated in his infantile megalomania and is always in debt to his ego ideal. As a result, he does not feel guilty, but feels shame for not being that which he is or of claiming to be more than he is. Moral narcissism concerns the subject's honor, his level of being, rather than guilt for having comitted some transgression. In moral narcissism, the punishment (shame) takes place through an insatiable redoubling of pride. Honor is never safe. All is lost, because nothing can wash away the pollution from soiled honor, unless it is a new and further renunciation of object relatedness for the sake of this narcissism. Hence narcissists are needy, despite their wish to be so godlike and independent. The ego ideal of the moral narcissist is built on the vestige of the ideal ego—on an omnipotent idealizing power of satisfaction which does not know the limitations of castration. Moral narcissism thus has less to do with the oedipal conflict than with that which denies it. The inevitable failure of such a clinical stance leads inexorably to depression. Green links his concept of moral narcissism to the clinical entity described by Pasche (1961/1969) as the "depression of inferiority."

There are close connections between this moral narcissism and the other types of narcissism, according to Green. Intellectual narcissism is a form of self-sufficiency and solitary validation which fills in and makes up for human desire and longing by intellectual mastery or intellectual seduction. It involves a hypertrophy of desexualized cathexes which are ordinarily occasion for the displacement of pregenital partial, scoptophilic, exhibitionistic, and sadomasochistic impulses. They turn against an instinctual life which must be not merely repressed or controlled, but totally extinguished. The shame is for being human and endowed with an instinctual life. Intellectual work is a displacement for this instinctual life. But even this displacement is doomed to failure, for the ever-vigilant superego detects, behind this intellectual activity, the strong eroticization involved. The work is sensed as shameful, and intellectual efforts may be accompanied by headaches, insomnia, difficulties in concentrating or reading, and the impossibility of utilizing what is acquired. It is shameful because the subject senses the link to sexuality and to masturbatory activity.

Moral narcissism has especially strong links to body narcissism as well. The body as appearance, as source of pleasure, of seduction and conquest of the other, is forbidden. For the moral narcissist, hell is not others, it is the body. The body is the other he thought to be rid of. In spite of the narcissist's attempt to efface all trace of the other, it rises again in the body. The body is limitation, servitude, finitude. For that reason the illness is preeminently a bodily illness: being-ill-in-one's-skin. Intestinal sounds, vasomotor reactions, sweating, sensations of cold and heat which occur in therapy sessions are a torture for narcissists because they can control their fantasies but before their bodies they are powerless, defenseless. The body is their absolute master, their shame.

## *SHAME AND THE EGO IDEAL*

Discussions of shame are to be found in the French psychoanalytic literature linking shame and the ego ideal. The work of Nicolas Abraham and Maria Torok (1972, 1972/1980) provide several reflections on the subject of shame, the other, and the ego ideal, together with important clinical considerations. I will concentrate, however, on an important essay by Janine Chasseguet-Smirgel on the ego ideal (1973/1985). In this work she delineates the pregenital elements in the ego ideal and sketches the development of the ego ideal and its pathology. She traces the linkage of the ego ideal to narcissism and to homosexuality. The same libidinal positions seem to her to be involved in shame.

Chasseguet-Smirgel alludes also to Piers and Singer's discussion (1953) of shame and the tension between the ego ideal and the superego. While the relationship between shame and exhibitionism was noted by Freud and further developed by Nunberg, she applauds the insight of Piers and Singer in making the link to narcissism. On the basis of this linkage she develops a quite interesting theory involving shame, the "homosexual double," and anality. She points out that we fear being seen in situations that are narcissistically unsatisfying. We fear being seen in these situations by our "counterparts" (*nos semblables*), who play the role for us of a mirror reflecting our ego with its possible faults. Everything takes place as if our feelings of personal worth, our self-esteem, the tension or harmony between our ego and our ego ideal depended, for a large part, on the image that our peers send back to us. Only through our *semblables* do we seem to have proof of the worth or the absence of worth of our ego. We have no proof of reality of our internal and external perceptions except in these mirrors that reflect our psychic self. Her thesis is that our perception of how our narcissistic, and thus homosexual, doubles perceive us permits us to gauge our own self. The manner in which we are seen and perceived by others is the equivalent of a projection onto the external world of our psychic self; it represents an essential, perhaps the only, mode of submitting our psychic self to the proof of reality. There is then a relationship between this evaluation of our psychic self and homosexuality; it is of course a homosexuality normally inhibited with respect to aim, and more or less perfectly desexualized, responsible for our social instincts as well as our sense of self-validation.

Chasseguet-Smirgel sees a complementarity between her formulations on the homosexual double and Freud's views in the Schreber case, (Freud, 1911/1958), as well as Victor Tausk's discussion of the influencing machine (Tausk, 1919/1933). Since the psychic self has no representative in the external world, it uses the body self with which it is identified to represent it. The body ego is a double, a homosexual double. In Tausk's theory, it becomes the influencing machine, that is, a homosexual object as the place of projection and of persecution.

The difficulty, of course, in submitting our ego to this test of reality is that our view of ourselves is never really stabilized no matter how much we may be gratified by this reflection from others. For the observing other is never entirely good, and there is always some dissatisfaction between the self and the ego ideal. When exhibition before these homosexual doubles fails to obtain a narcissistic satisfaction, a feeling of shame results. In Chasseguet-Smirgel's view the following sequence is involved: the desire to receive a narcissistic confirmation from one's likeness, and thus to diminish the margin between the ego and one's ideal, leads to an exhibition of the self before the homosexual doubles. If this exhibition fails to provide satisfaction but instead produces a narcissistic wound or a social rebuff, there is an immediate resexualization of homosexuality, which assimilates the narcissistic wound to a castration, with a fear of passive anal penetration. Shame represents the proximity of this sexual desire.

Chasseguet-Smirgel notes the curious fact that many authors who write about shame rarely discuss the blushing so closely associated with shame. The linkage between erythrophobia and paranoia has long been known. She believes that blushing indicates the presence of this sexual fantasy. The fear of blushing is thus linked to the nearness of the emergence of anal desire, a desire that risks being guessed by the observer and interpreted as a passive offering of oneself. To lose face—the final fear among certain patients, and in certain civilizations called shame civilizations—thus implies the humiliating exposure of the behind. It is also evident that the more fragile and insufficiently desexualized these social instincts are, the more violent and pathogenic will be the resexualization of the repressed passive homosexual impulse, and the deeper will be the narcissistic regression.

This mode of reality testing and the dangers of homosexual resexualization it produces have implications for analytic technique. In delegating reality testing to his peers or likenesses, the subject is not looking for the ego to achieve a moral ideal—this would be a matter for the superego—but rather hopes that he conforms to what the group expects of him. He hopes for the reflection of a satisfying image that lets him approximate his own ego ideal. In analytic, as opposed to psychotherapeutic, technique, the analyst cannot say, for example, to a patient manifesting guilt about his masturbatory practices, "But everyone does that." For the analyst has then not analyzed the transference and has abandoned his neutrality. In addition he has given favor to a regressive ego ideal, one which pushes the ego to conform to the desire of the group to escape from shame, and as a consequence, to escape from the resexualization of homosexual impulses. The analyst would thus thwart the integration of the patient's homosexuality, an integration that would have reinforced the narcissism of the ego, permitting the patient to acquire a greater autonomy with respect to his peers by diminishing in reality the margin between the ego and the ego ideal.

## *SHAME, GUILT, AND DEPRESSION*

Jean Guillaumin (1973) has amplified Chasseguet-Smirgel's discussion of shame in a paper published in response to her report. I shall attempt to give a brief précis of this tightly argued paper, for it continues our theme of shame and the other. Guillaumin emphasizes, as did Chasseguet-Smirgel, the voyeuristic-exhibitionistic dimension and the constant role it plays in the process leading to shame. All shame is spectacle, he points out, and, potentially at least, public spectacle. This underscores the role of the gaze as much in the setting up of the phallic ideal for all to see and to admire, as in its opposite, the public disparagement and rejection by the disappointed observers.

The ego experiences shame when the current ego state fails to find the anticipated narcissistic reinforcement from conduct which was to have brought it into proximity to its ideal model. The ego is brusquely decompensated when something that is thought to be beautiful, noble, and glorious, and presented as such to others, is suddenly revealed as ugly, infamous, and degrading. Shame expresses specifically the manner in which the ego tolerates this denunciation and failure. Instead of realizing its hope to benefit in and share the megalomaniac completeness of the ideal, the ego is shown up as inadequate and lacking. Shame could even be considered as a qualitative and quantitative index of the stability of the relations between the ego and ego ideal.

Guillaumin classifies Chasseguet-Smirgel's viewpoint as a *dynamic* interpretation of shame, while his own remarks focus on the *economic* aspects of the process. In particular, he stresses the suddenness and the radical shock involved in the process of shame, which Chasseguet-Smirgel also emphasized. Guillaumin feels this harks back to a primitive, all-or-nothing function. The suddenness is present in all cases. Even when shame appears to develop progressively or to be a continuing affect, even when it only concerns a limited aspect of behavior, one invariably observes that an initial surge of shame has occurred at a very precise moment. The extreme suddenness of the reversal indicates to Guillaumin a fragility of the instinctual organization and its diverse supports in the somatopsychic space, which have not arrived at a complex, mediated, secondary integration, capable of assuring a constancy and consistency. This all-or-nothing shift to extremes is often observed in idealization, because of the archaic defensive mechanism (splitting) involved.

The rapidity of the affective change involved in shame, Guillaumin argues, is probably correlated with an instability of the unconscious fantasy. The unconscious fantasy involves the two poles elaborated by Chasseguet-Smirgel. One can see a phallic narcissistic aspect in which the self desires validation from others, as well as the opposite, the anal, degraded, rejected self. According to Guillaumin, the two poles are simultaneously but unstably cathected. When narcissistic validation fails to occur, the archaic transitivity of the self and the other is not sufficiently overcome, self and object boundaries cannot be maintained, and the subject is all too vulnerable to experiencing passively in the moment of shame the opposite of what he had wanted to bring about actively in others. Instead of causing admiration in others, he becomes himself the object of their disgust. Such fluctuations also involve a narcissistic fragility, which implies an important need of realimentation by the other and merging with him, a need that expresses itself in a lability of identifications.

Guillaumin proposes the following dual explanation for this process of reversal. The rapidity of the shame experience is so sudden and its somatic concomitants so evident, that it has sometimes been regarded as an archaic physiological reflex (cf. Otto Fenichel, Herman Nunberg, and even Freud). In particular it has been held to be a function of the autonomic nervous system involving the deep circulation and the superficial vascular supply. These somatic concomitants sometimes are so prominent that they obliterate any other aspects of shame and make it difficult in treatment to make the patient conscious of the *meaning* of his experience of shame. This physiologic description of the mechanisms underlying this process is still appropriate, Guillaumin feels, for the shock that develops at the onset of shame can without doubt be thought of in the light of classic works such as those of Cannon or Selye. The abandonment of the primary *active* fantasy position may be viewed as triggering the sudden collapse or release of a group of tension-controlling mechanisms with the function of alerting the organism. Shame is the disorganizing result of this collapse. In Guillaumin's view, this dual analysis of shame, psychological as well as physiologic, is required to explain the rupture in narcissistic equilibrium. It is as if the image that one has of oneself, of one's place, even of one's limits, were threatened and shaken. Guillaumin compares shame to guilt, depression, and disgust, finding important differences in terms of their functions, meanings for the ego, and relations to the ego ideal, as well as important interrelationships in the shift from shame to depression.

Finally Guillaumin discusses the normal function of shame. In his study of shame he suggests that there is a very precise relationship between shame and the loss of reality testing. In the normal subject, with a sufficient hold on reality, shame would seem perhaps to protect against seduction by megalomaniac fantasies, and correlatively against depression. Shame in the normal person is well compartmentalized and quickly compensated for with a supple displacement of object cathexes, which improve the relationship to the ego ideal. The moment of shame then remains brief and discrete, and never diffuses massively through the ego.

## SUMMARY AND CONCLUSIONS

We have traced the interrelationship of the concept of shame and intersubjectivity in the development of French psychoanalytic thought, beginning with the philosophic recognition of the importance of shame for the intuitive perception of intersubjectivity. This theme was continued by Lacan in his seminal papers on the development of the sense of self in the mirror stage. The theme is found in his notions of the Other as a system of signifiers to which the subject belongs and in which he participates, and the other as an object to which he relates at the same time that he comes to differentiate himself as self-conscious subject. We have seen the close connection of these themes to perversions, especially in relation to issues of control, dominance, and submission, and, in the visual sphere, the meaning and implications of the gaze. We have examined some closely argued psychoanalytic papers dealing with theoretical questions concerning narcissism, dominance, and control in the anal object relationship, and the themes of abnegation and otherworldliness characteristic of the moral narcissist. Chasseguet-Smirgel considered the relation of shame to the ego-ideal, while in Guillaumin's paper the economic aspects of shame were discussed, and shame was linked to physiological processes as well as to subtle but sudden shifts in the cathexes of unconscious fantasies. Shame was differentiated from its cognate affective categories, and its role in the normal subject was explored.

What conclusions can we draw from this survey? For one thing, shame has been an important theme in the French psychoanalytic literature in spite of its relative lack of prominence in French bibliographies. Though shame has not moved into a central theoretical position in contemporary French psychoanalysis, we can see a hint of an important role for shame in organizing many psychoanalytic concepts concerning object relations, the ego ideal, and the attenuation of the narcissistic and megalomaniacal claims of primitive psychological life. In a sense, as this review shows, the concept of shame underlies all these issues of intersubjectivity, narcissism, and the ego ideal.

In pursuing such a survey, I feel there is much to be said for a look at how another intellectual tradition and another culture handle the same problems we are attempting to explore in our own. We come back to our own concerns with heightened awareness and insight, and our own hard-earned solutions and seemingly brilliant deductions sometimes seem to have left out something important. What we believed to be obvious turns out to be quite problematic and fraught with difficulties, while solutions that we thought would escape us are found available and close at hand. We resume our own researches with a sense of contrition, and a resolve to become more aware of our own blind spots, prejudices, and shortcomings. Such, I hope, has been one of the results of this cursory survey of some French theorists.

Perhaps contrition is the keynote here. I do not think we have understood the role of shame as yet. The attempts to channel the theme of shame back into psychoanalysis are among the vibrantly important efforts going on in psychoanalysis today. Shame may eventually come to play as crucial a role theoretically in understanding object relations and intersubjectivity as the role now occupied by anxiety in psychoanalytic theorizing about individual intra- or intersystemic conflict. But it would seem that at this point in time the subject of shame, or of affect in general for that matter, is disorganized and inchoate. It may well be that affect theory is the shame of psychoanalysis. We have begun to see over the past decade, along with the interest in shame and narcissism, a flurry of attempts to clarify psychoanalytic affect theory. There have been many attempts to revise Freudian theory, critiques of metapsychology, and so on, which have their origin in a recognition that something is missing in Freudian theory. We have at least two theories, perhaps several competing theories. There are certain concepts and phenomena left out of the Freudian scheme, as writers on empathy, affect, narcissism, and object relations have long recognized. We will see many attempts to revise psychoanalytic theory, from the efforts of Heinz Kohut to build a whole new theory for narcissism, to such hybrids as the "shame anxiety" of Léon Wurmser and Andrew Morrison. But perhaps the recognition that something about affect is lacking in Freudian theory is really what is troubling the anti-metapsychologists, who want to "humanize" our field at the expense of its scientific foundations. Perhaps this is the basis of such grandiose reformulations as those of Kohut, who attempts to graft uneasily onto the Freudian framework the creaking scaffold of a new theory. For something is missing in Freudian theory as we now have it. It is a beautiful and intellectually gratifying theory that somehow has failed to reflect the complexity and humanity of its subject. Perhaps it was well summed up in an aphoristic *pensée* of Pascal, Descartes's contemporary, when he wrote, "The heart has its reasons, that reason does not know" (1958, Sec. 4,

277, p. 85). Trying to find the reasons of the heart may perhaps lie at the base of this intense contemporary interest in affect theory.

## REFERENCES


Abraham, N. (1972). Pour introduire *L'instinct filial,* de Imre Hermann [Preface to *The filial instinct* of Imre Hermann]. Paris: Denoel.

Abraham, N., & Torok, M. (1980). Introjection–Incorporation: Mourning or Melancholia. In S. Lebovici & D. Widlöcher (Eds.), *Psychoanalysis in France* (pp. 3–16). New York: International Universities Press. (Original work published 1972)

Badouin, C. (1972). *Psychanalyse de Victor Hugo* [Psychoanalysis of Victor Hugo]. Paris: Colin. (Original work published 1943)

Bonnet, G. (1981). *Voir–être vu* [To see–to be seen]. Paris: Presses Universitaires de France.

Brentano, F. (1973). *Psychology from an empirical standpoint.* (L. McAlister, Ed.; A. Rancurello, D. Terrell, & L. McAlister, Trans.). New York: Humanities Press. (Original work published 1874)

Casey, E. S., & Woody, J. M. (1983). Hegel, Heidegger, Lacan: The dialectic of desire. In J. H. Smith & W. Kerrigan (Eds.), *Interpreting Lacan: Psychiatry and the Humanities* (Vol. 6, pp. 75–112). New Haven: Yale University Press.

Chasseguet-Smirgel, J. (1985). *The ego ideal.* (Paul Barrows, Trans.). New York: Norton. (Original work published 1973)

Clancier, A. (1973). *Psychanalyse et critique littéraire* [Psychoanalysis and literary criticism]. Toulouse: Privat.

Descartes, R. (1953). *Oeuvres et lettres* [Works and letters] (A. Bridoux, Ed.). Paris: Gallimard, Edition Pléiade.

Descartes, R. (1955). *The philosophical works of Descartes* (2 Vols.; E. S. Haldane & G. R. T. Ross, Trans.). New York: Dover.

Descombes, V. (1980). *Modern French philosophy.* Cambridge, England: Cambridge University Press.

Dodds, E. R. (1951). *The Greeks and the irrational.* Berkeley: University of California Press.

Freud, S. (1900). *The interpretation of dreams. Standard Edition, 4 & 5.* London: Hogarth Press.

Freud, S. (1911). Psychoanalytic notes on an autobiographical account of a case of paranoia. *Standard Edition, 12*; 3–82. London: Hogarth Press.

Freud, S. (1921). *Group psychology and the analysis of the ego. Standard Edition, 18*; 65–143. London: Hogarth Press.

Green, A. (1983). Logic of Lacan's objet (a) and Freudian theory: Convergences and questions. In J. H. Smith & W. Kerrigan (Eds.), *Interpreting Lacan: Psychiatry and the Humanities* (Vol. 6, pp. 161–191). New Haven: Yale University Press. (Original work published 1966)

Green, A. (1983). *Narcissisme de vie, narcissisme de mort.* [Narcissism of life, narcissism of death]. Paris: Minuit.

Grunberger, B. (1979a). Preliminary remarks for a topographical study of narcissism. In B. Grunberger, *Narcissism: Psychoanalytic essays* (pp. 90–117). New York: International Universities Press. (Original work published 1958)

Grunberger, B. (1979b). Study of anal object relations. In B. Grunberger, *Narcissism: Psychoanalytic essays* (pp. 143–164). New York: International Universities Press. (Original work published 1960)

Guillaumin, J. (1973). Honte, culpabilité et dépression. [Shame, guilt, and depression]. *Revue française de psychanalyse, 37:* 83–100.

Husserl, E. (1960). *Cartesian Meditations* (D. Cairns, Trans.). The Hague: Nijhoff. (Original work published 1931)

Kerrigan, W. (1983). Introduction. In J. H. Smith & W. Kerrigan (Eds.), *Interpreting Lacan: Psychiatry and the humanities* (Vol 6, pp. ix–xxvii). New Haven: Yale University Press.

Kojève, A. (1969). *Introduction to the reading of Hegel* (A. Bloom, Ed.). New York: Basic Books.

Lacan, J. (1977). The mirror stage as formative of the function of the I as revealed in psychoanalytic experience. In A. Sheridan (Trans.), *Écrits: A selection* (pp. 1–7). New York: Norton. (Original work published 1949)

Lacan, J. (1978). *The four fundamental concepts of psychoanalysis.* (J.-A. Miller, Ed.; A. Sheridan, Trans.). New York: Norton.

Laplanche, J. (1976). *Life and death in psychoanalysis* (J. Mehlman, Trans.) Baltimore: Johns Hopkins. (Original work published in 1970)

Lussier, A. (1983). Les déviations du désir: Étude sur le fétichisme. [The deviations of desire: A study of fetichism]. *Revue française de psychanalyse, 47:* 19–142.

Mannoni, O. (1982). *Ça n'empêche pas d'exister.* [That doesn't mean it doesn't exist]. Paris: Seuil.

Merleau-Ponty, M. (1962). *The phenomenology of perception* (C. Smith, Trans.). New York: Humanities Press. (Original work published 1945)

Merleau-Ponty, M. (1963). *The structure of behavior* (A.L. Fisher, Trans.). New York: Humanities Press. (Original work published 1942)

Merleau-Ponty, M. (1968). *The visible and the invisible* (A. Luyier, Trans.). Evanston: Northwestern University Press.

Morrison, A. P. (1984). Working with shame in psychoanalytic treatment. *Journal of the American Psychoanalytic Association, 32*: 479–505.

M'Uzan, M. (1973). A case of masochistic perversion and an outline of a theory. *International Journal of Psychoanalysis, 54:* 455–467. (Original work published 1972)

Neu, J. (1977). *Emotion, thought, and therapy*. Berkeley and Los Angeles: University of California Press.

Pascal, B. (1958). *Pensées: Thoughts on religion and other subjects* (W. F. Trotter, Trans.; H. S. Thayer & E. B. Thayer, Eds.). New York: Washington Square Press. (Original work completed 1662)

Pasche, F. (1969). De la dépression [On depression]. In *À partir de Freud* (pp. 181–199). Paris: Payot. (Original work published 1961)

Pasche, F. (1980). Antinarcissism. In S. Lebovici & D. Widlöcher (Eds.), *Psychoanalysis in France* (pp. 153–168). New York: International Universities Press. (Original work published 1965)

Piers, G., & Singer, M. (1953). *Shame and guilt: A psychoanalytic and a cultural study*. Springfield: Thomas.

Sartre, J.-P. (1956). *Being and nothingness* (H. E. Barnes, Trans.). New York: Philosophical Library. (Original work published 1943)

Scheler, M. (1970). *The nature of sympathy* (P. Heath, Trans.) Hamden, CT: Archon Press. (Original work published 1913)

Schroeder, W. R. (1984). *Sartre and his predecessors: The self and the other.* Boston: Routledge & Kegan Paul.

Smirnoff, V. (1980). The fetishistic transaction. In S. Lebovici & D. Widlöcher (Eds.). *Psychoanalysis in France* (pp. 153–168). New York: International Universities Press. (Original work published 1970)

Spiegelberg, H. (1960). *The phenomenological movement: A historical introduction.* The Hague: Nijhoff.

Starobinski, J. (1961). *L'oeil vivant, essai* [The living eye, an essay]. Paris: Gallimard.

Starobinski, J. (1971). *J.-J. Rousseau: La transparence et l'obstacle, suivi de sept essais sur Rouseau* [J.-J. Rousseau: The transparence and the obstacle, followed by seven studies on Rousseau]. Paris: Gallimard.

Tausk, V. (1933). On the origin of the "influencing machine" in schizophrenia. *Psychoanalytic Quarterly, 2:* 519–556. (Original work published 1919)

Ver Eecke, W. (1983). Hegel as Lacan's source for necessity in psychoanalytic theory. In J. H. Smith & W. Kerrigan (Eds.), *Interpreting Lacan: Psychiatry and the humanities* (Vol. 6, pp. 113–138). New Haven: Yale University Press.

Vergote, A. (1983). From Freud's "other scene" to Lacan's "Other." in J. H. Smith & W. Kerrigan (Eds.), *Interpreting Lacan: Psychiatry and the humanities* (Vol. 6, pp. 193–221). New Haven: Yale University Press.

Wurmser, L. (1981). *The mask of shame.* Baltimore, Johns Hopkins.

6

# A Mature Sense of Shame

CARL D. SCHNEIDER

*Somewhere in our training we are encouraged to believe that on becoming a psychotherapist we are granted privileges akin to those of the inquiring reporter—the right to intrude into the personal lives of others without reprisal. In this chapter, and in his (1977) book Shame, Exposure & Privacy, Schneider reminds us how we shudder instinctively when someone wracked with sobs and contorted with grief is exposed to public view on the evening news. There are, he says, certain central privacies—birth, death, eating, elimination, sex—moments in which exposure arouses shame, moments therefore* protected *by shame.*

*We live in an era that treats shame itself with disrespect, a phenomenon which Schneider associates with an increasing disrespect for privacy. The attitudinal set of the therapist must include profound respect for privacy along with the far better known respect for the workings of the unconscious.*

*During periods of radical change in social and political forms, shame may be devalued. This is natural because we are embarassed to break from conformity and must overcome our own shame boundedness to conceive and direct revolution. Yet, shame is not a disease. Rather,*

Carl D. Schneider. Senior Pastoral Psychotherapist and Director, Divorce Mediation Service, Pastoral Psychotherapy Institute, Parkside Human Services Corporation, a member of the Lutheran General Health Care System, Park Ridge, Illinois.

*it is a mark of our humanity. We are valuing animals, and shame plays an important role in our system of values, despite the fact that what is valued changes from generation to generation. The importance of shame cannot be overlooked, for we cannot afford to throw out the mechanism when we alter its target. It is shame that protects privacy, just as the sense of shame can draw us more deeply into our own spaces to determine if our actions and attitudes are acceptable to our personal morality.*

*If shame is demeaned, we restrict and deny feelings of uneasiness and reticence, private feelings which are inchoate and usually left unspoken. This is a dangerous tendency in our society, for if such feelings are overridden or discounted, life is reduced to the public and the explicit, to what can be programed into a machine. The central privacies of friendship and love, sex, birth and death, and prayer are demeaned. Without our vulnerability we are less human.*

*It is part of the cynicism of our contemporary culture that we value the techniques of "seeing through" another's defenses, ignoring the shame thereby evoked. Ruthless denial of the inner needs of the other is preferred to tact and loving sensibility. A deeper form of knowledge of the other allows seeing to be a private experience. What is inner to another may be his or her faith. Shame protects faith, and we must protect shame. The anonymous donor, the anonymous author deserve privacy lest the sentiments that animate their creative acts be inappropriately exposed and reduced by shame. Those who uncover in the spirit of "revealing truth" may be acting not only from sentiments of science but also out of voyeuristic and rapacious instinct.*

*Religion, which has been called "intimate and ultimate concern," also demands privacy. It provides a mask, a covering, for some of our most crucial personal decisions. Schneider calls attention to Ricoeur's (1973) suggestion that myths and parables are so powerful because they keep parts of their message hidden. There must be a dynamic interplay between the hidden and the shown, between covering and uncovering, between a respectful sense of shame before the "opaque transparency of an enigma" and a shameless deciphering of religion as a mask.*

*Schneider asks us to wonder why we intrude into the world of the patient. Are certain parts of the patient's life perhaps best left private? He suggests that inner growth necessitates a process of working on something* inside *oneself rather than under what may be the glaring light of the therapeutic interaction, and thus analogous to the processes which take place in the photographic darkroom, where premature ex-*

*posure is equivalent to destruction. We must encourage the patient to have a private life even within the therapeutic relationship—the patient has the* right *to disclose, not the obligation.*

Perhaps the title of this essay should be followed by a question mark. Many thoughtful persons would answer in the negative if asked whether there could be such a sense in a mature person. Shame is frequently seen to be the epitome of an immature form of experience, a leftover from a period earlier in development. Its appearance is seen to mark a lapse in, or a failure on one's journey towards maturity.

Clinical discussions of shame often reflect this image in ways both subtle and not-so-subtle. Like the early literature of anthropology which focused on "primitive" people (aborigines, South Sea Islanders) much of our discussion on shame seems to reflect our assumption that we, as clinicians, are not involved in all this. For the most part, we prefer to study the pathology of shame and the vicissitudes of shame in children and patients. There is an alternative way of viewing shame, and in this essay I invite the reader to consider the role of the therapist's sense of shame and how that sense can enhance our work in the clinical setting.

The task is to refine our understanding of maturity and to identify what is meant by a "sense of shame." We will then understand its indispensable role in the maintenance of an integrated self, and be able to discuss the therapist's mature sense of shame.

Aristotle thought shame "ran a developmental course, so that shame was an appropriate deterrent in the young but was inappropriate in the old. . . . If shame persists into mature life," he wrote, "one must regard it as indicative of a faulty character, lacking in proper self-control" (Aristotle, 1941).

Many would agree with Aristotle that it is a contradiction in terms to speak of a *mature* sense of shame. This is a debate that belongs to our whole culture, and is not just a disagreement within the disciplines of psychology and personality theory. Immediately one encounters quite disparate views of how we construe maturity and the nature of our humanity.

Our modern culture and our contemporary psychology

abound similarly with expressions of the sentiment that the eradication of shame is a mark of maturity. In California (that vanguard of a new humanity) shame has been identified repeatedly as the enemy: Fritz Perls, founder of Gestalt therapy and sometime resident therapist of Esalen Institute, called shame and embarrassment the "Quislings of the organism" (Perls, 1969).

In his book *Shyness*, social psychologist Philip Zimbardo (1977) has been an advocate of "shyness clinics" to help people overcome what he sees as an affliction. In yet another instance, published in *Psychology Today* (now an official publication of the American Psychological Association) Sam Keen asked Herbert Marcuse, "If shame and guilt cut us off from our sensitivities, doesn't it follow that a revolutionary form of therapy would have to de-shame the individual?" Marcuse, however, refuses to follow:

> Marcuse: I think you have brought up the decisive point. I would say that shame is something positive and authentic. There are qualities and dimensions of the human being that are . . . his own and he shares them only with those whom he chooses. They do not belong to the community and they are not a public affair.
>
> Keen: But you seem to be implying that only shame would protect privacy. Surely it is possible for an individual—a human being—to have privacy without shame.
>
> Marcuse: I don't see how.

Marcuse seems to have gotten through to Keen, who later writes a review of Zimbardo's book, now arguing that shame indeed has a proper end. Shyness, that cousin of shame, he argues, "is a special grace to be celebrated, rather than a disease to be cured. . . . Shyness guards the sanctuary of our privacy. . . . To value shyness is to cherish the interior life it protects."[1]

It is a widespread assumption that we would all be better off if there were less shame in the world. But the contemporary debate on this issue is all too often a shallow one which fails to recognize its own roots. Those authors who lament the lack of attention to shame are usually speaking of contemporary psychoanalytic literature—they fail to note the important writing on shame of the last century. Since the Enlightenment many of the best minds of the nineteenth century—Darwin (1969), Scheler (1957), Nietzsche,[2] Havelock Ellis[3]—wrestled with the significance of shame for our understanding of ourselves as human beings. Nietzsche, for example, defines us as "the creature who blushes." The climactic chapter of Charles Darwin's seminal work, *The Expression of the Emotions in Man and Animals*, is a chapter on shame in which he writes, "Blushing is the most peculiar and the most human of all expressions."[4]

The earliest sustained reflection on shame comes from the pen of Thomas Burgess, a member of the Royal College of Surgeons. In his 1839 essay, *The Physiology or Mechanism of Blushing*, he makes clear how much to the fore was the anthropological question of the nature of the human. Quoting Humboldt, he asks: "And how can those be trusted who know not how to blush? says the European, in his inveterate hatred to the Negro and the Indian." Christopher Ricks (1974) comments on this passage: "Establishing that the dark-skinned races do indeed blush was not just a foolishness or a pedantry since it was involved in a sense of their full humanity."

Much of the confusion over shame in our culture results from our failure to distinguish between two kinds of shame, "the sense of shame" and "being ashamed." We all know the hot blush of "being ashamed"—what Wurmser (1981) calls simply "shame about" or, more formally, "shame affect proper as a complex reaction pattern."[5] This is the feeling to which George Bernard Shaw referred when he wrote: "We live in an atmosphere of shame. We are ashamed of everything that is real about us: ashamed of ourselves, of our relatives, of our incomes, of our accents, of our opinions, of our experience, just as we are ashamed of our naked skins."[6]

Despite the fact that many commentators deal only with such shame-as-disgrace, this is inadequate, for almost all languages have at least *two* words for shame. One is for being ashamed, but the other is for the sense of shame[7]—this latter more akin to a sense of modesty or discretion. It is what Wurmser calls, "shame protecting," or perhaps more technically, shame as a reaction formation.[8] This is the sense in which we implore someone, "Don't you have any shame?"

The two root cultures of Western civilization, Hebrew and

Greek, are especially sensitive to the concept of shame as discretion. In a beautiful passage of the *Talmud* we read: "A sense of shame is a lovely sign in a man. Whoever has a sense of shame will not sin so quickly; but whoever shows no sense of shame in his visage, his father surely never stood on Mount Sinai" (Talmud, Nedarim, fol 20a, cited in Andrae, 1918, p. 198). Plato (1892) in the "Laws," also speaks positively of shame, referring to "that divine fear which we have called reverence and shame." Perhaps the modern figure who most clearly recognized the import of both kinds of shame is Friedrich Nietzsche. While he never failed to rail against false shame, he also recognized that there is "true modesty" as well as false. He was equally passionate in his affirmation of our need for freedom *from* shame, as he was toward our need *for* a sense of shame. One should "unlearn the shame that would like to deny and lie away one's natural instincts."[9]

Gained only out of long experience, however, was awareness of a need for the sense of shame:

> We no longer believe that truth remains truth when the veils are withdrawn; *we have lived too much to believe this*. Today we consider it a matter of decency not to wish to see everything naked, or to be present at everything, or to . . . "know" everything . . ..
>
> The shame with which nature has concealed herself behind riddles and enigmas should be held in higher esteem.[10]

"We have lived too much to believe this": Nietzsche is speaking of a sense born only out of long experience—a *matúre* sense of shame.

The two forms of shame—being ashamed and the sense of shame—share a common element, for *at its core, shame is intimately linked to the human need to cover that which is exposed.* This common element is apparent in the Indo-European root*(s)kem-; *(s)kam-, meaning "to cover," which gives us not only our English word *shame*, but the Italian word *camera* (a little room, and therefore something hidden) which becomes the English *camera* (a little room which reveals); the French *chemise*, and the German *Hemd*, all involving covering or protection. Even more fascinating, the word for shame in Lithuanian derives from a second Indo-European root **(s)que-; *(s)qewa-*, also meaning "to cover," from which root have descended our English words *custody, hide, house, hut, shoe,* and *sky.*[11]

Does a healthy human being need covering? Some think not, and equate "covering" with "hiding," and "hiding" with that which is disgraceful, devalued, or discredited. I propose that there are times and places in all phases of human life where covering is appropriate—indeed, needed—not because something is amiss, awry, or wrong, but because it *is* appropriate, that is, "fitting," "proper." Human beings are, in Bachelard's lovely phrase, "half-open beings," always partly exposed, partly covered. Human experience, always vulnerable to violation, needs protection. Thus an element of reticence is always present and appropriate to human relationships, including one's relation to oneself. To ignore or to deny this is to be shameless.

Unquestionably there is much shame that is pathological and unconscious, involving rigid and brittle defensiveness. Our clinical literature is replete with documentation of this aspect of shame. But much as psychoanalysis focused on pathology in its early years, only much later developing a general and normative psychology, so too have studies of shame traced the pathologies of shame without simultaneously bearing witness to the constructive role played by shame in normal development.

Wurmser identifies that role as follows: "shame guards the separate, private self with its boundaries and prevents intrusion and merger. It guarantees the self's integrity. . . . More specifically, it shields the self against overexposure and intrusive curiosity.[12] Stated more technically: "Shame is thus the social protection mechanism in expressive-communicative and perceptual-attentional interchanges.[13]

"Teleologically," Wurmser suggests, "shame may be important as the protector of primary process thought—the language of the self [just as] guilt . . . fulfill[s] the same purpose for secondary process thought—the language of object relations.[14] Wurmser's work is the most refined in the field but similar descriptions of the role of shame can be found in the other major commentators on shame, including Warren Kinston, Helen Merrell Lynd, and Helen Block Lewis.[15]

Essential to our comprehension of the role of such protective shame is recognition that this integrity is not a static "thing" to be preserved; rather, the achievement of a sense of self is an ongoing process, a dynamic balance of the many parts of ourselves and the identifications we have made.

The maintenance of a sense of self is much like a juggling act. Once, in my youth, I attempted (briefly) to learn juggling. I found it impossible to do in front of others initially—I could not maintain the necessary concentration on these new skills while distracted by my self-consciousness. I needed to practice, to have space to myself within which I might develop before I could maintain my balance in front of others.

Each of us needs some time offstage, a private space, before we are ready to go public. Rehearsal is a process which becomes more sophisticated and differentiated as we mature, but throughout life it is a human need.

The sense of shame protects this process. This protection is in relation to ourselves as much as against others, for what is sheltered is not something already finished but something in the process of becoming—a tender shoot. Like a darkroom, shame protects against premature exposure to light that would destroy the process. It functions like a protective covering during the period of gestation until the embryo—whether seed or soul—has come to full term and is ready to emerge.

Let me illustrate this with an example taken not from a clinical setting but from the life of a Protestant minister who felt there was a period when her own religious development and her emerging sexuality were linked as intensely private experiences. She says:

> Looking back at my childhood religious experiences what stood out most vividly in my mind was the experience of identification I had with a group of nuns that lived in a convent on the way to church. I remembered when I was in middle elementary school, probably about early puberty age, playing in my bedroom and acting out what I thought was going on in the convent. One of the things that intrigued me about the convent was . . . the drawn shades, and always wondering about what was going on behind there. So what I did in my bedroom was to dress up as a nun, with a skirt, bobby-sox, and kind of made myself a habit out of a towel. And I would celebrate communion by punching commun-

ion wafers out of a piece of bread with hair rollers, and dry them out in my underwear drawer, and then I would put on my Catholic . . . holy cards and a rosary, and different things like that that some of my girlfriends had sneaked to me because I was a Protestant and if my mother had caught me with any of these things I'd have been shot at sunrise, I think, and I would take these either into my bedroom with the door closed, or sometimes back into a big walk-in closet and would pray the rosary, and would celebrate communion.

This was all going on at the same time that I remember going through some of the early explorations of myself as I began to change and develop sexually. It wasn't masturbation that was involved there, but simply finding out what changes were going on with me genitally as I developed. And I remember these experiences being very close; and they weren't only close in terms of the time that I was acting them out, but they were also close together emotionally. . . .

In addition to that, I know that . . . I'd have been very ashamed if my mother caught me in either one of those things; . . . this was just very, very personal . . . a highly personal experience.[16]

Normally this woman did not have to hide things from her mother. But at that time, while exploring processes which were both new and largely unspeakable, she needed privacy. Anna Marie Rizzuto (1980), speaking of the psychic processes involved in the development of religious faith, invokes the importance of "what Winnicott calls 'silent communication' with our objects of the past and the present."

When the child becomes able to hide some aspects of [herself] from [her] parents, [she] still needs the company of an adult in the privacy of [her] world. God . . . [she adds] is the supreme being whose constant presence is available to the child in case of need: God knows the child internally and is a constant witness of [her] experiences.[17]

Children's author Judy Blume spoke of the reason such experiences need protection. Many people had protested that in her book *Deane* (the story of a handicapped girl who begins to explore her body and to touch herself) the author had been writing about masturbation. Blume observed that she didn't *know* the word masturbation when she was a 12-year-old. In

Blume's nice phrase, this young woman knew only that "she had a *special place*, and that it was pleasurable when she touched it."[18] Such experiences deserve protection from intrusion and from premature exposure. Shame thus plays its most prominent role during childhood and adolescence, the times of formative growth and vulnerability.

The emerging values and half-formed commitments of these periods need time to mature. To intrude on that process, to yank up the roots as if to see how they are growing, can destroy the plant. Shame protects our inwardness and the integrity of the self. Perhaps it is closer to our actual experience to use the verb form rather than the noun: shame protects that *ongoing process of integrating* our selves.

Katie, a 26-year-old graduate student, looking back at her preadolescent years, describes how destructive it was to be in an intrusive family that lacked a sense of shame and violated a young girl's need for privacy:

> My family lacked a sense of rules and regulations. . . . Lacking a sense of shame my family was ruled by lust and desire. . . . I was introduced into puberty by my stepfather who used to get into bed with me when my mother was sleeping. I enjoyed it so much when he would come to me. . . . He was my first sexual encounter.
>
> Because the experience had been so enjoyable to me, I felt no shame initially. . . .
>
> When I was fourteen I began to see my friends hide and cover their heads when he would begin to seduce them. I saw the shame of my friends with their heads covered. Somewhere in my mind it must have registered, but I didn't understand it.
>
> When I was still fourteen my stepfather came home one day. He grabbed me to kiss me. It wasn't really lust, it was desperation, but still I wanted to be fourteen. I pushed him away. I wanted to be wholesome. Leave me alone, let me be, let me grow. I wish you were dead!!!! I had an exam to study for. He killed himself that day. I was the last person to see him alive. I heard him close the back door. I smelled the gas. I saw him slumped over in the back seat of the car. I was only fourteen; I didn't know what to do.[19]

Katie went off to college, went through a series of relationships, more trauma, and was finally hospitalized. Later Katie identified her capacity to experience shame as one of the signs that demonstrated her real progress toward recovery:[20] "I remember when I used to have intercourse with fellows, I would walk into work almost embarrassed. I remember how good it felt to blush. How good it felt to have someone care enough about me to tell me in a nice way I was doing something wrong." She concludes: "I've developed (a) proper sense of privacy and have learned to cherish and adore that privacy because someone finally accepted that private part of myself. And with that proper sense of shame I no longer have to share myself with lots of people."

Respect for a private realm of experience, and for a person's right to have control over that realm which Katie describes, is an indispensable component in the process of achieving an integrated self and in the dynamics of maintaining healthy relationships.[21] At heart, our meeting and relations as humans are always simultaneously disclosing and concealing. In meetings both participants make contact yet are separate. The sense of shame involves respect for the reality of our separateness and the space that is there between us. Language both discloses and covers in all encounter. The sense of shame implies respect for this depth and resonance of human meeting.

Perhaps the most relevant example of a mature sense of shame is its role in *the therapist's sense of shame in clinical practice.* So much is vulnerability to exposure and violation heightened in therapy that our awareness of shame becomes indispensable. Indeed, many of our clients remain shamed for years even that they are coming to therapy.

There are at least three structural components to the vulnerability of clients. First of all, clients are enjoined to speak whatever comes to mind. As Gary Thrane (1979) notes, this "injunction to tell all is the injunction to be shameless." At that same time that a client is involved in ongoing disclosure, however, the therapist maintains a studied neutrality. Normal relationships involve a process of mutual, measured self-disclosure: this break in the pattern of normal relationships is both unsettling and threatening for most clients.

This is understandable, for some measure of anxiety must

be expected in asymmetrical power relationships (of which therapy is a classic example). But at issue is not only the imbalance in the degree of self-revelation involved, but also the disclosure of a diminished sense of self. Therapy is an event in which a client, previously unknown to the therapist, presents in circumstances that one way or another reflect a damaged or uncertain self.

This sense of damage supplies the very motivation to come to therapy in the first place. In this respect therapy is like chronic illness: people are forced to encounter others when they are less than they know they are. And as such, they are specially vulnerable to intrusion, violation, and degradation. The client is at the mercy of the therapist's sensitivity and sense of shame. The therapist must be able to respect the client at a time when the client may himself be unable to experience, maintain, or claim such self-respect. The therapist's capacity to extend a protective covering is critical if the client is not to be shamed. A mature sense of shame functions to prevent us from shaming others.

How shall we describe the mature sense of shame appropriate to our work as clinicians? Leon Wurmser, following Freud, has spoken of it as a sense of "analytic *tact*" which he defines as the capacity "to protect the patient's narcissism from undue hurt and thus to enhance his curiosity."[22] If tact seems like a synonym for politeness and mere restraint, a static term to use for our work in a dynamic setting, it is rather, I believe, an activity requiring the utmost skill and discernment. Far from being a simple trait, tact involves the capacity to balance several dynamic elements. I will suggest two such aspects of therapeutic tact.

First, therapeutic tact involves *the ability to balance the tension between surface and depth*. As therapists, our task is to see below the surface. Indeed, "depth therapy" is a synonym for dynamic or psychoanalytic therapy.

Freud thought of therapy in such terms. Writing about his famous patient Dora, Freud (1905) sets out his own vocation as excavator: "I set myself," he says, "the task of bringing to light what human beings keep hidden within them." In biblical language, Freud urges that "he that has eyes to see and ears to hear" can participate in "the task of making conscious the most hidden recesses of the mind." Yet in pursuing his work of uncovering, Freud immediately encountered resistance by his patients to being thus uncovered. Dora, indeed, gave multiple indications to Freud that she saw him as a dangerous, violating and seductive figure from whom she felt a need to flee for self-protection.

It is not enough, then, simply to uncover the truth and present it to clients. Freud (1910) himself labeled this "wild" analysis and required that we deal with clients in a spirit of tact and consideration. The capacity to monitor and match interpretations to what clients themselves are ready to hear and "discover" is an integral part of this requirement. Freud thought that "a fairly long period of contact" was needed to achieve a working alliance with a client. It was, he thought, "bullying" the patient and "reprehensible" to attempt to short-circuit this process by "brusquely telling (the patient) the hidden things one infers behind (the patient's) story."[23]

We must not simply work to uncover: such an approach has earned us our popular image as "shrinks"—people who want simply to *see through*, to penetrate and reduce the full reality of our clients' experience. Nietzsche aptly described the violating and voyeuristic qualities of such a "science," which, he wrote, "offends the modesty of all real women. It makes them feel as if one wanted to peep under their skin—yet worse, under their dress and finery."[24] As a counter-image to this, Nietzsche offered a description of the artist, which I believe we might entertain as a model for the mature clinician. In the face of those who would want to penetrate, uncover, and go beyond the surface, art requires, he said, a *respect* for appearance, for the surface, and for the clothing in which it is presented.[25] To uncover everything, Nietzsche thought, was an act of indecency. A therapist's mature sense of shame involves sensitivity to a client's need to save appearances while making it possible for a client to reveal himself or herself in depth.

Second, a mature sense of shame, of analytic tact, involves the capacity to handle sensitively *the interplay between the public and the private in our clinical work.* The paradox of our profession is that we invite and, in analysis, require that people talk of what is most private with us, who are professionals—public figures. A friend who is in analysis said it well: "God! I feel like

I am constantly exposed, like there is a big gaping wound that never closes. I can't wait for the time when I can close myself up again."

Wurmser observes: "analysis . . . is a situation of almost ruthless exposure and intrusion into privacy. It is the art of self-revelation met by disciplined respect; yet shame is an unavoidable companion, inherent in this inevitably "shameless" procedure.[26] This character of therapy is so many-layered and so pervasive that James Anthony (1981) has spoken of analysis as "an arena of shame."

The potential for shaming is present in the very name of our enterprise: psychotherapy. "Therapy" comes from the Greek word "therapeia," meaning "to attend" to the psyche, the soul of another. But, as Wurmser has made clear, the very function of attending and the experience of being paid attention can be shame-laden. And this is so for therapist as well as client: Analytic lore says that we have the ritual of the couch in analysis because Freud didn't like the strain of people sitting and staring at him all day. Focused attention—never mind whether negative or positive—can be overwhelming to most of us. Witness, for example, the discomfort of most persons at the focused attention they receive at birthday parties. In therapy that discomfort is intensified as another human being devotes himself or herself solely to attending to us.

How then does one handle a setting so potentially charged with shame? We do not have to reinvent the wheel: *the fundamental rules of technique in analytic therapy can be understood* (though they seldom are) *as roles for how to conduct therapy in the face of the ever-present potential for shame.* The cardinal shift in technique from an emphasis on the uncovering of repressed material to a focus on "interpreting defense before content" was a recognition of the shaming potential of uncovering therapy.[27]

A corollary of the rule that "interpretation of resistance precedes interpretation of content"[28] is the rule that "one should always work from the side of the ego and, more specifically, start very carefully from the surface."[29] Freud himself stated this rule in his discussion of "wild" analysis and of the dilemma faced by the analyst in communicating to patients things they do not know about themselves not simply out of ignorance, but because they have repressed them. If a client is not simply to flee such interpretations and break off therapy, "[F]irst, by preparatory work," says Freud, "the repressed material must have come very near to the patient's thoughts, and secondly, he must be sufficiently firmly attached by an affective relationship to the physician . . . to make it impossible for him to take fresh flight."[30]

Freud proposed these requirements out of his own painful experience. Earlier, in the case of Dora (long before he had an alliance with his client) he moved beyond the surface and forced upon her the knowledge that she was not simply the victim of sexual advances by Herr K, an older married man, but that she herself was in love with him and fantasied having an affair and a child with him. Freud tells us that "Dora disputed the fact no longer." But, he reports, she opened the next session "with these words: 'Do you know that I am here for the last time today?' "[31]

Ignoring repeated warnings by Dora that she was being overwhelmed by such interpretations, Freud still plunged ahead to insist further that Dora even hoped Herr K would divorce his wife and marry her. At the end of his comments, Freud reports, "Dora said good-bye to me . . . and—came no more."

Such experiences led to a revision in technique toward greater sensitivity to the pacing of interpretations. Fenichel articulates the shift in technical terms: "Often the question should more correctly be put: 'How could I have interpreted more superficially?' . . . For we must operate *at that point* where the affect is actually situated *at the moment*."[32]

Other ground-rules of interpretation also relate to shame. That "transference interpretation has priority over other material" (Muslin & Gill, 1978) is also, I believe, frequently a rule that functions to monitor and keep at tolerable levels a client's shame-proneness.

We may say this less technically. Correct interpretations are not necessarily good interpretations. As we see so clearly in the Dora case, a correct interpretation can be experienced by a client as an attack and a humiliation. Thus we come to the core of the psychoanalytic contribution to our understanding of the clinical task: information, data, and correct theory are not enough. In an age that has largely lost any sense of this, psychoanalysis reminds us that truth is inseparably *personal.*

Freud gave us a "talking cure." But it is only in the context of a personal relationship that a client may overcome shame about speaking. A therapist risks shaming a client every time an interpretation is offered. Freud helped us see the depth in our speaking. Personal speech is not flat and linear, except when used as a defense. Human speech always refers beyond itself. Speech is the symbolization of our experience. Personal speech has an inherent doubleness, for human consciousness is not transparent to itself but is "at the same time what reveals and what conceals" (Ricoeur, 1973).

Thus, at the same time that our speaking gives explicit expression to our experience, it also reminds us how much reality's fullness remains unvoiced and implicit. In articulating some themes, it remains mute to others.

This *hidden–shown* character of both consciousness and language places a special burden on us as clinicians. We practice a strange discipline in which we simultaneously affirm the disclosive, revelatory power of human speech while knowing also and always the capacity of language to obscure and cover. This dialectic cannot be eliminated, for it is the essence of our humanity.

We are called on to maintain a mature sense of shame because we practice in a field marked by the dynamic interplay between covering and uncovering, between the tacit and the explicit. The ancient Greeks knew the deeply religious dimension inherent in a mature sense of shame. Their concept of *aidos* meant both shame and awe. The proper therapeutic stance is finally one of awe and deep respect, for we stand on holy ground—we engage in an encounter that involves doubleness—the experience of both mystery and revelation, of reticence before the indescribable and of the revelation of that which was concealed.[33] Or, as I have written elsewhere, (Schneider, 1982) "Shame symbolizes our mutual involvement. It also reminds us of the dividedness and estrangement that characterize that involvement. To refuse to acknowledge this broken character of our lives leaves us open to that which is demonic and destructive. Because we know ourselves incapable of living together in a community of complete trust and openness more than momentarily, shame is and will be always in order as the mark of our vulnerability as selves both separate from and belonging to a larger whole."

## NOTES

1. Keen, S. (1978, March). Deliver us from shyness clinics. *Psychology Today*, pp. 18 ff.; Keen, S. (1971 February). An interview with Herbert Marcuse. *Psychology Today*, pp. 37–38.
2. For example, see, Nietzsche, F. (1966). *Beyond good and evil: Prelude to a philosophy of the future*. (W. Kaufmann, Trans.) New York: Vintage Books.; (1974). *The gay science*. (W. Kaufmann, Trans.) New York: Vintage Books.; (1954). *Thus spake Zarathustra*. (In *The Portable Nietzsche*, W. Kaufmann, Trans.) New York: Viking.; (1967). *The will to power*. (W. Kaufmann & R. J. Hollingdale, Trans.) New York: Vintage Books.
3. Ellis, H. (1936). The evolution of modesty. In *Studies in the psychology of sex* (3rd rev. ed., Vol. 1, Part 1). New York: Random House. See also the work of the great 19th century philosopher Vladimir Soloviev. Soloviev, V. (1918). *The justification of the good: An essay on moral philosophy* (27: 135–138). (N.A. Buddington, Trans.) New York: Macmillan. This work places shame at the heart of philosophical anthropology and ethics. Soloviev writes: "The feeling of shame is a fact which absolutely distinguishes man from all lower nature."
4. Darwin, C. (1965). *The Expression of the emotions in man and animals* (p. 309).
5. Wurmser, L. (1981). *The mask of shame* (pp. 48, 59).
6. Shaw, G. B. (1903). *Man and superman*, cited by Wurmser, L. *The mask of shame* (p. 60).
7. This has been noted by, among others, Schneider, C.D. (1977). *Shame, exposure and privacy*, (pp. 19ff). Boston: Beacon Press, Kinston, W. (1983). A theoretical context for shame, *International Journal of Psychoanalysis, 64*: 213; Wurmser, L. *The mask of shame*.
8. Wurmser, L. *The mask of shame* (pp. 48, 49; 84–85).
9. Nietzsche, F. (1967). *The will to power* (sections 326, 327, pp. 178–179).
10. Nietzsche, F. *The gay science* (Preface of the 2nd ed., section 4, p. 38; emphasis added).
11. See Klein, Ernest, (1971). *A comprehensive etymological dictionary of the English language* (Vol. 2), New York: Elsevier., s.v. "shame," "hide," "sky." See also s.v. "shame" *Oxford English Dictionary*, E. Partridge, *Origins: A short etymological dictionary of modern English* (4th revised ed.), s.v. "shame." See also Malvezin, P. (1924). *Dictionnaire des racines celtiques* (2nd ed.), s.v. "chemise."
12. Wursmer, L. *The mask of shame* (p. 65; see also pp. 48, 62).
13. Wurmser, L. *The mask of shame* (p. 65).
14. Wurmser, L. *The mask of shame* (p. 67).
15. Lewis, H. B. (1981). Shame and guilt and human nature. In S. Tuttman, C. Kaye, & M. Zimmerman (Eds.), *Object and self: A developmental approach* (p. 245). New York: International Universities Press. See also Wurmser, L. *The mask of shame* (pp. 65, 67). Thrane, G. (1979). Shame and the construction of the self, *Annual of Psychoanalysis,* 7: 336, 339, 340. Warren Kinston puts it succinctly: "The price of individuation is shame." Kinston,

W. (1983). A theoretical context for shame. *International Journal of Psychoanalysis, 64*: 219.

16. Personal communication. April, 1984. For an analogous literary example see Dalsimer, K. (1986). *Female adolescence: Psychoanalytic reflections on literature* (p. 37) New Haven: Yale University Press.
17. Rizzuto, A.M. *The psychological foundations of belief*, p. 133.
18. Radio interview on the Studs Terkel Show, WFMT-FM, Chicago, March 1984.
19. Written communication to author.
20. See Kinston's remarks on the capacity to experience shame as a component of a mature personality: "an analysand does not, as Loenfeld (1976) and Levin (1971) suggest, work through shame to the point of being unshamed. If the analysand commences shameless, he must be brought to the experience of shame."
21. Cf. an analogous account of Dawn, in Schneider, C.D. (1977). *Shame, exposure and privacy* (pp. 73–74). Boston: Beacon press. The experience of both Dawn and Katie illustrate R.D. Laing's statement that all persons need an "area of experience which is private in an unqualified sense." Laing adds: "The loss of the experience of an area of unqualified privacy, by its transformation into a quasi-public realm, is often one of decisive changes associated in the process of going mad." Laing, R. D. (1961). *Self and others* (2nd rev. ed.) (pp. 20–21). New York: Pantheon.
22. Wurmser, L. *The mask of shame*. Wurmser describes the exercise of analytic tact as follows: "To know the right time and the right form of saying it is a good part of what we would call analytic tact. Above all, it means to be in touch with the affect of anxiety, pain, or grief that is on the surface at any given moment and to fit one's comments as closely as possible to this feeling. It also means not to overlook the positive affects within the patient, those of expectant discovery and of opening up new links in the course of associations, to recognize and respect the patient's increasing freedom to say what he has pushed aside before, to connect what had been disjointed before. Still more important is saying it in the right way and at the right time so that the patient is neither unnecessarily hurt nor unnecessarily spared and so no material that can be connected is overlooked by silence" (pp. 285–286).

    From a very different theoretical framework, Thomas Scheff makes a similar analysis of the need for a mature sense of theme on the part of the therapist in his discussion of treating a client with "respect." See Scheff, T. (1987). The shame–rage spiral. In H. B. Lewis (Ed.), *The role of shame in symptom formation*. Hillsdale, NJ: LEA.
23. Freud, S. (1910/1957), p. 226. "Bully" and "reprehensible" are the translations in Philip Rieff's edition. See (1963), *Freud: Therapy and technique* (p. 94). New York: Collier Books. The translations in the *Standard Edition* are "rash" and "objectionable."
24. F. Nietzsche, *Beyond good and evil* (Section 127, p. 87).
25. Art involves what Nietzsche calls "the good will to appearance." F. Nietzsche, *The gay science* (Section 107, pp. 163–164).

26. Wurmser, L. *The mask of shame* (p. 265).
27. Levin adds that "The analysis of resistance must also be conducted with extreme tact; for example, if the analyst calls attention to the blocking created by the patient's primary shame, this may precipitate intense secondary shame of being an 'analytic failure'." Levin, S. (1971). The psychoanalysis of shame. *International Journal of Psychoanalysis, 52*: 355–362.
28. Fenichel, O. (1941). Problems of psychoanalytic technique. (D. Brunswick, Trans.) *Psychoanalytic Quarterly*. Cited by Wurmser, *The mask of shame* (p. 288).
29. Wurmser, L. *The mask of shame* (p. 268).
30. Freud, S. Observations on "Wild" psychoanalysis (p. 226).
31. Freud, S. Fragment of an analysis of a case of hysteria (p. 105).
32. Fenichel, op cit.
33. Léon Wurmser has written on this theme of the fundamental doubleness of experience, and the implications this has for our clinical practice. L. Wurmser, The Janus face of psychiatry: An editorial. *Journal of Nervous and Mental Disease, 164*(6): 375–379. In this report, Wurmser argues for the indispensibility of the two "faces" of human science, the "explaining psychology" of logical-mathematical method, dealing predominantly in horizontal truth, and able to achieve "a particular lucidity and regularity, a shining clarity," and the "understanding Psychology" (Dilthey), employing metaphor and myth able to portray vertical truth, "revealing hidden depths," a mode in which "no concept is sharply delimited" but all have a cloud of connotations, implications, and meanings." Wurmser argues that rather than setting these two modes in opposition, the "richness and vitality" of science and psychiatry rests on maintaining both "together."

    See Wurmser, L. (1983). Things are not always what they seem: The nature of doubleness in Dickens. *Psychoanalysis and Creativity,* October 1983. Wurmser speaks eloquently of "the antithesis between the manifest significance of all reality and every communication—and the abyss of meaning behind" in a fine exposition of this theme. He concludes: "as to the doubleness of all experience: I think the sudden incongruity between expectation and outcome, the shock of the unsuspected, is broader even than shame, breach of trust, and disillusionment, though encompassing all these. It could perhaps be called the absolute ultimate incommensurability of the world of *inwardness* of the soul, of the self—and the world of *adaptation,* of objectivity, of social and historical demands." (p. 27, 42).

# REFERENCES

Andrae, T. (1918). Die Person Muhammeds in Lehre und Glauben Seiner Gemeinde (Archives d'Etudes Orientales, J. A. Lundell, Ed., No. 16). Stockholm: P. A. Norstedt & Soner.

Anthony, E. J. (1981). Shame, guilt, and the feminine self in psychoanalysis. In S. Tuttman, C. Keye, & M. Zimmerman (Eds.), *Object and self: A developmental approach.* New York: International Universities Press.

Aristotle. (1941). *Nicomachean ethics.* In R. McKeon (Ed.), *The basic works of Aristotle* (pp. 1001–1002). New York: Random House. (Original work ca. 330BC)

Burgess, T. (1839). *The physiology or mechanism of blushing.* London: John Churchill.

Darwin, C. (1969). *The expression of the emotions in man and animals.* Chicago: University of Chicago Press. (Original work published 1872)

Freud, S. (1905). Fragment of an analysis of a case of hysteria. *Standard Edition, 7:* 77–78. London: Hogarth Press.

Freud, S. (1910). Observations on 'Wild' psychoanalysis. *Standard Edition, 9:* 222. London: Hogarth Press.

Muslin, H., & Merton, G. (1978). Transference in the Dora case. *Journal of the American Psychoanalytic Association, 26*(2): 312.

Perls, F. S. (1969). *Ego, hunger and aggression* (p. 178). New York: Vintage Books.

Plato. (1892). *The dialogues of Plato* (B. Jowett, Trans.; Vol. 5: "Laws;" 3rd rev. ed.; p. 51). London: Macmillan. (Original work ca. 340BC)

Ricks, C. (1974) *Keats and embarrassment.* London: Oxford University Press.

Ricoeur, P. (1973). Two essays by Paul Ricoeur; The critique of religion and the language of faith. *Union Seminary Quarterly Review, 28*(3): 206.

Rizzuto, A.M. (1980). The psychological foundations of belief in God. In J. W. Fowler & A. Vergote (Eds.), *Toward moral and religious maturity: The First International Conference on Moral and Religious Development.* Morristown, NJ: Silver Burdett.

Scheler, M. (1957). Uber Scham and Schamgefuhl. In M. Scheler & M. S. Frings (Eds.), *Schriften aus dem Nachlass* (Vol. 1: *Zur Ethik and Erkenntnislehre*). *Gesammelte Werke* (Vol. 10). Bern: Francke Verlag.

Schneider, C. (1977). *Shame, exposure and privacy.* Boston: Beacon.

Schneider, C. (1982). *The end of shame.* Concilium, 156: 38.

Thrane, G. (1979). Shame. *The Journal of Theory of Social Behavior, 9*(2): 162.

Wurmser, L. (1981). *The mask of shame.* Baltimore: Johns Hopkins University Press.

Zimbardo, P. G. (1977). *Shyness: What it is, what to do about it.* Reading, MA: Addison-Wesley.

7

# The Shame of Narcissism

WARREN KINSTON

*In a previous communication Dr. Kinston (1982) suggested that the concept of narcissism, flawed as it may be, is an irrevocable, ineradicable part of our literature best accepted as an "ideogram" incapable of precise definition. Concentrating our attention on two aspects of narcissism, he suggests that "self-based experience has a peculiar characteristic: an attempt to exclude or reject a part of experience leads to loss of awareness more globally. So, in order to remain in contact with one's own feelings and therefore those of others, it is necessary to tolerate and manage negative feelings about the self." He points out that traumatic experiences lead to the activation of modes of self-protection, which in certain cases can produce states which Freud referred to as "the stone wall of narcissism."*

*Noting that psychoanalysts are divided over whether their focus is on self-esteem or on self-protection, he introduces the concepts "self-narcissism" and "object-narcissism," interlocking mental states to which he attaches a unique theory of shame. Central to his thesis is Lichtenstein's (1963) idea of shame as a boundary function, in which the person is seen as living in a state of constant tension between identity maintenance and the temptation to abandon psychic reality altogether.*

Warren Kinston. Institute of Organisation and Social Studies, Brunel University, Uxbridge, Middlesex, England.

The case material is reprinted with permission from Kinston, W. (1984). Clinical illustration of a theory of shame. In T. Tamminen (Ed.), *Theories of narcissism: Clinical applications.* Helsinki: Foundation for Psychiatric Research in Finland.

*It is as if identity is maintained only at the cost of constant energy consumption, with the desire to renounce identity analogous to the physical concept of a return to entropy. Kinston discusses the relationship between shame-propensity and narcissistic vulnerability and suggests that some narcissistically vulnerable people defend against shame by retreating to a state of object-narcissism. Clinical examples are included which demonstrate the utility of this theoretical position in the treatment of a variety of shame experiences.*

## INTRODUCTION

To understand a feeling is to empathize with another experiencing that feeling; it is to recognize the contextual factors associated with that feeling; it is to appreciate the subtle blending and linkage with other feelings; it is to play with multiple metaphors of the feeling. To understand a concept is to place it in a theoretical framework of interlinked concepts; it is to use it in a consistent and coherent fashion; it is to develop predictions that can be checked; it is to be able to use the concept in situations for practical benefit. This latter (scientific) understanding encompasses but does not replace the former. Indeed the former may invalidate the latter. Shame refers to a feeling and it is also a concept. Determining the nature of the shame experience, that is, the empirical referents of the shame concept, only goes part of the way in offering understanding. It is necessary in addition to place the concept of shame within a theory.

To date psychological theory has not made an adequate place for shame. Indeed some leading psychoanalysts have argued that shame is of no importance. Other psychoanalysts have defined shame in a limited way so as to fit it into the straitjacket of current theory. However, such an approach blocks appreciation of the shame experience. Understanding the experience, as it turns out, uncovers a need for new theory. Modern psychotherapy, which is at last reconsidering shame, appears to be handling this difficulty by ignoring theory and simply letting analysts get on with describing human experience as best they can.

The problem with such a pragmatic and theoretical approach is that a comprehensive and consistent account of shame should not rest only on clinical psychoanalytic observations, but must consider and integrate, or purposefully exclude, much written by others. To do otherwise is to impoverish our understanding by basing it on a partial sample of disturbed individuals in a most unusual setting. Psychoanalysts are in a unique position to study certain personal aspects of shame, like the absence of shame in perversions, the links between shame and other disturbing emotional states, and the phenomenon of shame propensity; but perhaps this is why psychoanalysts have taken such a negative view of shame (Wurmser, 1981).* In contrast, the Bible viewed the acceptance of shame as the ultimate in commitment; and Shakespeare associated shame with truth and honor. These social aspects of shame have been less amenable to psychoanalytical study.

The two-sidedness of shame, its personal and social aspects, is less clear in English which has one word for shame, than in languages such as German and French which have two or three words. "Shame" does however have two antonymic forms in English which correspond to these meanings. The origins of the word "shame" are obscure, but scholars believe it derives from the Teutonic root *(s)kem* meaning "to cover oneself" (*Oxford English Dictionary*). The meanings that have come down to us are as follows:

> *Shame-unashamed* (German: *Scham,* French: *pudeur* or *vergogne*) refers to modesty, chastity, shyness, bashfulness. In Biblical usage it refers to genitals. The emphasis in this meaning is on inner personal experience.
>
> *Shame-shameless* (German: *Schande*, French: *honte*) refers to disgrace, scandal, criminality (cf. deeds of shame). The emphasis in this meaning is on social customs and standards.

## REVIEW OF THE LITERATURE

It may be useful to scan rapidly the various approaches to shame in the psychoanalytic literature. This literature is a substantial body of inquiry, and is pertinent to the chapter because it reveals my own background and prejudices.

*This text, the most extensive recent psychoanalytic account, which manifests a negative view of shame, can be contrasted with the positive views in the texts by Lynd (1958) and Schneider (1977), neither of whom are psychoanalysts.

As mentioned earlier a common response of psychoanalysts has been simply to ignore shame or mention it only in passing, or perhaps link it in with some other feeling like inferiority, failure, or guilt as if the complex feeling had primacy or was more explanatory. Indeed leading scholars like Hartmann and Loewenstein (1962) asserted that shame was so similar to guilt both in scientific and common usage that the two terms could be considered together. Freud certainly never made shame an object of detailed study as he did in the case of anxiety and guilt. Another equally dismissive response is to assign shame solely to the realm of social interaction, implying therefore that it does not really belong to psychoanalytic discourse which focusses on the purely intrapsychic.

The most significant theoretical model in psychoanalysis to date, known as the structural model, refers to a tripartite division of the mind into agencies: id, ego, and superego. Various authors have tried to place shame within this model. For example, one suggestion was that shame appeared when the ego recognized that the individual had failed to live up to his or her own ideal standards as established in the superego. Another version of the ego–superego model of shame was that shame was based on the ego's fear of contempt and fear of abandonment by the superego. There are many problems with such suggestions, but the most important is the way that they select from the range of phenomena which are part of the shame experience. For example, the fact that many shame-prone people do not possess strong ideals suggests that ego–superego tensions are not necessary for shame. Such individuals are markedly ambitious and exhibitionistic and ideals linked to ambition are connected with ego goals rather than the superego; furthermore, exhibitionistic causes of shame suggest the involvement of the id. Problems of the same sort continue when an attempt is made to fit shame within the other major psychoanalytic theory, the theory of instincts. Shame as a component of, or defense against, the sexual instinct is difficult to accept and use given the contextual responsiveness of shame—its connection with rejection, exposure, failure and so on. In addition, defining shame as a wish or as a defense bypasses its characteristic unpleasurable nature.

Most importantly, existing psychoanalytic theories rarely explain why shame often fails to appear in the face of the suggested triggering agent whether it be love, attention, exposure, failure, contempt, or whatever.

Those authors who most incisively describe the phenomenology of the shame experience tend to ignore theory altogether. However the central message they offer is clear: shame is associated with the notions of identity, narcissism, and sense of a separate self.

## *PHENOMENOLOGY*

Recognition of the importance and singular nature of shame is not new. Otto Rank (1968) was an early writer who suggested that shame was "an emotional reaction to the realization of difference, of separation (between people)." However, the detailed development of this insight has only come in recent decades.

Erikson (1968) named his second psychosocial phase "autonomy versus shame and doubt" and referred to the crucial conflicts as "will to be oneself versus self-doubt" and "self-certainty versus self-consciousness." He saw shame as deriving from helplessness and loss of self-control and connected it with being seen and the impulse to hide. He wrote "the obligation to achieve an identity . . . is apt to arouse a painful overall ashamedness . . . over being visible all around to all-knowing adults." He carefully and explicitly avoided the usual confusions by labeling the third phase "initiative versus guilt" and the fourth phase "industry versus inferiority."

Lynd (1958) has offered a careful and comprehensive description of shame that makes a simple equation with awareness of short-coming, wrong-doing, or exhibitionism difficult to accept. The sense of exposure in shame is of "sensitive, intimate, vulnerable aspects of the self" and it is primarily exposure to one's own eyes—hence involving the discovery of identity and uniqueness. She noted an element of unexpectedness, a feeling of inappropriateness or incongruity, and related this to the discrepancy between what is felt from within and what is apparent from without. Shame is accompanied by confusion (more generally recognized by psychoanalysts in association with blushing) and in her existential analysis this is explained as a loss of identity which one thought one had. She highlighted the threat of trust in oneself and the world and instanced the child's shame when an adult treats casually or indifferently an event that is highly significant to the child. She also observed that shame is portrayed in literature as not just agonizing and painful but also revelatory and rapturous. Finally she referred to the involvement of the whole self in the act of shame. Unlike the guilty act for which one can make confession, expiation, penance, or reparation, the shameful act requires an alteration of the person. The person thinks, "I cannot have done this. But I have done it, and I cannot undo it because this is I." Shame is provoked by experiences that question our preconceptions about ourselves and compel us to see ourselves and society; it is a necessity for personal growth.

Lewis (1971) has suggested that shame functions as a protection against the loss of self-boundaries and helps to maintain the sense of separate identity and emotional relatedness. This description distinguishes it clearly from guilt. Among other things she noted that the experience of shame is directly about the *self* and its negative valuation and gives rise to "identity imagery," whereas in guilt, the self is negatively evaluated with respect to some activity and is not itself the focus of the experience.

Lichtenstein (1963) also postulated a boundary function for shame. He suggested that a person lives in a constant tension between identity maintenance and the temptation to abandon his or her identity as human altogether, and he claimed that people oscillated between identity and loss of identity. Shame, Lichtenstein suggested, was associated with a breakthrough of yearnings to yield to the ever-present temptation to abandon our unique experience of the world and sense of ourselves. More recently, Schneider (1977) has incorporated phenomenological analyses of shame from sociology, anthropology, philosophy, and religious studies as well as psychology. His work is wide-ranging and subtle but his message is concordant with that of the authors in this section. In Chapter 6 he speaks for himself. In view of the theory to be proposed in the next section, it is as well to note that he puts shame at the dividing point between on the one hand the demonic and destructive in human nature and on the other that part of ourselves that is most sensitive, vulnerable, and dependent on mutual emotional involvement.

## A NEW THEORY OF NARCISSISM

If, as appears to be the case, the experience of shame is to be implicitly or explicitly located within the field of self-psychology and narcissism, then an adequate theory of narcissism will be necessary. The psychoanalytic literature here shows an interesting phenomenon—it is divided into two camps that use the term "narcissism" for different psychological and interpersonal phenomena. One of these camps frequently mentions shame, while for the other it does not appear to exist theoretically or clinically. My own theory, briefly summarized below, reveals that the two camps are looking at different sides of the same coin.

Healthy self-esteem is not so much feeling perpetually good and worthwhile, but is rather the ability to manage feelings like inadequacy, weakness, incompetence, or guilt. Such feelings have their roots in those universal experiences and fantasies of childhood in which a person is bad, sick, crippled, ugly, deformed, repulsive, vicious, unlovable, and so on. Within limits, the less satisfactory the childhood the more significant and potentially intrusive such disturbing experiences will be in later life. In other words, when we see self-esteem disturbance, we find an individual who is being overwhelmed by negatively valued early experiences, and in that state cannot think or act as the current situation demands.

Self-based experience has a peculiar characteristic: attempt to exclude or reject a part of experience leads to loss of awareness more globally. So, in order to be in contact with one's own feelings and therefore those of others, it is necessary to tolerate and manage negative self-feelings. As a child this can be difficult, and even as an adult it is no mean task. The experiential correlate of such a state of mind is a sense of vulnerability, openness, sensitivity, and willingness to experience mental pain. A person benefits from self-awareness through a deep sense of aliveness, a feeling of personal continuity and integrity, and a powerful coherence in feeling, thought, and action. However these benefits are less tangible and usable in childhood and do not outweigh the suffering, terror and risk associated with traumatic experiences. Traumatic experiences therefore lead to the activation of modes of self-protection. In adult life, any form of painful self-feeling or negatively valued self-image may produce a similar and now thoroughly counterproductive response.

Self-protection differs from (ego-) defense. Defenses are aimed solely at some component wish or affect, whereas self-protective devices attempt to wall off experience, and hence relationships, globally. The self-protective state implies that the outer world, mainly other people, is dangerous or overwhelming. However, social situations must still be handled if the individual is not to die or be locked up; this is achieved through production of acceptable behaviour, saying the right things, avoiding intimacy, and generating emotion if this is likely to be useful.

This state of self-protection, which Freud referred to as "the stone wall" of narcissism, has a number of interesting features. The adjective "mindless" fits well, because idiosyncratic meaning cannot be assigned to situations, and sensitivity to feelings is replaced by social convention or absent altogether. The individual may therefore act in ways that show his or her lack of consideration of others or a lack of concern for himself. Such behavior destroys relationships. In the self-protective, mindless state, a person cannot grow or develop insofar as this refers to the enrichment and increasing complexity of emotional understanding. The immediate consequences of self-protection are equally serious: continuity and persistence in efforts is weak because actions are not driven by the inner coherence of the self; commitment cannot be given or counted on; decisions concerning the person's own life or future are avoided; and all significant activity is driven by expedience, wishes to fit the expectations of others, and social conventions. The individual inevitably denies his or her own needs, experiences confusion, and becomes confused with those about him or her.

The two theoretical camps in psychoanalysis have divided on whether their focus, broadly speaking, is on self-esteem or self-protection. I have labelled the two positions "self-narcissism" and "object-narcissism" respectively, and as described above they are interlinked mental states (Kinston, 1982). Self-narcissistic disturbance activates object-narcissistic maneuvers, and object-narcissism covers self-narcissistic pathology. For practical purposes, the two states can be seen as mutually exclusive. They do not correspond to conventional distinctions within many discussions of narcissism like "healthy–pathologic," "primitive–developed," or "benign–malignant." Self-narcissistic feelings of well-being and ill-being may be more or less primitive or developed and more or less healthy or pathologic. Object-narcissism, too, though its description above seems fearsome, has its healthy correlate in custom, politeness, manners, and social skills, and may exist in a more primitive or more developed state.

The well-functioning individual is able to make transitions from self-narcissism to object-narcissism and vice versa in an appropriate fashion as the situation demands and is able to operate effectively and efficiently in either state. The poorly functioning individual may find himself or herself in the wrong state at the wrong time, may be unable to manage the states well when s/he does get it right, or may be restricted primarily to one state of mind. For example, some psychotherapists appear to drown themselves in intimacy and avoid public events because of a poor capacity for social intercourse. Correspondingly some successful businessmen and politicians are highly successful socially in managing people and situations but their intimate lives are chaotic.

Transitions between these two states of self-narcissism and object-narcissism are of great interest. We indicated above that in the face of self-narcissistic disturbance there is an inherent tendency to move to object-narcissism. This move severs emotional interrelatedness and may therefore release mindless destruction. It is, however, impossible to thrive in this state and so a move back to self-narcissism often occurs. The destruction and its consequences are then witnessed and must be handled, but if this feels unbearable a move back to the protection of object-narcissism is likely and so on in an oscillatory fashion. Circumstances may result in an individual remaining permanently in a state of object-narcissism with dire consequences to the personality.

The alternation between self-narcissism and object-narcissism can be traced back to childhood. It develops in those situations when the mother accepts the child only insofar as the child is an extension of herself and serves her needs. The child is therefore being rejected in terms of its uniqueness—that is to say, its own particular constellation of feelings, needs, and wishes. This leads to two states within the early dyadic relationship, states that the child himself can observe and eventually manipulate (Figure 7-1). The interpersonal relation is painful, horrible, and traumatic for the child. Should s/he exist as himself or herself, the child is subjected to rejecting and invalidating attitudes and finds that s/he causes pain, depression, rage, or resentment in the parent. Should the child comply with the parental projection, s/he must destroy his or her own experience. The former course is clearly associated with low self-esteem, identity disturbances, and problems of self-regulation. The latter course results in a spurious sense of well-being due to the receipt of (false) approval and love, and the absence or psychic destruction of personal need, frustration, or conflict. Interpersonal contact then becomes a reaction or a deliberate production without root in personal desire or spontaneous gesture.

Figure 7-1. The schema of narcissistic development.

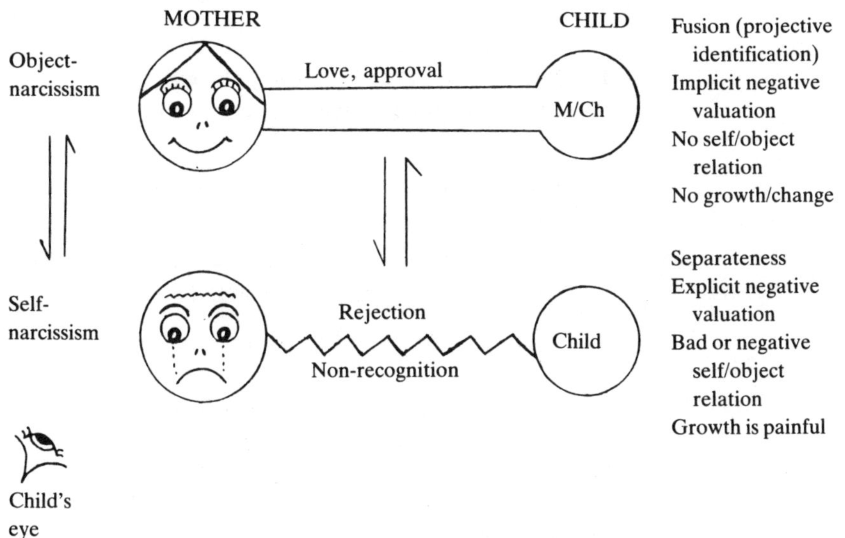


*Note.* Reprinted from Kinston, W. (1983). "The positive therapeutic reaction," in *Scandinavian Psychoanalytic Review, 6*:111–127. Copyright 1983 by Scandinavian Psychoanalytic Review. Reprinted by permission.

*THE CONCEPT OF SHAME*

Having briefly specified the theory, I can now propose a formal definition of shame. Shame is defined as the experience that signals that a transition from self-narcissism to object-narcissism is imminent. The emotional experiences surrounding shame will therefore be expected to be associated with self-narcissistic, object-narcissistic, and transitional phenomena.

The crucial question is how this conceptualization of shame can be validated. There are two main approaches. First, it must be asked how well the theory explains the various clinical and nonclinical observations and descriptions. This after all was the fundamental criticism levelled at previous theoretical efforts. Second, and perhaps more persuasive for the clinician, it must be asked how helpful the theory is in daily psychotherapeutic practice. Most of the rest of the chapter will be taken up in answering the first question. The latter question is best demonstrated via detailed examination of clinical material, preferably during review or supervision of ongoing therapy. However, some illustrative material from two different types of patient will be offered with commentary at the end of the chapter.

## THE PHENOMENOLOGY OF SHAME AND THE NEW THEORY OF NARCISSISM

I believe that the existing observations and descriptions fit in nicely with the view that shame appears in the state of self-narcissism associated with the urge to move to object-narcissism. In his description of shame, Erikson (1950) writes:

> there is a limit to a child's and an adult's individual endurance in the face of demands which force him to consider himself, his body, his needs, and his wishes as evil and dirty, and to believe in the infallibility of those who pass such judgment. Occasionally, he may turn from things around, become secretly oblivious to the opinion of others, and consider as evil only the fact that they exist. (p. 245)

Erikson crucially places shame within the phenomenon of negative valuation, and links it to the problem of evil. Obliviousness to others is a manifestation of object-narcissism and is seen as a response to the type of parent–child interaction described in the previous section. Shame is the signal experience that the individual, faced with painful self-awareness and still with the capacity to relate meaningfully to another, wishes to abandon this and to adopt a state of mind that is sensed as evil, that is to say, characterized by a denial of all that is human: need, dependency, conflict, meaning, imperfection.

Once the person has moved to object-narcissism, the experience of shame recedes. Indeed, destructive behavior in this state often gets described as shameless. The move to object-narcissism is expedient and reflects a cynical triumph over the pain and effort involved in the commitment to truth. This manifests in a later psychotherapy as an unwillingness to know what occurred in childhood or to re-experience it with the therapist. The violation of the young child's mind in order to preserve parental well-being exacts a terrible toll in later life. Self-containment and self-regulation become difficult; and disgraceful, scandalous, or criminal activities result, recreating the negative valuation of the self.

Given an infancy where the parents responded positively to spontaneity and self-assertive struggles, a person feels in the main "unashamed," that is, self-awareness is not overly painful and there is relatively little urge to fusion and object-narcissism. Self-exposure is then associated with a sense of modesty, humility, and reticence because of an awareness, at a tolerable level, of sensitivity and vulnerability. A perspective of one's significance and place in the order of things develops and precludes pretentiousness and bouts of wounded rage.

In this view, a person in therapy does not work through shame to the point of being unashamed. Rather, if s/he commences shameless, s/he must be brought to experience shame. The alleviation of excessive shame depends on core self-images losing some of their intense negative valuation. As the possibility of returning to a solution of human problems by returning to object-narcissism does not disappear, shame always remains.

Shame propensity and narcissistic vulnerability are related but distinct notions. All shame-prone individuals are narcissistically vulnerable but the reverse is not true. This is because many narcissistically vulnerable people lock themselves into defensive invulnerability by becoming more or less committed to a shame-free (shameless) state of object-narcissism. This group includes both ostensible failures (psychopaths, perverts) and highly successful persons who are withdrawn or chaotic in their private lives. In contrast, the shame-prone person is on the brink of behaving in an unfeeling or inhuman way. For longer or shorter periods s/he is aware of himself or herself, but with an awareness loaded with negative connotations. S/he may try to counteract this by obtaining public acclamation and admiration, but the shame reflects a longing for the easy escape into object-narcissism, and s/he periodically succumbs.

## *IS THERE AN "UNCONSCIOUS SENSE OF SHAME"?*

Emotions have some human action as part of their definition: for guilt it is the need for punishment, for anxiety it is the urge to run away. These action components provide a fantasied relief for the experience and may be acted upon in various ways. If only the action is observed, psychoanalysts speak of an "unconscious" experience. The action component of shame is the wish to hide. This may be expressed in a more obvious fantasy form such as a wish to sink into the ground. In this action, both aspects of narcissism are evident: withdrawal and protection of the self are self-narcissistic; becoming part of the ground (mother) is object-narcissistic.

During analysis, patients with narcissistic disturbance are often "not there." Their associative and dream material commonly reveals that they are hiding and attempting to relate by either putting up a facade or sending a delegate to speak for and about themselves. Direct relating is felt to be messy or sordid and unacceptable and when it occurs shame is felt.

Freud's longest discourse on shame is in *The Interpretation of Dreams* (1900) in which he examines dreams characterized by the conjunction of nakedness, shame, and the wish to hide (pp. 242–248). Such dreams epitomize the shame experience by including its three components: the precipitating event (nakedness—self-exposure, self-awareness), the affect (shame), and the action (hiding). Although he links such dreams to the desire to exhibit, Freud quotes at length a literary reference to Homer that is remarkably pertinent to our theme.

> If you are wandering about in a foreign land, far from your home and from all that you hold dear, if you have seen and heard many things, have known sorrow and care, and are wretched and forlorn, then without fail you will dream one night that you are coming near to your home; you will see it gleaming and shining in fairest colours, and the sweetest, dearest and most beloved forms will move towards you. Then suddenly you will become aware that you are in rags, naked and dusty. You will be seized with a nameless shame and dread, you will seek to find covering and to hide yourself, and you will awake bathed in sweat. This, so long as men breathe, is the dream of the unhappy wanderer. (pp. 246)

If we take the story as a whole then we may add to Freud's interpretation. The unhappy wanderer is the rejected miserable child who has to face the world alone. His dream is not a wish-fulfillment spoiled by the emergence of instinctual strivings, but one "beyond the pleasure principle," that is, a repetition of a traumatic event. The exposed vulnerable child desires his or her parents (their positive valuation glows) and suddenly finds himself or herself (including his or her instinctual wishes) not valued. In that state of awareness s/he experiences shame. The unhappy wanderer lives out an unconscious sense of shame.

## *INDIVIDUATION AND VOLITION*

The price of individuation is shame. Andreas-Salome (1921/1962) put this poetically: "Now the profoundly racking illness—the primal hurt of all of us—had ended its long course, the uncomprehending self-abasement of becoming an individual." Because shame is located at this developmental and adult dynamic focus, it has an important connexion with volition.

The child's dilemma, as described above, is either to gain approval, love, and pleasure by submitting passively to interaction which denies its own existence or to reject the parental object-narcissism and assert individuality and autonomy, both at the cost of a negative response from the parent and with the responsibility for producing pain and depression in the parent. Turning from an autonomous existence, abandoning choice, and losing volition are existential crises based on being a thing for the other.

Nietzsche wrote (1937): "Shame occurs where man feels that he is nothing but a tool in the hands of a will infinitely greater than is his own within his separate individuality." Hermann (1943), a Hungarian psychoanalyst, wrote that "man is capable of being shamed by anything that shows him to be enslaved by laws and necessities impervious to his own will." These insights receive some confirmation from experimental studies that reveal the existence of an acute distress state associated with the infant's inability to influence, predict, or comprehend an event when s/he expected to be able to do so (see Broucek, 1979). This distress seems to be the experience of shame.

Human functioning in health is characterized by decision (judgment and valuation), purpose, and a sense of free-will—all manifestations of self-narcissism. The object-narcissism counterpart is activity that is reactive, confused, artificial, mechanical, or automatic. The classic defense of inhumanity is that of Eichmann, namely "acting under orders." Erikson (1950) wrote: "A sense of self-control without loss of self-esteem is the ontogenetic source of a sense of *free-will*. From an unavoidable sense of loss of self-control and of parental overcontrol comes a lasting propensity for *doubt* and *shame*." When the child allows himself or herself to function as an extension of a parent, s/he has lost self-control and has abandoned himself or herself to the parent. Parental overcontrol is most compulsive and coercive when parental narcissism is at stake, in contrast to overcontrol related to habit or ignorance. Parents who bring their child to a psychiatrist often refer to this struggle for control in identity terms: "It's him or me."

## *GUILT AND FAILURE*

How did shame get mixed up with notions like shortcoming or wrong-doing? One explanation might be that experience is complex and, because painful experience is reacted to and defended against in many ways, there is a wealth of psychological data that allow ordering in a number of ways. It is possible that the inability of psychoanalytic theories to accept the concept of shame naturally made it easier for analysts to conjoin shame to concepts like guilt or inferiority that did fit the models well. The destructiveness of object-narcissism does, of course, commonly lead to experiences of guilt or failure, so shame experiences do have temporal links to these experiences.

The developmental perspective may again be helpful. As described earlier, in the narcissistic child–parent relation, every assertive step of the child that proclaims "I am separate . . . I am different" results in parental pain, depression, and resentment. These intersubjective meanings of individuation have two prominent characteristics. First, self-assertion is an attack on the parent and the consequent loss of love, approval, and well-being is experienced by the child as punishment. Second, the (child-in-the) parent is being failed by the child. These meanings are not specific to a particular act but color the child's total existence. The individual in later life is said to be riddled with guilt or feelings of failure. The common understanding of shame as the anxiety aroused by failure to live up to internalized parental ideals under the unconscious threat of abandonment can now be reformulated as follows: Shame is associated with the urge to live up to parental expectations that disregard or violate a unique personal identity; but that offer a sense of closeness, love, or approval.

It is worth noting that every child goes through this type of experience and has to face these issues during development and the process of socialization. The universal impact of parental narcissism on infant narcissism is too large a subject to be covered here. We may, however, touch on the transition from intimate relations to social relations in the disturbed family. When narcissistic impact goes wrong within the intimacy of family life, problems often do not appear until this environment is left for the wider social environment. In such a family, independent existence and awareness of the parental behavior and its intersubjective meaning (self-narcissism and genuine interpersonal relating) are unpleasurable and unwished-for in the context of readily available relief and ease through fitting in (object-narcissism). As a result, shame is often felt and experienced as an additional source of suffering. In later life, however, object-narcissistic functioning is frequently realized to be undesirable and shame may then become a valuable ally of the person's efforts to maintain meaningful interpersonal relations. In this way shame appears not so much as a guardian against instinctual undesirables but rather as a device to ensure the use of instinctual drives in the service of reality, relating, and core values.

Guilt-shame cycles have been noted by many psychoanalysts who explain them as follows. An instinctual impulse arises and leads to guilt and inhibition; passivity and inaction generate feelings of inferiority and shame; these evoke acting out which in turn leads to guilt. Guilt-shame cycles are explained differently in the current theory in the light of developmental considerations. Narcissistic phenomena are about the option of moving backward and forward between self-narcissism (with genuine interpersonal relating) and object narcissism. Moves in the direction of self- to object-narcissism are associated with shame, while moves in the other direction result in an awareness of the destruction produced while in the object-narcissistic state and consequent guilt. This only increases the urge to move back to object-narcissism. The cycle is liable to be instigated in any personally important activity as the individual must then make decisions that commit himself or herself and this activates a self-narcissistic state of mind.

## *EXPOSURE, KNOWLEDGE, REJECTION, EXHIBITIONISM*

Shame, it has been emphasized, is related to knowledge: self-knowledge and the knowledge of psychic and external reality. The development of empirical knowledge is rooted in visual metaphors such as "observation," "speculation," "contemplation," "insight," and "imagination." Knowledge of the inner world is expressed symbolically predominantly in terms of visual experience in myth and dreams. The conjunction of shame, knowledge, and seeing is well illustrated in the biblical story of creation. When Adam and Eve ate from the Tree of Knowledge, they knew they were naked, they knew shame, and they were expelled from Eden. This marked the beginning of the human race. Similarly, individuation, commencing from knowledge of separateness and consciousness of one's humanity, means the loss of blissful responsibility-free states of fusion and the appearance of shame. The myth clarifies the problem of who is seeing or knowing whom: it is the person seeing and knowing himself or herself.

This conclusion deserves some further consideration. The "social behavior" theory of shame, which focuses on being seen, criticized, or rejected by another person, is superficial, not just because it fails to explain why criticism, rejection and so on often do not generate shame, but also because it avoids any links to infantile fantasy or childhood experience. For example, the "other person" in later life could be either the mother or the child, or a part of the child—his or her ego or superego. Lynd (1958) believed that the shame exposure was primarily to one's own eyes and she related it to self-knowledge and self-awareness. It is a recurrent observation that the human being's capacity for self-knowledge and self-observation is not great, but the psychoanalytic method bases itself on the fact that it can be developed and reinforced by mirroring. Lynd wrote: "When you look at yourself in the mirror, someone stares at you who is not you and yet it is—this is the form of exposure in the shame experience."

Nietzsche (1937) described the futility of revenge on the witness in *Thus Spake Zarathustra:* the ugliest man has murdered God who saw everything but if the superman, the perfect being, is unattainable, then there is no point killing God, it is better to have killed shame; only shame is not another but the individual, himself or herself. In other words the other who observes one's defects and "causes" shame is none other than one's own self, and shame is an expression of the individual's humanness. Shame-prone individuals are liable to self-consciousness; this must be some form of internal scanning connected with the awareness that self-images that define one can enter into someone else's mind as part of a relationship. Self-awareness, in contrast, is not an ego or ego-ideal scanning phenomenon but is the active presence of self-images, related to early and current experience, in unconscious and conscious mental life.

The importance of exposure for the shame experience is consistent with the theory offered because exposure implies a coming into awareness of what was formerly hidden as well as a wish to hide or avoid. However, an individual aware of himself or herself and his or her characteristics is not shamed when these are pointed out or criticized, nor will s/he have an urge to protect himself or herself by denying or ignoring the reality of the situation. It is therefore insufficient and confusing to say that shame is produced by exposure to others who have negative reactions or who can be imagined to have such reactions. Rejection does surround the disturbed narcissistic parent–child interactions but it is a complex phenomenon made up of a variety of parental rejections, self-rejections, talion fears, and defenses. In adult life, the experience of shame when a move toward someone is rejected (or during the move when fear of rejection is a fantasy) is related to the urge to move to object-narcissism so as to banish feelings and conflicts, to deny one's own basic characteristics, and to fit in rather than to maintain full awareness of the interpersonal tensions.

Similarly the exhibitionistic instinct may be important in shame-laden experiences but to define shame in its terms seems most incomplete. The phenomenon of adult exhibitionistic activity is not solely instinctual but a complex, mainly defensive, activity. For example, it attracts attention and admiration of criticism that deals with the self's nonexistence or negative valuation; it externalizes self-images so that others see and know rather than oneself; it may have a repetition-compulsion quality related to the coercion of the child to show something for the benefit of the parents; and it may be a counterreaction to the wish to hide.

## *SHAME, LOVE, AND SEXUALITY*

The narcissistic pleasure of parents in their children can be very great indeed, and during fusion the child shares in this in an especially intense way. Shame therefore becomes connected with self-abandonment, rapture, ecstasy, and sexuality. Even in adulthood, sexuality is associated with experiences of fusion and contains an element of treating the other as a thing. In view of this and the bodily intimacy and exposure, sexuality can never be totally divested of shame. Stendhal (1822/1947) wrote: "Modesty (i.e. shame) is the mother of love." Intimacy and sexuality can only be rendered shame-free by dehumanization which results in perversion and pornography.

The assertion that positive feelings release shame is not generally true and misses the point that *any* form of personal relating is potentially linked to shame. Affection leads to shame when the child discovers that his or her parents will only accept a particular form of affection: the child must love the parent the way the parent wants to be loved and in return the parent will do the same for the child. In this battle, the child may surrender or may choose to fight on. It is the urge to surrender that activates shame. Unfortunately, surrender does not usually lead to safety but rather to further encroachments on to the child's own existence and self-valuation. Hence hostility toward the parent comes to have ego-strengthening functions and is crucial for growth. In later therapy, contact with and release of hostility serves a similar purpose.

## *SHAME AND AGGRESSION*

Shame is often talked about as if it causes aggression and the phenomena of object-narcissism. Movement between states of object-narcissism and self-narcissism does result in characteristic experiences and behavior that include aggressive and hostile components, but shame, rather than being the cause of these releases, is an independent phenomenon. Perhaps a reinterpretation of an example of Stierlin's (1977) may further explicate the present viewpoint. Stierlin reports that the patient had attacked the analyst outside the session and came feeling guilty about this. He tried to justify the attacks by looking for faults in the analyst. This was interpreted and the patient cried. Stierlin then writes: "Yet while he cried, he was overcome with shame. He called his crying a despicable show of weakness and blamed me for having triggered it. Out of his humiliated fury he attacked me again."

My understanding of this would be as follows: the patient

experienced guilt over his attacks and tried to evade it as described. The interpretation of this led to a depressive response and awareness of responsibility. The patient is then faced with a choice. Either he looks at why he is attacking and hurting the other at the cost of guilt and a sense of weakness, or he blindly and inhumanly continues to attack and remain unaware of its origins. At this point of choice, in touch for a moment with the negatively valued weakness, he experiences shame. He goes on to choose attack, using his reaction of despising himself as a weapon and an attempt to restore his self-value. In addition to shame, the patient was probably experiencing a sense of inferiority as evidenced by his initial search for faults in the analyst. This latter state can be seen as based on ego–superego tensions and does have a tendency to stimulate aggressive release.

## *MECHANISMS FOR DEALING WITH SHAME*

A person may defend against painful guilt or allow himself or herself to experience remorse and deep regret. The experience of guilt must still be dealt with and methods for this operate internally and have been institutionalized in religion, law, and custom to enable their enactment. These include atonement, confession, penance, punishment, repentance, reparation, and forgiveness. Much has been written in the psychoanalytic literature about these topics.

Much less has been written on methods for dealing with painful shame states following self-exposure; indeed it is often asserted that they are few or ineffective. A recent major compendium of defenses has a full index column of references to guilt while shame is not mentioned at all. Shame, like any experience, may be defended against with the usual variety of mechanisms. In addition, completing the transition to object-narcissism will immediately extinguish shame. Lewis (1971) described one typical form: bypassing the affect and watching the self from the viewpoint of the other. Maintenance of a permanent state of object-narcissism will prevent the experience of ever moving to object-narcissism and hence results in the absence of shame: this is shamelessness. Being secure within self-narcissism and self-object relating also results in an absence of shame: this is unashamedness.

The move to object-narcissism, it has been suggested, involves the subjection of the whole person (including his or her mental apparatus) and replacement of spontaneous directed awareness by stereotyped or ritualized activity. In childhood, self-expression produced parental pain so it is not surprising that methods for subduing such activity have been developed by the human mind and institutionalised in society. These methods include mortification, taking refuge, hypocrisy, dishonesty, incognizance, and hiding.

Mortification originally simply meant the destruction of vitality and vigor. The experience following exposure is sometimes described this way and a popular expression for it is "I could have died:" Mortification was a specific religious activity for subduing one's self and body by using self-denial and self-discipline, often with austere living and the infliction of pain and discomfort. In addition to the surface masochistic aspects it is possible to conjecture the existence of an active recreation of childhood activity: the child controlling and subduing his or her own impulses in the face of parental coercive demands.

Religions have often advised withdrawal from life and the entering of a retreat. This may be solitary as in hermitages or in groups such as monasteries; and the retreat may be temporary or permanent. In group living, solitude is usually emphasized, even prized, and communication kept at a minimal level or predominantly ritualized. In modern life, arrangements to ensure privacy or certain types of holiday fulfill similar functions.

Social life requires that the individual submit to the group and restrain his or her unique and personal urges. Manner, custom, and ritual assist the individual but to the degree that they are insufficient they are modulated with hypocrisy. Freud believed that social cohesion was more dependent on hypocrisy than guilt. However, the "white lie" of social hypocrisy may be insufficient to maintain poise and self-protection, and it then shades into flagrant dishonesty. The threat of social exposure of personal actions is the power behind blackmail. This blackmail may be found at the psychological level as the cost in thought and action of covering up or fraudulently misrepresenting one's experiences to oneself. Indeed the main emotional energies of some patients are expended directing a stream of lies and propaganda at themselves to prevent internal exposure.

A common protest of the narcissistically vulnerable patient in analysis is "I don't want to know!" This "incognizance" is distinguishable from "denial." It reflects a deliberate ostrich-like attitude of burying one's head in the sand, and saying, as in the child's game: "I can't see you so you can't see me." The person feels that admitting something will be overwhelming to him or her and takes the position "even if I know something is there, if I don't say it is and if I act as if it's not, then I don't have to take it into account." This mental mechanism may itself be subject to elaboration or secondary hiding maneuvers.

Simply hiding, as described earlier, remains a final possibility for dealing with shame. These mechanisms are united by their reference to the whole person, not to any particular act. For example, one patient was ashamed to acknowledge that she lived in a rented flat which she explained in terms of status, but she also found that she wished to hide her age of 26 years, and the only explanation we could find for this was that it was her and she just did not want anybody to know. Hiding avoided a painful sense of discomfort, embarrassment, and overall self-awareness. As has been frequently noted, shame and the wish to hide can be associated with the self-exposure of others with whom one is identified.

Other people may find it very difficult to hide. Communication with these in analysis may be just as difficult as with those who hide. One analysand said that whatever she said to me would be a lie: she meant by this both that she felt trapped in object-narcissism and that she could not communicate her wholeness (self-narcissism). When she did speak, her sentences were like crystals whose faces reflected innumerable meanings each illuminating an aspect of her whole self.

## CLINICAL ILLUSTRATIONS

Clinical material can never prove a theory to be true. However, it can help convey what the theory is supposed to be about. Good theories in psychoanalysis have two characteristics. First, they increase sensitivity to important psychic phenomena that otherwise would be neglected. Second, they enable clinicians to see patterns or order where previously there had been confusion. Inevitably, no examples can provide more than a glimpse of the enormous variety of experiences that are relevant to our theme. The two case illustrations below are drawn from quite different therapies. The man of average intelligence presented with characteristic neurotic features and a settled ordered life. The woman of superior intelligence presented with narcissistic features and a chaotic life. Both were successful in careers which suited them and both were married with children.

## *CASE 1: MR. S*

Mr. S presented with an acute anxiety neurosis but refused to attend more than once per week with a variety of excuses. It became clear that this was part of an attempt to exert control over his experiences. He initially insisted on sitting up and carried on a social conversation much as if I was his physician. My nonacceptance of this role was ignored by him and he behaved in a compliant and polite fashion, filling the session with meaningless words below which his terror could be sensed. (This stone-wall type of object-narcissism often destroys almost any possibility of therapeutic interaction. Only not coming at all is more difficult to handle.)

He tried the couch once and was left in a state of inarticulate pain and terror alternating with states of blankness. In this act the patient gave himself and me a glimpse of what he was protecting himself against. Some months later he returned permanently to the couch but the sessions were largely unproductive. As his initial fear decreased, so did the compulsive talking; but we were not much nearer his inner world. Neither dreams nor fantasy elaborations were available and my interpretations seemed to be seized on often more in an effort to comply than to gain insight. Eventually he reported that his external situation was much improved and that he felt comfortable and safe in therapy. Compliance had led to a new object-narcissistic pattern of pseudo-cooperation as the patient tried to adapt to the analyst's expectations. Sessions then became characterized by long silences. The sessions to be reported were generated by an accidental error of mine, a phenomenon that often leads to contact with reality.

Two consecutive sessions will be reported in detail. In the first session, Mr. S describes how a strong sense of embarrassment preceded a move to object-narcissism ("blankness"). In the next session, he refers to shame rather than embarrassment and is deeply involved in understanding it. He recognizes that shame is both part of being in touch with himself (a manifestation of self-narcissism) and therefore positive, and part of an urge to turn away from reality (a manifestation of object-narcissism) and therefore negative. He then finds himself reliving an early experience of disappointing his parents, just prior to the end of the session. At the third session (not reported in detail) he reveals a way he disappointed them that goes to the core of his being. As object-narcissism is about fitting in with parental expectations, the patient's linking of shame to awareness of disappointed expectations is further confirmation of the theory of narcissism within which the concept of shame is being placed.

*Session 1*

(Mr. S had been given a monthly bill the session before.)

MR. S: After leaving last session, I wanted to come today with a blank mind. When I walked in then, I felt anxious and I wondered what I would think if I had no thoughts in my mind. (There followed comments about the day's activities which trailed off into a silence.)

Things in this room seem to have a tinge of red on them. Red is danger—in that sense you are white. I've got another strange thought—I don't know why—it's as if red is associated with punishment. (*Silence*) When I'm silent, I think that you're going to criticize me.

(We had noted frequently his repression/suppression of a critical and complaining attitude to my silence, mainly from a fear of a massive retaliation. He felt the analyst was not playing the game and not being supportive and helpful as expected.)

DR. K: Could it be that you want to criticize me and it's easier to think of me criticizing you.

MR. S: Yes, as we've said before, it seems that I don't want, don't like to criticize you. I've just remembered something. When I walked out of the last session, I looked at the bill and I saw you had charged me for one session too many. I immediately felt guilty—even after checking my diary to confirm I was right. I realized it would be sorted out. (He then spoke about his own scrupulousness, wishes to avoid criticism, and his dislike of finding me not perfect.) My main memory of seeing the bill is feeling embarrassed. I don't know why. (*Silence*)

DR. K: When you saw the bill you became aware that a mistake had been made and knew that this meant there would have to be a personal interaction with me. For a start I would have to be confronted with the error and would have to respond and just possibly show you that you were wrong. In any case there would be a variety of emotions and experiences including particularly your criticism of me and sense of guilt for mentally attacking me. The best solution was to blank out your mind and you decided to do this, as you explained at the beginning of the session. The embarassment after seeing the bill was the signal that you were about to avoid personal contact by going blank—at which point you went blank.

MR. S: I don't remember the matter about the bill at all from that moment of embarrassment till it suddenly came to me in the middle of this session. (End of session)

*Session 2*

MR. S: After the pangs of embarrassment and the directness of last session, I feel introverted. I want to recoil into myself. The feelings so obviously outweigh—are so out of proportion to the substance of the event. It's as if there is something wrong about them. I want to get small—or sneak into a corner. It's so as not to feel shame. I feel a lack of confidence in my abilities. I recriminate against myself for having mentioned the thing at all. I'm telling myself I should have shied away from it. But I was, and I am, very bothered that I didn't, don't, want to face up to it. You know—I feel that it would have been better to have paid the extra session and say so what. It's not right. (*Silence*) It was amazing the way the feelings emerged three-quarters way through last session. Now I feel small.

DR. K: Could one connection with feeling small be the fact that when you were small you avoided facing things a lot?

MR. S: I used to live in a fantasy world. I had a vivid imagination but was a loner. I stuttered and was very shy. Contact with people was embarrassing. I used to enter novels. Science fiction—the escapist sort. Since coming here I've been reading disaster novels. It's my mood. When I was a child, my parents weren't there (he spoke on about this and gave anecdotes of not facing new ideas or situations).

DR. K: By the way, I checked my diary and it was my error.

MR. S: I still feel guilty. I knew I was 100% correct—if I hadn't thought that, I would never have mentioned it. This is what I am trying to face up to. Coming here in the car, I felt small. I need reassurance, mothering. I lack confidence. I must tell myself over and over again that I did the right thing. I have this very strong sense of shame tonight. It runs very deep: connected with feeling inferior. Why is it in my character like this? And why so much tonight?

DR. K: It seems tonight as if you are moving between two poles: telling yourself that you should never have raised the matter, and telling yourself that you must face reality.

MR. S: Well I think that the session and the events and tonight are constructive—something seems to be happening. I'm feeling shame intensely, partly because I am getting somewhere—but I do have this inner turmoil telling me to get away. Shame seems to be negative and controlling trying to get me back to the fantasy world and away from the real world.

I understand shame—it's direct contact with the real world that I don't understand. (*Silence*) That's the negative side. I can also feel shame in a positive way—as a genuine emotion, an involuntary feeling which just wells up.

DR. K: Perhaps a feeling can tell you something.

MR. S: It's possible. When things happen like with the bill, I make a decision, then I change it and I oscillate in a state of indecision. This is connected with shame. I'm ashamed of being the sort of person I am.

DR. K: It's impossible for you to face reality if you are not you.

MR. S: When I came here in the past, I often was physically here but not really here. Not in my mind. I never felt shame.

I'm saying I don't want to be me. (*Silence*) Someone wanted me to be someone else. (*Silence*) There's a sense of disappointment about. Not mine. It's more like a feeling of expectations disappointed. It's linked to this constructive shame. I must come to terms with the fact that I am what I am (*silence till the end of session*).

At the next session, he revealed for the first time that his parents wanted him to be a girl.

## *CASE 2: MRS. P*

Mrs. P came to me 9 years after the completion of a successful analysis. In the final phase of this analysis she had got married and sometime later had a boy. Her difficulties recurred with the birth of a girl a few years later. However it was several years before she became seriously concerned about the distance she had put between herself and her family. After an initial period of settling into the analysis and feeling comfortable about being understood, she went into a prolonged phase of continual arguing, denying meaning in what I said, putting up barriers to contact and getting confused by interpretations. The first long holiday was very difficult for her but on return she was pleased to be back. She rapidly developed a warm soft relation which soon turned into an anxious inability to talk which resolved with interpretations of her fear of spoiling the analysis. It became clear that, except within her family, Mrs. P operated with a social facade under which lay intense and primitive infantile experiences and much confusion. For example, an important piece of work just preceding the sessions to be reported, focused on her confusion between her mouth and her vagina and their associated sensations. This seemed to be important in enabling her to take from the analyst, as interpretations were being experienced simultaneously as nourishing feeds and exciting penetrations.

Again, the pattern we are concerned to examine extends over two sessions. In the first, the patient is in a state of self-narcissism, in touch with her emotions and the value of the sessions. At the end of the session she refers to an experience of embarrassment and locates it in the waiting room. The waiting-room is the transition area between her different contexts—out of her social milieu but not yet fully in the analytic milieu. As a final comment in the session, it is part of her transition to the outside world (which she usually makes by looking at her watch about 5 minutes before the end of the session), and a transition, possibly, between one session and the next. There was no time for any interpretation, but, as I had expected in the next session the patient presents in a florid state of object-narcissism; false, confused, and blocking out assistance from and relation to the analyst. This is interpreted using my theory of narcissism.

*Session 1*

She attended in a very distressed state. The previous evening she had had sexual intercourse without taking any precautions against conception. She was panicky about being pregnant. She was uncertain about whether she wanted a baby, particularly as she was aware that she just wanted a baby, and not a child destined to grow up. I commented that the uncertainty concerned whether she would accept the baby part of herself and that she had a strong wish to locate this part outside herself as a solution to having to own it at all. She went on to talk about going to a gynecologist friend to have a coil (intra-uterine device) inserted. She hated this procedure and referred to the previous interpretation which was equated to herself, to the baby, and to a penis. My interpretation simply referred to her baby experiences. She replied thoughtfully; "I feel so vulnerable in the analysis . . . (*silence*) . . . in the waiting-room, I feel embarrassed."

*Session 2*

Mrs. P arrived 20 minutes late. Though she frequently had come a few minutes late, this was the first time lateness was substantial. She offered an apology couched in social terms though fully aware that lateness is to be analyzed, not to be pushed aside with politeness. She then described having forgotten to put the alarm on and rapidly became confused. Her sentences were ungrammatical and their sense jumbled. She said she did not understand my ideas about baby feelings but insisted that she wanted to come to the analysis. She also spoke about problems at work. During these associations, I made two interpretations which I thought might be helpful. On both occasions she said that she had been thinking about something else while I was talking. In both cases, the something else referred to uncertainty as to whether or not she should participate enjoyably and cooperatively in some group activity. I reflected to her that she had ignored the contents of my comments and connected it with her uncertainty as to whether she should participate in the analytic process. When I pointed out the way she stopped herself taking anything in, she replied: "I don't want something inside me. I went and had the coil removed. I often don't listen to people." I replied: "If your social facade is not on, you feel so vulnerable—you are sensitive to being affected, like a baby." She was silent for a while, and then said: "Your arrangements make it all so impersonal. A series of patients come in . . . the common entrance . . . the door bell and electrical opening." I responded: "You make it impersonal because if it's personal, then you would be irritated or annoyed by these things. You would want to criticize me. These are the sorts of experiences you think are horrible and that you don't want to have." The session ended here.

## CONCLUSION

The unalterable nature of a person's childhood and the basis and limitations of his or her psychic constitution in those experiences means that each person has an urge to abandon psychic life altogether. The resulting freedom is illusory and destructive. I believe that shame developed as a signal that such an urge is about to be given in to. Once contact with psychic reality is abandoned shame is no longer felt, and the most prominent inner experience is confusion. Typically, self-abandonment is hidden by social adaptation or the artificial production of experience. As the tendency to abandon oneself increases, shame appears initially as a wish to hide and eventually painfully and intensely as an affect. At this point reassertion of the value of psychic reality and human relations is possible. This means tolerating a self-image with negative tonings, that is to say, feeling inadequate, pathetic, crippled, hideous, or whatever. No one finds this pleasant or desirable, but narcissistically damaged individuals find it so intensely painful and very difficult to bear, they come to prefer object-narcissism. Unfortunately, once a state of object-narcissism is established in the mind, it may be difficult to shake off.

The main implication of the approach to shame offered here therefore is that the "capacity for shame" is as crucial as the "capacity for concern (guilt)." Guilt implies that we realize our aggression hurts others whom we care for and who have the power to punish in retaliation. Shame implies that we realize we have the choice, the personal option, to be artifical or mindless and act destructively, or to be authentic and thoughtful and act creatively.

## REFERENCES

Andreas-Salome, L. (1962). The dual orientation of narcissism, *Psychoanalytic Quarterly, 31:*1–30. (Original work published 1921)

Broucek, F. (1979). Efficacy in infancy. *International Journal of Psychoanalysis, 60:*311–316.

Erikson, E. H. (1950). *Childhood and society,* Harmondsworth: Penguin.

Erikson, E. H. (1968). *Identity: youth and crisis.* London: Faber and Faber.

Freud, S. (1900). The interpretation of dreams. *Standard Edition, 4.* London: Hogarth Press.

Hartmann, H., & Loewenstein, R. M. (1962). Notes on the superego. *Psychoanalytic Study of the Child, 17:*42–81.

Hermann, I. (1943). *Az Emberiseg Osi Osztonei* [*The primordial instincts of man*]. Budapest: Pantheon.

Kinston, W. (1982). An intrapsychic developmental schema for narcissistic disturbance, *International Review of Psychoanalysis,* 9:253–261.

Lewis, H. B. (1971). *Shame and guilt in neurosis,* New York: International Universities Press.

Lichtenstein, H. (1963). The dilemma of human identity: Notes on self-transformation, self-objectivaton and metamorphosis, *Journal of the American Psychoanalytic Association, 11:*173–225.

Lynd, H. M. (1958). *On shame and the search for identity.* New York: Science Editions.

Nietzsche, P. (1937). *The philosophy of Nietzsche,* New York: Modern Library.

Rank, O. (1968). Emotion and denial (from *The Genetic Psychology*). *Journal of the Otto Rank Association, 3*:9–25.

Schneider, C. D. (1977). *Shame, exposure and privacy,* Boston: Beacon Press.

Stendhal, H. (1947). *On love.* New York: Liveright Publishing. (Original work published 1822)

Stierlin, H. (1977). Shame and guilt in family relations. In *Psychoanalysis and family therapy,* New York: Jason Aronson.

Wurmser, L. (1981). *The mask of shame,* Baltimore: John Hopkins University Press.

# 8

# Shaming Systems in Couples, Families, and Institutions

DONALD L. NATHANSON

*When, in 1983, I shifted my attention from the general matter of emotional resonance and the study of its underlying affect mechanisms toward the specific emotion of shame, I was struck (startled) by the pervasive disavowal of shame conflict in the psychotherapy profession. Tomkins (1962) explains the affect surprise-startle as a resetting mechanism—data have entered our system so rapidly that the central assembly is momentarily cleared, allowing us to focus attention on a new source of information. The result of that clear, new focus was a decision to alert my colleagues, culminating in the symposium "Shame—New Clinical and Theoretical Aspects" at the May 1984 meeting of the American Psychiatric Association, and the present volume.*

*Joining me in Los Angeles were Drs. Wurmser, Will, and Schneider (whose contributions to this volume are extensions of those papers) and E. James Anthony. So much has shame been the ignored affect that, according to the American Psychoanalytic Association, which cosponsored the symposium, this turned out to be the first meeting in the history of psychiatry/psychoanalysis (European or American) to focus exclusively on shame. The following chapter is based on my own presentation at that symposium, a paper that looks at the interpersonal*

Donald L. Nathanson. Senior Attending Psychiatrist, The Institute of Pennsylvania Hospital; Clinical Associate Professor, Mental Health Sciences, Hahnemann University, Philadelphia, Pennsylvania.

*manifestations of shame—the disturbances in relatedness caused by the use of shame as a mode of interpersonal control.*

*What I would like the reader to carry away from this contribution is the understanding that our personal experience of shame, of the transient destruction produced in us by a moment of embarrassment, plants the seed of a realization that we too can disable someone by using shame as a weapon system. I think that we therapists tend to ignore the existence of such warlike interpersonal systems, despite their importance in the lives of those we counsel.*

Have we not all experienced failure in our work as therapists? We read the published reports of our colleagues to learn from their successes and their failures, review again and again the texts of our training, group with friends to study issues, attend conferences hoping to remain abreast with the pack; and, if we ourselves are not currently in some therapeutic relationship, seek out a trusted advisor to find whether the problem arises from within us or our patient. Occasionally we wish secretly that this palpable evidence of our incompetence would just go away and haunt a colleague, while from time to time we accomplish this freedom by mutually agreed upon referral to another. If the patient does well with this new therapist we say that they deserved each other; if poorly, we feel vindicated. But most often the patient chooses to stay with us in what becomes an atmosphere of stagnation within which any tiny change, however unrelated to our work, is greeted as a milestone.

One such patient, whose complaints had become so entirely predictable that I felt I could finish her sentences, surprised me not long ago, and this volume is the direct result of my reaction to the overwhelming nature of that surprise.

In the initial sessions, a decade earlier, she had told me about something she called "The mantle of hate." At all times, she said, there would be one person who was the object of her rage. "It can be either one of my daughters; frequently it is my husband; if you and I continue to work in therapy it will occasionally be you. But whoever I designate as the wearer of the 'mantle of hate' is the recipient of all my anger. During that period of time everybody else is safe, at least until I choose another target." And do not think that she was exaggerating about the degree and intensity of her negative affect. I did come to know her tirades. These outbursts were the closest thing to pure hate that I have ever encountered.

You will have to take my word for the fact that in working with her I used a number of therapeutic modalities, including varying intensities of insight-oriented psychotherapy, couple and family therapy, eventually a wide range of medication (the violence of the anger was reduced by lithium, but not its pattern), sexual counseling, and behavior modification. We dealt with her flimsy sense of self ("There's no 'me'," she said many, many times) and with her narcissism. Each approach contributed a bit to her general welfare. Nothing altered this basic theme—that she lived with the propensity for coruscating rage. Therapy helped her become a more effective person, a more consistent mother, a happier divorcee, a better-integrated person except during these outbursts.

I cannot identify what sparked my curiosity one day—the session seemed at first only another listing of complaints about life in general, somewhat incongruous now that she and a lover were living together and happy. Perhaps she paused when describing one of the outbursts, as if she no longer wanted absolution for her actions, but felt capable of thinking about the rage and what might lie underneath it. She took up the issue of the outbursts as if I were a new therapist, and therapy itself, on this level, something she had never tried before. Now, in this happiest period of her life, it did not feel logical to her that these outbursts could occur.

Since she had decided to deal with me as if I were a new therapist, I decided to deal with her questions as if she were a new patient. I asked her, as an assignment for the following session, to keep a journal in which she would record each episode of rage and something about the moments which immediately preceded it. She brought in a list of interactions. As near as I could tell, each seemed to involve some sort of guilt. I asked, as the next week's assignment, for journal entries describing each experience of guilt, even those that were not associated with outbursts of anger.

And this is where I began to wake up. She did bring in a list, but as she and I examined it, each and every incident we were about to approach as guilt, turned out to be an example of embarrassment. And suddenly I was seized with a terrible feeling of inadequacy. I realized, suddenly, that I did not know anything about the affect shame. Yet now we came to understand that the bursts of rage that characterized her for husband, children, and neighbors could be seen as stemming from severe and crushing shame, an emotion against which she could defend only by returning the favor and humiliating those whom she blamed for her embarrassment.

In the nearly 20 years I had been a psychiatrist I had not heard a single lecture on shame; through the infinitude of case conferences for which I had stayed awake there had been no mention of it; no senior colleague had recommended a reference on shame; nor had one discussed a case of his or her own that involved it. My own personal library contained in toto less than half a page that illuminated this aspect of the dynamics of her case, so I called on the resources of our hospital library and mounted a months-long search of the literature for competent reference works. I learned a great deal that allowed me to revise my treatment of that signal patient, and, as you might expect, I began to see everywhere shame and its cognate states of embarrassment, ridicule, put-down, contempt, humiliation, and mortification.

## THE PHENOMENOLOGY OF SHAME

Leon Wurmser (1981), in his superb book *The Mask of Shame*, considers shame a layered affect. Using his language, we can consider its content as the topmost layer—shame reveals us to be defective, weak, inadequate, a loser in competition, dirty, infantile, unable to control our bodily functions. It engenders a characteristic action, that of hiding, avoiding being seen, averting gaze. (Indeed, the Indo-European root from which shame is derived, *skem*, or *sham*, means "to hide.") This hiding may serve the function of breaking a link with the one who has seen our weakness. Shame has a sudden onset and a slower resolution; it always involves a moment of discovery. There are two modes of uncovering, as well—we are embarrassed when, suddenly, *we* are revealed; and when we are caught looking at someone else. This is why Peeping Tom is unpopular, and accounts for some of the reasons the voyeur lives in such a peculiar state of tension.

The shame experience is one of utter isolation. It is all those moments in which we felt like crawling into a hole and disappearing forever. It involves sudden, unexpected separation; no matter what our age, shame resonates with the worst of our fears of abandonment. And shame can shape a character. We can live in fearful anticipation of embarrassment, experiencing shame-anxiety; or develop a perfectionistic style to avoid shame.

Shame differs from guilt, although these two affects are frequently confused (Alexander, 1938; Lewis, 1971; Wurmser, 1981). In guilt we are punished for an action taken; in shame we are punished for some quality of the self, some unalterable fact. Guilt limits action; shame guards the identity. Shame is the affect associated with narcissism.

We tend to label what (or who) we do not understand, and by these labels achieve personal comfort denied the bearer of the label. Terms like "borderline illness" and "inaccessible narcissism" are in danger of becoming nosologic wastebaskets to which we can consign certain of our most frustrating cases. Yet much can be retrieved from such storage to become understandable and useful once we begin to appreciate that shame affect accompanies these states, and help the patient work through the layers involved.

When we think of shame at all, most of us therapists think of it from the standpoint of personal, intrapsychic experience. No matter what our therapeutic discipline, from the most staunchly psychoanalytic to the undaunted student of pure transaction, despite our devotion to the techniques and philosophical bases of our work, we must from time to time link arms and admit the relatedness of our fields. (Each person in an interaction has an unconscious, each unconscious resides in a person who interacts.) It is fascinating to see what happens when we shift our focus away from the one experiencing shame and take the position that wherever there is shamed there is a shamer, that even when we blush while sitting alone with our memories, we have in that moment relived the exposure of some hidden "fact" before another person.

## INTERPERSONAL ASPECTS OF SHAME

From my study of shame as an internal experience I have been led to an understanding of the interactional aspects of embarrassment, to what shame does in a relationship, and how shame can be used to affect, even to control relationships. This has led me to an investigation of the public as well as the private aspects of shame, of the social and cultural aspects; and from the inner experience of shame as an unexpected event to shame as the intentional product of conscious action on the part of the shamer.

Take a pencil and a pad of paper in hand, as I have done, and watch the comedies and dramas that cross your television screen; note how frequently shame occupies center stage. Just as we tend to forget the content of dreams unless we are trained for recall, we are quite unlikely to remember the content of an embarrassing experience, whether our own or that of someone else. And as our defenses make even a remembered dream increasingly vague or simplistic over time, we remember the laughter rather than the antecedent affect. It may be true that jokes involve hostility, but it is important to recognize than an astonishing number of them involve embarrassment. A paradox—we are ashamed about shame. A corollary—professionals though we all may be, old hands with case histories, the clinical examples that form an integral part of this study may produce discomfort of unexpected intensity—we are unused to thinking about shame.

It is this ubiquity, this everywhereness of embarrassment that has made it difficult for us to understand that so common a feeling that permeates our existence also affects our lives. Think of the air around us. We do not notice, we do not discuss nitrogen, despite the fact that it makes up 80% of the gaseous envelope of the planet. It is inert. Nitrogen is all around us, and it disturbs nothing. So we have been led to consider embarrassment (Lewis, 1981).

How could we be expected to grapple with dynamics when we were living ignorant of our own involvement in shame? Like the protagonist in Moliere's *Bourgeois Gentilhomme*, who said; "Until today, I had never heard of prose, and now I find I have been speaking it every day of my life," we ourselves are rarely without embarrassment, rarely unaware of the possibilities for humiliation, the opportunities to make a fool of ourselves. We study hard and work hard in order to avoid embarrassment. We even distort facts at times—who among us has not exaggerated now and then? What else is a fish story but an attempt to deny our embarrassment that we have nothing to show for a day of fishing, to bias the listener into ignorance of what we fear may be seen as our lack of skill. The degree of embellishment is a good measure of our mortification, or of our anticipation of ridicule.

Of course it is not possible to grow up without having experienced the affect shame. It must be basic to the human condition, else how do we explain the fact that it has its own neurological pathway leading to the blush? And if all of us have felt its paralyzing force, then we know what a weapon it might be. From earliest life we remember feeling destroyed by a remark that exposed us unmercifully; not only did we remember the incident, but we stored away the knowledge that we too could produce that degree of paralysis merely by using the shame-weapon.

There is some debate among scholars of shame as to the source of the power inherent in the shame experience. Since shame produces temporary separation, or instant insecurity, logic suggests that somewhere near its core, shame has to do with separation anxiety, the emotion calling to the attention of the child that he or she is in danger because the mothering, protecting person is unavailable. Lewis (1981) suggests that the blush is a signal indicating awareness of this separation. Since the shamer is quite aware that separation has deadly implications for the shamed, seeing the other blush, the former can bestow on the latter a forgiving smile and undo the threatened exile, now that the levels of dominance have been redefined.

Shame is about eye contact. We lower our eyes, avert our gaze when embarrassed. This certainly interrupts whatever had been going on between the participants. The act of hiding from the shaming stimulus may represent an attempt to escape from the experience, to pretend it never happened. But it does more than that. The eyes are the window of the brain, and in the language of primary process, we may feel people can look in on our thoughts almost as well as we can see out. It is as if when we avert our eyes we hope to prevent the other person from knowing what we are thinking. And what we are thinking, in such moments, is rarely friendly. As we will discuss in some detail a bit later, almost immediate to the experience of embarrassment is the fantasy of retribution, swift justice of biblical equality—as you hurt me, so must I punish you. Some decision must to be made as to how much of what we are thinking will be conveyed to the other person.

It is one of those little decisions that makes a lot of difference in the formation of a personality. One of my patients, Samantha, prefers to withdraw in the face of an embarrassing remark, or when she has been placed in an embarrassing situation, or even when she notices something that might embarrass the other person. All Samantha will do is half-lower her eyelids and dart a glance at the other person before turning away. Periodically she will complain of depression, characterized by reduction in her level of energy, a wish to sleep "all day," and a nearly global withdrawal from human contact. Over the years, before I became aware of the importance of shame, we had searched in therapy around issues of repressed anger, but none came to mind.

Antidepressants forced Samantha out of her lethargy, which effect she disliked especially because this made her more active. Most patients are grateful for a lift in their spirits, a lift that allows them to focus on the problems which they perceive as having driven them into the depression. Samantha prefers withdrawal to this chemically augmented level of activity. I have come to understand that this withdrawal, which we call depression, but which more closely resembles depersonalization, is a more or less voluntary state, a place to which she goes rather than respond to embarrassment as her nature might dictate. Shame, to her, is destruction, and she finds her own fantasies of retribution completely unacceptable.

As I studied shame, and shared with her some of my findings, Samantha began to open up about her own experiences. Now I could understand what it meant to grow up in the home of bitterly competitive parents, whose success never brought them confidence or joy, only fear that whatever ground they had gained in the game of life would be taken away from them by a meaner competitor. They remind me of the chess master, Bobby Fisher, who said that "the object of playing chess is not to win a game. It is to crush the opponent's ego" (Steiner, 1972). In normal human interaction, losing a game is instructive. You learn from your opponent's moves, learn more about strategy, learn how much to trust your intuition, and end up filled with ideas for the next encounter. The degree of embarrassment is minimal. But in the kind of system Fisher described, and within which Samantha grew up, defeat is humiliation.

It is, however, quite a different thing to be the recipient of a shaming attack from your mother than to be the deliverer of one. Although the child may be mortified, that is, shamed near death, it would be another matter indeed to deliver back to mother such a blow. The child knows s/he has already survived this particular attack. To say something to mother of equal violence invites two opposite sorts of disaster. If the shaming blow is of mortal intensity, and delivered to a vital spot, mother may die, leaving the child bereft and just as abandoned as s/he felt when s/he was attacked. On the other hand, if the blow is not mortal, mother may get very angry, and loose even more punishment on the child's head. In most families a child learns to suffer humiliation in silence. It is even possible that this early experience of repressing shame anger acts as a training ground for the later development of depression.

My patient Samantha is such a person. Since childhood, her personality has been characterized by acts of selfless, smiling devotion to the needs of others, performed with worried concern, and vicious jabs of a verbal dissecting knife wielded with savage intensity and astonishing accuracy. Frequently, she chooses to remain silent rather than trust language; at such moments her eyelids close slightly as she darts a glance at the offending other before turning away. Her own children call that half-lidded reaction the "laser look." She is stuck simultaneously in the two opposite extremes of a shaming syndrome—Samantha lives to avoid conflict, but abjures her own response to it.

During the verbal fighting that preceded their divorce, her husband would complain that he never learned to anticipate her anger, feeling as if he had been swept into her storm. Shame anger, what Lewis (1971) called humiliated fury, the accumulated unspoken rejoinders to a thousand perceived insults, would store up in her until they reached critical mass, and explode almost without control. And the atomic analogy is apt, for these arguments proceded in chain reaction of specific form.

Family arguments can be divided into process and content, both of which are amplified by affect. It may be interesting at this juncture to break into a narrative about the specific affect shame to make some general comments about the nature of affect itself, and then return to my argument about arguments.

## AFFECT PSYCHOLOGY

Although the community of psychotherapists describes its mission as the various approaches to "emotional illness," we spend a disproportionate amount of our time and energy involved with cognition. For the most part, "emotion" itself is treated as "that which interferes with cognition." We search for the historical antecedents of such interference, devise behavioral strategies to loop around and avoid it, we come ever closer to ascertaining its biochemical nature the better to prevent its effects; but like the air we breathe or the planet we inhabit, we ignore it (and those who illuminate our ignorance) because we prefer to take "the emotions" for granted. Texts, compendia, handbooks, and such devote the merest fractional percent of their bulk to the nature of emotion, and the remainder to our work in handling its effects.

In Chapter 4 of this volume you will have an opportunity to read something about affect psychology written by one of its giants, Silvan Tomkins (1962, 1963); here I will only sketch some of his ideas. Tomkins sees the affects as a group of innate, biologically programmed mechanisms, present at birth and clearly visible on the face of the newborn. The primary affects (surprise, interest, joy, distress, anger, fear, disgust, dissmell, and contempt) are produced in response to stimulation of specific receptors or to patterns of stimulation. Thus, the word "disgust" carries the root *gustare*, and clearly implies that it is the signal indicating that the organ of taste has detected danger and advised the organism to take evasive action protecting it from whatever chemical has caused this taste. Tomkins calls disgust a drive auxiliary because it modifies the drive hunger, which otherwise might lead us to eat something dangerous. We are protected similarly by a nose-centered drive auxiliary, which appears in adult life in the expression "turning your nose up" at something.

Tomkins demonstrates that, in the infant, it is the rate and intensity of the flow of data along input pathways (what he calls "neural stimulation") that determines which of the following affects is triggered: a slowly rising input produces "interest"; which can amplify itself to produce "excitement"; a steady, higher than optimal level of stimulus produces "distress"; an even higher steady state level of input triggers the subcortical program for "anger"; and a rapid reduction in stimulus input causes "enjoyment" or "joy." It is not the channel along which these data are transmitted that is important in eliciting affect (sight, hearing, touch, memory, and the like) but the gradients of increase or decrease in stimulation. "Shame" and "guilt" are considered auxiliary affects because they require other affects and modulate other affects (like interest or enjoyment). In the adult, usually they require the presence of another person, of a relationship, in contrast to the remainder of the innate affects, which can occur in the isolated organism.

This theoretical position is so logical, so amenable to experimental testing, yet so different from any of its predecessors that when it was introduced (between 1954 and 1963) it created a great deal of stir in the world of psychology, and was kept in that special place reserved for something we know is important but which we do not dare accept lest it upset our cherished understandings. In the generation between its introduction and the present time, Tomkins's work has begun to nag at the corners of our consciousness (not to mention conscience) and excite the interest of the burgeoning field of "infant research."

Tomkins states that the affects function as a system of amplifiers that call attention to the needs of the organism as indicated by its physiologic data inputs. Affect is what tells us which input deserves attention, else how would we discriminate among the many data tracks running simultaneously? Affect is how the organism first learns about rank ordering and "importance"; affect works by producing urgency.

Basch (1976, 1983), building on Tomkins's work, defines "feeling" as our awareness of an affect, and "emotion" as the gestalt of an affect (or combination of affects) together with our lifetime of associations to each affect. To Basch, the emotions are highly complex, remarkably personal phenomena, not capable of duplication from person to person because of the inherent differences in our lives; the situations in which we have experienced each affect are so various that this rich gestalt can never be the same for any two people. Affect and emotion interrelate not as "brain" and "mind," but as biology and biography.

This clear separation between affect and emotion makes it possible to explain certain mostly ignored interpersonal phenomena. When infectious disease was the frontier of science, Scheler (1913/1954) described "contagion of emotion": "We all know how the cheerful atmosphere in a 'pub' or at a party may 'infect' the newcomers, who may even have been depressed beforehand, so that they are 'swept up' into the prevailing gaiety. . . . The process of infection is an involuntary one" (p. 15). "When someone says that he wants 'to see cheerful faces around him,' it is perfectly clear that he does not mean to rejoice with them, but is simply hoping for infection as a means to his own pleasure" (p. 17). "Infection by other's emotions . . . occurs in its most elementary form in the behavior of herds and crowds. Here there is actually a common making of expressive gestures in the first instance, which has the secondary effect of producing similar emotions, efforts and purposes among the people or animals concerned; thus, for instance, a herd takes fright on seeing alarm in its leader, and so too in human affairs" (p. 12).

Freud (1921), amplified by Basch (1983), later suggested that when we are in the presence of another person who is experiencing affect, we tend to mimic the facial display of the other, producing in ourselves the same affect. This, of course, is followed by our associations to that affect, which are experienced as our own emotions. Affective transmission of this sort accounts for infectious laughter and gloom, for audience reaction and mob violence. Basch points out that this form of empathic communication is not the same as what he correctly calls "mature empathy," which involves an intentional awareness of or learned sensitivity to the affect of the other, and which he rightly associates with maturity or a high level of intrapsychic growth.

I find it useful to postulate the existence of a separate ego mechanism which I have called the "empathic wall" (Nathanson, 1986) which functions dynamically, much in the manner of the living cell membrane, to protect (insulate) us from the affect of the other, allowing us to remain ourselves in the face of the other person's mood. This concept helps me understand why children are more susceptible to the affects in their millieu than are adults (ego mechanisms develop over time) and has helped me understand those patients who seem frequently to be taken over by the affect of other people, as well as those who seem almost unaffected by the emotions of others. This concept bears brief mention here to explain the connection between affect psychology and family arguments.

## ARGUMENTS

One of the little discussed phenomena of family dynamics is our willingness to accept the mood of the dominant member, to decrease our level of insulation from the affect of someone we love, trust or need. Within the family we resonate with the affect being broadcast by the more powerful other. An anxious parent makes an anxious family, as an angry parent makes an angry family.

It is clear from the phenomenology of shame affect, discussed earlier, that the experience of embarrassment sets up its own sort of tension. A parent who returns home after a blow to his or her self-esteem is likely to attempt recovery from this reduction by looking around for someone else to shame. In battles for dominance and fights for position, shame is our constant companion. Most of Adler's work needs to be reexamined today in terms of our new understanding of shame. His concepts of superiority and inferiority are much more immediate when their affect is added. The cartoon (Figure 8-1) shows this quite well. And whatever intensity and style of emotional expression characterize this dominant parent alters the affective climate of his or her family. The mood of an argument is in itself infectious, and (as I will demonstrate) amplifies both its process and its content.

The process is frequently a battle over levels of dominance,

Figure 8-1.

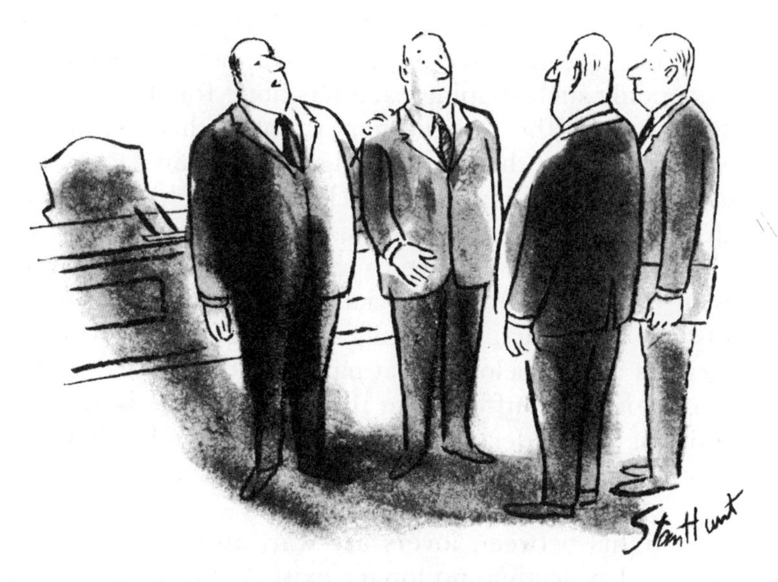

*"And this, gentlemen, is Mr. Quodley, my immediate inferior."*

*Note.* Drawing by Stan Hunt; © 1972 The New Yorker Magazine, Inc.

over the position each partner perceives or takes as his or her own, a battle which goes on until the combattants have achieved either a feeling of equality, or at least reestablished the balance characteristic of that relationship. The content is always the definition or nature of those levels. At the most primitive, shown beautifully in Goodall's (1971) observations of chimpanzees in the Gombe Strip, is the behavior of threat and display, from arm waving and chest beating to bragging. Underneath, the content of this behavior is "I am big. You are little," with "big" and "little" taken at their most literal. The degree of modulation of affect utilized by the participants varies remarkably, and in itself conveys messages about levels of dominance.

In the run of the mill family argument most of the ground to be gained by bragging has long ago been used up, and competition is joined not by raising the self but by reducing the other. The material for this sort of battle is always at hand, for its source is in the realm of the happy and normal.

One of the benefits of living with others is the tendency of social relationships to limit the expansion of the self by bringing into the open the unfounded portion of a member's self-image, and through the resultant embarrassment, move this member toward a more realistic self-appraisal. Happily married couples discuss openly such shaping each has done for the other. The subtle contracts, the unwritten portion of the marital rules, frequently require that we each ignore certain facets of the personality of the other. Sullivan (1953) called love the state in which another person's welfare is as important to us as our own. For the sake of love we agree to ignore certain foibles or attributes of our loved ones, especially those which, if discussed, might hurt or embarrass. Equally do we agree to overlook certain actions of our beloved that have caused us discomfort—a certain amount of suffering in the name of love is acceptable to all of us. These decisions are part of our higher consciousness, part of the altruism that characterizes mature relationships.

But fights between lovers are war, and the restraints of decency and peacetime no longer exist. What we hurl at each other during arguments are precisely those comments that we withheld out of love but (guilty as we may be about this) stored up because of some secret mistrust, comments guaranteed to produce stinging shame, allegations that reduce the self-esteem of the partner for no other reason than to elevate the relative self-esteem of the attacker. The choreographed interchanges we call "fights" proceed in chain reaction, each volley of insults provoking another of just slightly greater intensity. And as Wurmser (1981) has explained, the difference between shame and guilt is that shame guards the boundaries of the self, while the guilt we have taken action and aggressed on the territory of another. We can create embarrassment by pointing out that the other person is not what s/he thinks s/he is, and we can create guilt by pointing out the untoward results of his or her actions. To the best of my knowledge, the verbal portion of a fight is only either shaming or "guilting."

This explains the peculiar phenomenon that rarely do people discuss in therapy what actually was said in a quarrel. We had been trying to repress our knowledge of our own defects and of our crimes, and the phrases hurled at us during a fight break through this denial only long enough to make us feel terrible. We defend against this negative affect by becoming increasingly angry, and when we feel our self-esteem has been reduced beyond our ability to tolerate this new view of ourselves, not infrequently we move from verbal to physical action. There is a Chinese proverb about this: "He who lands the first blow was the first to run out of insults." Contempt is much less bearable than anger or hate.

From here a fight moves in one of four directions, depending largely on the intensity of affect involved and the ability of the combattants to handle it. One point of this compass involves withdrawal into the more peaceful silence of a depressive position rather than continued dispute with its certainty of escalation; while another possibility is for one individual to become so guilty at the pain evoked in the other that the hostilities cease. (I think that this guilt, amplified by anxiety accompanying a perhaps unexpected degree of separateness, is chief among the reasons couples kiss and make up after a fight and why fighting, in some couples, leads to sex. Stoller (1979) showed that the secret scripts of sexual excitement allow us to reexperience and triumph over earlier emotional trauma. Shame certainly provides many of the scenes for this process.) A third alternative is for one of the battlers physically to walk out of the fray ("I'm going home to mother!"), while the final solution is a fight that defines the levels of dominance in terms of bodily power.

## NORMAL BANTER

It seems reasonable to mention that there is such a thing as normal banter, which toys at the border of embarrassment, but which is modulated by tact. O'Henry said that love means knowing what will hurt the other person and not using it. In a healthy family the shaming thrusts are playful and of mild intensity; they serve to keep within bounds the self-esteem of each member of the system. After all, if one member of the family wins a prize, or does well in competition, it is perfectly reasonable for him or her to feel proud, for the family to share in and reflect that pride, and to adjust its view of the victorious member to take into account this new attribute. Of course, there is a limit to the amount of change any social system can handle per unit time. Occasionally even the healthiest of families may feel incompetent in the face of one member's success, experience shame, and withdraw from or even shun him or her for a while.

Nevertheless, if 12-year-old Johnny hits a home run in sandlot baseball, it is acceptable for him to glow about it for a day or so. If he wears this triumph for too long a period of time, or uses it to extend his self-image to that of a homerun hitter for one of the professional teams, this extension of his identity beyond consensually validated limits begins to affront his social network, which brings him back to reality by exposing his thinking process and producing embarrassment. Nobody wants pain, nobody wants shame. But just as you wouldn't want to go through life without pain fibers, you really wouldn't want to go through life without shame fibers.

Notice the number of opportunities for this system to go wrong. If the family is too eager for a child's success, and fails to use the embarrassment tool to shape a realistic self-appraisal, it makes the child into a narcissistic extension of itself, of its own dreams and fantasies of what it might be, of what it should have been. By doing this, it predisposes this child to ridicule outside, and fosters the later development of a defensively narcissistic identity which functions more to maintain his or her perceived place in the unwieldy fantasy structure of this nuclear family than it does to allow integration with the immediate surround. If the family is very brittle, made up of people with chronically low self-esteem who see themselves as failing always in competition, and who live therefore always at the border of shame, the real rise, through achievement, of one member may upset this fragile system, producing profound shame affect in the others, who must therefore use bitter shaming technique to prevent any permanent change in the identity of the successful member. Elsewhere I have discussed the interpersonal and sociologic aspects of such interactions as the phenomenology of the shame/pride axis (Nathanson, 1987). Shame guards the boundaries of the self, sometimes nipping and barking at them. When it promotes integration of fantasy with reality, this limiting action is a positive force in the growth of an individual. Sometimes, however, it can be used to prevent a person from using true talents and real gifts toward their possible peak potential.

It is into such a family that Samantha was born. Both parents are entertainers who reached for stardom, but lacked that special something needed to propel them to the top. They have, instead, become teachers, albeit teachers of stars. Since they are well-known public personages I have been able to observe them for many years. They wear the stigmata of the shame syndromes—her lean, athletically conditioned father is kindly and chronically self-effacing, and her mother, now nearing 70 years of age, is a hawkishly thin, cruel, jealous, and angry woman who wears black leather clothing and carries a thin black umbrella, which in her hands seems to be a combination of a Field Marshall's swagger stick and a small whip. And, more coincidence, long before I met Samantha I lived in an apartment next door to a couple who were contemporaries of her parents. From them I had heard a wealth of stories about how this mother ridiculed and demeaned Samantha's considerable talent as a painter simply because it was embarrassing that a daughter might not carry on the tradition of her parents' profession. Nothing became of this talent, which was effectively blunted and stunted by shame. Samantha simply could not expand or realize her wished-for concept of her self without risking total rejection by her mother. Throughout her therapy, until I began to work in the arena of shame, she described dreams in which she was on stage, alone, poorly prepared for a recital she did not want, anticipating the derisive reaction of an audience she had not invited.

Coincidence clusters for me around this family. More than a decade ago, long before I knew the implications of these stories in the language of shame, I treated a man who had dated Samantha in college. What made their relationship memorable for him was neither the degree of intimacy nor the thrill of their adolescent sexual explorations. It was a single scene he could not erase. One night, while they were embracing on a sofa in her parents' drawing room, he trying valiantly to achieve the conquest of her virginity, this young man felt a strange sense of another presence in the room. Torn between his curiosity and his wish not to disturb the mood of the moment, he managed to scan the room with nonchalant caution. Framed clearly in the small window of the swinging door barring entry from the next room was her mother's face, watching calmly.

I told Samantha this story in our second psychotherapy

session, many years ago, as soon as I made the connection myself. She laughed quietly, recalling more about her adolescent struggles to preserve her virginity than about her mother, and wondered wistfully about whatever fun she might have missed. Should she have taken that lusty friend for her first lover? Then the enormity of her mother's intrusion hit with full force as she visualized this reversal of the primal scene. Recall too, as Schneider (1977) has discussed, that shame guards privacy—missing here is not merely the mother's lack of understanding of Samantha's need for (right to) privacy, but the absence of this mother's own sense of shame at seeing what should have been so deeply personal. Later in therapy Samantha commented that she had never been able to make her husband understand why she had become so enraged when he gave his own mother a key to their first apartment.

And finally, you may be interested to know that Samantha's youngest daughter, now 20, has escaped her grandmother's attention long enough to achieve recognition in still another art form, and is regarded by teachers, peers and audience alike as a rising star. Samantha commented that Jessica never seemed to need any validation of her talent, never really mentioned to the family that she was doing anything unusual, and treats her success with diffidence.

I asked Samantha to go over an early draft of this chapter, partly to enquire whether I had disguised sufficiently the cast of characters. (It was she who choose the name Samantha.) She said that I still did not understand shame. "Don't you see?" she said. "For all that they did to me I would have preferred that everybody know exactly who they were."

## OTHER SYSTEMS

In some families, other families, the stench of shame pervades, permeates all interactions to such an extent that no amount of perfumed trappings, of purchased elegance will contain it. In one such wealthy couple, the wife, whose fragile self-esteem was dependent on her sturdy fantasy of the power inherent in her beauty, and in her ability to convey the affective broadcast of sexiness, was enraged at her passively impotent and later overtly homosexual husband for his sexual inattention to her. She began to cruise the streets of their fashionable neighborhood, initiating a series of degrading, masochistic affairs in which she was treated like a streetwalker. One of these liaisons culminated in a pregnancy, the baby from which she kept for the equally powerful reasons that she wanted a child in order to compete with her happily married sister, and that the existence of this child would serve as permanent shame for her husband. It is remarkable how frequently the three musketeers of jealousy, competitiveness, and shame-proneness travel in consort.

Upwardly mobile families, constantly striving and doing, are constricted by guilt more than by shame, concerned that their actions will be limited by competitors or by some authority. The overwhelming majority of therapists and patients come from this setting. The more we are willing to learn about shame affect, the more we may be able to understand those in the upper reaches of society, whose wealth was established by an ancestor of the striving sort, but preserved by families that now have position and fight to prevent its erosion, which they see as shameful. One of the ways those with established power preserve their hegemony is to declare themselves normative, and all others less than normal. This is analogous to the Chinese nation which has always called itself the "Middle Kingdom," one step below heaven, but well above all the rest of us. Anybody who is not Chinese is demeaned by being defined as a barbarian. The therapeutic community is far more comfortable dealing with the stereotypical guilt-provoking "Jewish mother" than with the supercillious WASP whose certainty of social dominance makes us uncomfortable.

This tendency to control by shaming goes throughout the fabric of such old, wealthy families, in which fear of downward migration reaches remarkable proportions. As mentioned above, the content of family arguments is rarely discussed because its shaming style is so deeply repressed and because exposure of secrets to anybody, even the therapist, is embarrassing. Once the subject of shame has been legitimized by the therapist a patient from this milieu will begin to report, for example, exactly what her mother screamed at her, and exactly what she wanted to say in return, thus allowing therapy to move forward with some authenticity. But if the therapist, without understanding these mechanisms, touches on something that may produce shame, a door clicks shut and "social" defenses are raised to exclude him or her. We have all been struck by the sudden feeling of our own unworthiness when working with these patients. In a controlled study by Lewis (1971) those cases in which shame issues were introduced early seemed to go faster and fare better. Nowhere is this more true than in the treatment of the upper-class patient.

I have begun to wonder whether the presence of such shaming systems, to a degree that overshadows the importance of guilt, has anything to do with the disproportionate frequency with which we see substance abuse, especially alcoholism, in these families. It is interesting how little guilt or shame such people experience relative to the havoc they bring into the lives of those they touch. This behavior is consistent with our observations that memory of shame affect is repressed and denied. As families with a basic belief in the preservation of dominance rather than in the search for realistic self-appraisal, they are frequently loathe to admit the possibility that they may err in the direction of narcissistic overvaluation. Embarrassment does not work to correct drinking behavior; indeed, behavior that would have been mortifying under any other circumstance is the subject of bragging by the alcoholic. Alcohol augments shifts along the shame/pride axis.

Alcohol seems to work as a shame killer. We were always told that the superego was soluble in alcohol. We just sort of took it for granted that this meant that alcohol took away guilt. It works for shame, too.

In Alcoholics Anonymous (and remember that anonymity protects against shame) no one begins to improve until "hitting bottom," a state of profound shame for the condition to which one has been reduced by alcohol. If you study the written material of AA you will learn a great deal about shame (Kurtz, 1981; Nathanson, 1985). When AA says that the member must acknowledge alcoholism as a disease, a condition that he cannot control, it requires the admission that s/he is less powerful than something, which is a healthy shame experience. Accepting the existence of a higher power, another basic tenet of AA, is also a healthy shame experience—as Schneider (1977) has shown, it is shame that protects our relationship with deity, and guards our faith. A person who will not accept shame cannot lead a balanced life. One who grows up being attacked and manipulated by shame cannot learn its healthy function.

Exclusivity, whether in club, school, or professional society, is often achieved by shaming tactics as when the threat of rejection from membership, or of removal from the fold for being different, is used as blackmail. Much of the cachet achieved by certain products, ranging from highly visible, cleverly advertised name brands of clothing to extremely expensive luxury goods, stems from a sort of defensive conformity operating as a mode of shame avoidance. When membership or employment is denied for artificially designated reasons of incompetency and inadequacy like race, religion, or gender, shaming tactics are in use. Hazing is shaming, as is teasing, staring, debagging, or forcing one to behave in an undignified manner. When people complain about the conduct of law enforcement officers, the behavior most commonly cited is that which produces shame. When a police officer feels secure in his or her relationship to the populace s/he wields power with grace; when his or her dominance is ridiculed, s/he, like all of us, tends to react with contempt.

This relationship between shame and power exists at all levels. President Carter attempted to lead us in a mode of respect for human rights, discussing the essential dignity of each person. Awareness of the indignities perpetrated in other countries, as well as in our own, made us uncomfortable because it produced shame affect as well as guilt. This caused too much shift of national focus along the shame/pride axis and contributed to his lack of popularity. The nation, not willing to continue under his leadership, elected a man who proposed to make us so mighty we would never have to fear shame, shifting us toward a more comfortable range of pride.

Shame can backfire, boomerang to destroy the one wielding it as a weapon. Recently the 64-year-old mother of one of my patients, a born-again Christian, received an obscene telephone call. It took her a few moments to understand that a stranger was talking to her about intimate sexual matters in a taunting, familiar tone, calculated to paralyze her with embarrassment. She rose from her chair, holding the telephone, and told the caller firmly "In the name of Christ Jesus I bind thee." Completely flustered, he hung up, the shamer shamed into silence.

## WHERE DO WE GO FROM HERE?

It is the nature of our craft that we learn from our errors. Many of us who work in the arena of shame affect have been drawn to its study by the sober analysis of our own failures. Throughout the history of psychoanalysis and psychotherapy we have met the enemy to find that it is ourselves who must change before we can help others. As I have stated elsewhere (Nathanson, 1984):

> Wherever I have opened the study of shame among my colleagues it has produced striking outpourings of highly charged affective material. (It is not unusual to hear contempt and scorn in professional meetings—we laugh at anyone who tries to make a colleague feel guilty, but we do not comment about attempts to create embarrassment.) Pandora's box has another compartment, and I believe we therapists cannot work in it until we have become much more comfortable with its contents; until we have a generation of therapists as comfortable dealing with issues of shame as they are with other affects, shame remains, for the most part, veiled. (pp. 598–599)

So shame is all around us, part of the air we breathe. But it is not inert, not the benign and innocent source of humor it sometimes appears to be. As therapists we can learn its layers, learn to ask the questions that draw our attention beneath the surface as we have learned to do for other affects. It can be a weapon of the most insidious sort and of variable intensity. If we ignore its effect on the lives of those who come to us for help, we misunderstand such things as their failure to improve, and fall into diagnostic complacency, labeling their silence as the absence of symptoms, or as petulant withdrawal, instead of seeing it as an integral part of the experience of embarrassment. We begin to understand that the diagnostic labels that make us comfortable are in themselves a source of shame to our patients, and that a patient's refusal to perform a behavioral task may be out of unrevealed embarrassment rather than obsessional stubbornness. Let us reexamine the layouts of our offices and waiting areas, of the traffic within and around them, to see if we ourselves produce this affect, however inadvertently. We must be ever-sensitive to our own involvement in the shaming systems of everyday life, their appearance in the couples and families of our practice of therapy, and to the hidden ways shame is institutionalized. To change the old adage, we might do well to remember that "Sticks and stones just break your bones. Its names that really harm you."

## REFERENCES

Alexander, F. (1938). Remarks about the relation of inferiority feelings to guilt feelings. *International Journal of Psychoanalysis, 19*:41–49.

Basch, M. F. (1976). The concept of affect: A re-examination. *Journal of the American Psychoanalytic Association, 24*:759–777.

Basch, M. F. (1983). Empathic understanding: Review of the concept and some theoretical considerations. *Journal of the American Psychoanalytic Association, 31*:101–126.

Freud, S. (1921). Group Psychology and the Psychology of the Ego. *Standard Edition, 18*:67–143. London: Hogarth Press.

Goodall, J. (1971). *In the shadow of man.* Boston: Houghton, Mifflin.

Kurtz, E. (1981). *Shame and guilt: Characteristics of the dependency cycle.* Center City, MN: Hazelden.

Lewis, H. B. (1971). *Shame and guilt in neurosis.* New York: International Universities Press.

Lewis, H. B. (1981). Shame and guilt in human nature. In S. Tuttman, C. Kaye, & M. Zimmerman (Eds), *Object and self: A developmental approach.* (pp. 235–265).

Nathanson, D. L. (1984). Book review: *The Mask of Shame,* by Léon Wurmser. *American Journal of Psychiatry, 141*:598–599.

Nathanson, D. L. (1985). *Inadequacy.* Center City, MN: Hazelden.

Nathanson, D. L. (1986). The empathic wall and the ecology of affect. *Psychoanalytic Study of the Child, 41*:171–187.

Nathanson, D. L. (1987). The shame/pride axis. In H. B. Lewis (Ed.), *The role of shame in symptom formation.* Hillsdale, NJ: Analytic Press. pp. 183–205.

Scheler, M. (1954). *The nature of sympathy* (P. Heath, Trans.). London: Routledge and Kegan Paul. (Original work published 1913)

Schneider, C. D. (1977). *Shame, exposure and privacy*. Boston: Beacon.
Steiner, G. (1972, October 28). Fields of force. *The New Yorker*.
Stoller, R. J. (1979). *Sexual excitement*. New York: Pantheon.
Sullivan, H. S. (1953). *The interpersonal theory of psychiatry*. New York: Norton.
Tomkins, S. S. (1962). *Affect/imagery/consciousness* (Vol. 1). *The positive affects*. New York: Springer.
Tomkins, S. S. (1963). *Affect/imagery/consciousness* (Vol. 2). *The negative affects*. New York: Springer.
Wurmser, L. (1981). *The mask of shame*. Baltimore: Johns Hopkins University Press.

# 9

# The Eye Turned Inward: Shame and the Self

ANDREW P. MORRISON

*So much of one's view depends on where one stands. Freud saw the person as primarily individual and secondarily social, while Sullivan saw intrapsychic development as the internalization of the interpersonal. To exaggerate the differences between their positions, one might say that the Freudian baby is preoccupied with internal concerns, protected from maternal influence by a stimulus barrier, and is hardly capable of seeing mother as a person until s/he is quite mature; the Sullivanian baby is interactive from birth, always affected by mother on an empathic level, and limited in the sophistication of his or her involvement only by maturational factors. Each pole of observation allows a realm of understanding, and each is limited by blind spots.*

*Some of the most important alterations in psychoanalytic theory have been made possible by the work of Kohut, who pointed out that the infant* is *actively involved with mother from birth, but that when the infant looks at the mother s/he does not see that mother as we would see her, but as a reflection of the infant, the self mirrored on the face of the mother. The mother is a "selfobject," rather than an object because it is this* empathic quality of responsiveness, *rather than her own*

Andrew P. Morrison. Assistant Clinical Professor of Psychiatry, Harvard Medical School, Massachusetts Mental Health Center.

*unique personal qualities, that define her for the infant—the term "selfobject" refers to a* function *rather than to a person.*

*Empathy takes on special meaning in Kohut's work, and provides a new way of understanding the development of the self, or what is called "narcissistic development." Hovering always in the background of self-psychology is the affect shame. Morrison, one of the most astute observers of shame from the Kohutian standpoint, states that "Just as* guilt *is the central negative affect in classical (conflict/drive) theory, I suggest that* shame *occupies that position in problems of narcissism, in the psychology of the self and its deficits."*

*In this chapter he takes up the case material presented in Chapter 8 on "Shaming Systems in Couples, Families, and Institutions" and demonstrates a novel and powerful way of conceptualizing the case of Samantha. Recognizing and accepting the wealth of data on the classical, intrapsychic meaning of shame, on the* layers of meaning *brought out during analytic therapy, I had elected to concentrate on the interpersonal aspects of shame, noting (as might have Sullivan) that shame is usually experienced in the context of an interpersonal interaction. Morrison asks for a subtle shift in our attention from the at-the-moment effect of a shaming interaction (and how that transaction might affect personality development) toward the dynamic equilibrium of that transaction with the prior development of Samantha's self.*

*The therapeutic implications of his analysis demand significant alterations in the classical stance, which sees empathic support as akin to sympathy and therefore antianalytic. Morrison is right to point out that the shame weapon works only to the degree that we have experienced failures in narcissistic development; the shaming attacks to which people are vulnerable in adult life sting fiercely when they land on a structure earlier deprived of proper empathic support. No one is completely immune to contempt or scorn; but, in the language of self psychology, shame wounds to the extent that one is the bearer of a defective self.*

Donald Nathanson has served the psychotherapeutic community well by bringing together this selection of current papers on so important a subject as shame. As he has noted, given the importance of shame as an affective experience for our patients, as well as for ourselves, the absence of an extensive shame literature and the scant attention given the existing work are perplexing phenomena. In previous works (Morrison, 1983,

1984a, b) I have considered some of the historical reasons for this anomaly in psychoanalytic theory and practice. The literature on shame and shame-related subjects represents a wide diversity of theoretical orientations, including the works of Alexander, 1938; Broucek, 1982; Grinker, 1955; Hazard, 1969; Kaufman, 1974; Levin, 1967, 1971; Lewis, 1971; Lynd, 1958; Piers & Singer, 1953; Thrane, 1979; and Wurmser, 1981. Nonetheless, this volume represents the first collection of reports devoted exclusively to the study of shame, and thus addresses a deficiency in psychoanalytic literature.

In one of his contributions, Nathanson (Chapter 8) has outlined nicely many issues generated by a focus on shame. He brings to our attention the relationship between shame and embarrassment, humiliation, rage, aggression, and mortification, emphasizing the connection between shame and the *shamer*. For him, as for Levin, the threat from experienced shame is isolation, separation, and abandonment. Although he suggests that shame generates punishment "for some quality of the self," Nathanson focuses on the shame that is essentially "social," a product of interpersonal interaction necessitating the presence of a "significant other" (the shamer).

In this chapter I will suggest a complementary view of shame, one that does *not* require the presence of an external person, but that emphasizes rather the eye of the self gazing inward. Certainly, shame may occur in a social context (best characterized as humiliation or embarrassment) but it need not necessarily be so embedded. The contributions of ego psychology, with subsequent attention to the ego ideal, the self and its "ideal" configurations, and, ultimately, renewed interest in narcissism, have spurred investigation of the experience of shame (Morrison, 1983). It seems to me that the contributions of Kohut and of self psychology itself provide a framework for the optimal understanding of shame and its relationship to narcissism and the self, without necessarily invoking the presence of an external shamer. I shall review and question the relevent aspects of Kohut's writings as they relate to shame, and then will reconsider some points in Nathanson's chapter from the self psychological perspective. In particular, using this framework, I will attempt to offer a somewhat different view of the clinical material on Samantha.

## SHAME AND THE WRITINGS OF KOHUT

The self, and its supraordinate position in problems of narcissism, was the principal tenet in the evolution of Kohut's work. He felt that object relations and affiliation with other persons had been overestimated in psychoanalytic theory, to the detriment of attention to the self and its states of cohesion—particularly the various transformations of narcissism. For him, object ties should not be considered a "given" of the human condition, but must be regarded as part of the matrix of the self's many needs. Thus, Kohut emphasized the "self" side of the equation of the self's interaction with its objects. Just as *guilt* is the central negative affect in classical (conflict/drive) theory, I suggest that *shame* occupies that position in problems of narcissism, in the psychology of the self and its deficits (Morrison, 1983, 1984a). Patients with fundamental narcissistic problems experience shame as the core feeling about their self and its failings. Levin (1971) differentiated internal from external shame, defining internal (primary) shame as intrapsychic, an affect reflecting punishment imposed by the superego for the fundamental self-defect seen in the self's failure to live up to an internalized ideal. In contrast, the shame experienced in neurotic conditions is external and secondary, representing failure to achieve an external, reality-derived goal. This usually results from a defensive, passive retreat from intrapsychic (e.g., oedipal) conflict. Thus, it is primary, internal (self) shaming that characterizes the experience of the narcissistic patient.

What place does shame play in Kohut's writings? For him, shame is exclusively a reflection of the self overwhelmed by its infantile and split-off grandiosity (the "vertical split"; see Kohut, 1971). He explicitly rejected the view of shame representing the ego's failure to fulfill the expectations and demands of the superego/ego ideal (1971, p. 181). This (limited) view of shame is based, I suggest, on Kohut's conception of the bipolar self, in which a "tension arc" exists between the grandiose self and the idealized parental imago, between archaic ambitions on the one hand, and ideals on the other (Kohut, 1977). Implicit in this construct of a bipolar self is the notion that a person has two chances to attain self-cohesion. If the first chance fails, through inadequate mirroring of infantile, exhibitionistic grandiosity (usually by the mother), a second chance is provided through empathic acceptance of the child's idealization of, and wish to merge with an omnipotent, tension-regulating object (frequently the father). Take, for instance, the case of an energetic, gregarious infant who shrieks with glee at her newfound capacity to reach for a bottle on the table. Her depressed mother responds to this commotion as if it were a personal assault, rather than as her child's skillful triumph, and turns away in distress. In the language of self psychology, repetition of this sequence reflects inadequate mirroring, and may launch developmental difficulty in cohesive self-formation. However, a year later the child, now a toddler, turns to her father with admiration, imitating his gait as they walk together. In contrast to the mother's earlier empathic failure, the father accepts his daughter's attachment to him, encourages her to walk faster, and embraces her tenderly when she cries in frustration after falling. The father's presence as an accepting, comforting figure represents the "second chance" at self-cohesion through idealization and soothing.

Kohut rejects the proposition that the bipolar self implies an inherent developmental process (i.e., from the need for mirroring to a need to idealize) but asserts, rather, that mirroring and idealization represent parallel forms of narcissistic development. He views the tendency to consider the grandiose self as more primitive than the idealized parental imago as a reflection, again, of a cultural prejudice that assigns object love supremacy over narcissism. It must be remembered that in his early work Kohut viewed narcissism as having a line of development parallel to that of object love, and later included narcissistic development as part of the normal evolution of the cohesive self. A viewpoint relating shame to failure in attaining the expectations of the ego ideal would, therefore, come perilously close to assigning the idealized parental imago (with the self's quest for objects) a developmentally higher role than that of the grandiose self.

Nevertheless, in view of our observations about shame, and our recognition of certain inconsistencies in Kohut's formulations, I believe we must do just that. Clinical experience demands that our definition of shame involve more than the self overwhelmed by archaic grandiosity—it must also account for disappointment, failure, and deficit. Thus, Kohut's framework must accommodate failures of the self to live up to its ideals. I hope to demonstrate that the notion of an *ideal self*, and a developmental view of the idealized parental imago reflecting the self's movements toward its objects, allow us to incorporate a self-psychological perspective into our understanding of shame.

At this point in our consideration of shame in the work of Kohut, I shall turn to his construct of the *selfobject*, and how it assists in an attempt to place shame into a self psychological framework. While the selfobject does exist as a real person to whom the self is attached and from whom it is not clearly differentiated, it is not the selfobject's external, configurational qualities which are of primary importance to the evolving self (in contrast with the object-embedded oedipal transferences of more highly differentiated patients) but rather the *function* served by the selfobject. Thus, to the grandiose, exhibitionistic infant, availability of the age-appropriate mirroring function provided by the parental selfobject establishes the development of early self-cohesion. For instance, recalling our earlier vignette of the gleeful infant reaching energetically for the bottle, had the mother responded with enthusiasm to her child's effort, had she clapped her hands or smiled approvingly, she would then have provided an instance of what Kohut called the age-appropriate, mirroring selfobject function necessary to self-cohesion. It is the presence of the selfobject's responsiveness, rather than her configurational qualities, which delineate the selfobject function. The mother's actual distress and her lack of responsiveness to the infant's need for affirmation (in this vignette) reflected empathic failure, and inability to provide the appropriate mirroring selfobject function.

Similar to the toddler's need for merger with the selfobject's omnipotence and perfection is the facilitation of further "firming" of the self by parental openness to idealization. The vignette shows the father's acceptance of his daughter's need to admire his physical prowess, and his sensitivity and reassurance when she failed to emulate his gait—this represents the self-affirming presence of the idealized selfobject's function. I think this example illustrates as well the developmental movement toward the representational world of objects delineated by the idealized selfobject. While the selfobject function still predominates in this example, we can see that the differentiated, configurational qualities of the father were beginning to play a significant role in the child's cognitive development. Thus, although it is premature to view the facilitating function of the mirroring selfobject in an object-relations perspective, such an approach begins to gain importance in terms of the idealized selfobject. From this perspective, the "idealized selfobject's omnipotence and perfection" reflect early movement toward internalization of, and identification with, the (external) object. However, in Kohut's writings it is not the differentiated, object-representational qualities of the selfobject that lead to self-cohesion, but rather the self-affirming functions (of mirroring and idealization) which are important (i.e., the "self" side of the selfobject equation).

We might assume that each side of the bipolar self—the grandiose self, with its exhibitionistic need for affirmation by the mirroring selfobject, and the idealized parental imago, with its availability for infantile merger with the idealized qualities of the omnipotent selfobject—would allow for the experience of shame when the appropriate selfobject function is not available to the developing self. Why, then, did Kohut maintain that only the breakthrough of unmirrored grandiosity would account for shame? I suggest that this position reflected Kohut's commitment to the centrality of the self over its objects. Similarly, as I have suggested earlier, this same commitment forced him to deny a developmental progression from grandiosity to idealization, despite the fact that he implied such a progression at several points in his writings (e.g., Kohut, 1971, pp. 133, 140). The implications of these inconsistencies suggest, I believe, that there *is* a developmental sequence from grandiosity to idealization in Kohut's writings which reflects movement from primary narcissism toward the self's progressive affiliation with its objects. I have indicated elsewhere (Morrison, 1984a) that *idealization* represents initial movement outward from the self toward appreciation of objects, and that this movement reflects, in part, *projective identification* of the *ideal self* "into" the idealized selfobject.

If this is so, failure of the selfobject to respond to the self's idealizations leads inexorably to the experience of shame, and provides an anchor for our understanding of shame within a

Kohutian framework. Thus, shame occurs, not only in response to overwhelming grandiosity, but also when the self fails to attain its ideals through unresponsiveness of the idealized parental imago to projective identification of the ego ideal, or, in the language of this chapter, of the ideal self. Had the toddler's father (in the earlier vignette) ignored rather than hugged her after she tripped and fell, she would have experienced shame and humiliation. This formulation, then, brings us closer to a self-psychological appreciation of shame which takes into account unresponsiveness over a full range of selfobject functions.

We are still faced with the question of whether shame can occur in the absence of a social context (without the presence of a shamer). I suggest that Kohut is essentially right to maintain this possibility, for the absence of age-appropriate selfobject responsiveness to the self's needs for mirroring or idealization leads to an inherent vulnerability to shame. As I have noted above, this is the core affective vulnerability of the narcissistic personality. We have seen that the idealized selfobject represents the movement of a developing self toward affiliation with objects. Nevertheless, it is the intrapsychic effect of the available selfobject "function" that remains central as the influence on self-cohesion, rather than the object's interpersonal, configurational qualities. Thus, shame may be experienced by the vulnerable self in isolation—a reflection of disavowed, overwhelming grandiosity, or of failure or deficit with regard to the ideal self. Vulnerability to shame from these self-phenomena is particularly relevent to our understanding of narcissistic personalities.

In his description of self-pathology, Kohut differentiates two elements of disintegration of the self, those of *fragmentation* and *depletion*. Self-fragmentation relates to states in which the nuclear self has attained no core cohesion, as in certain psychotic and primitive borderline conditions. On the other hand, self-depletion reflects the failures of a self in the process of attaining tenuous cohesion, seeking to make up for enfeeblement through merger with the power of an idealized selfobject. Unresponsiveness of the idealized parental imago to the self's idealizing attempts leads to self-enfeeblement and depletion anxiety with resultant feelings of failure and emptiness in terms of ideals, and to shame sensitivity.

In *The Restoration of the Self* (1977), Kohut refers to shame directly only once, when he speaks of a time

> of utter hopelessness for some, of utter lethargy, of that depression without guilt and self-directed aggression, which overtakes those who feel that they have failed and cannot remedy the failure in the time and with the energies still at their disposal. The suicides of this period are not the expression of a punitive superego, but a remedial act—the wish to wipe out the *unbearable sense of mortification and nameless shame* imposed by the ultimate *recognition of a failure* of all-encompassing magnitude. (p. 241; my emphasis)

This statement by Kohut is an eloquent description of the guiltless despair and shame experienced by those who have not been able to realize their nuclear ambitions and ideals. However, I believe that the language of shame permeates the rest of that book as well when Kohut speaks of "mortification" (p. 137, 224), "disturbed self-acceptance" (p. 94), and "dejection" (p. 97, 224). These affective references appear in observations about the self's "defeat" in realizing its goals. However, these feelings reflect the experience of shame at the self's evaluation of its own performance, at not having achieved its own ambitions and ideals. I would suggest that a certain degree of self-cohesion must have been attained for one to register shame—this is *not* an affect experienced during the process of acute fragmentation. Again, the relationship between shame and self-depletion is underscored, as well as the relationship of shame to the "guiltless despair" which accompanies both overwhelming grandiosity and the failure to attain one's ideals.

Clearly, it is the qualities of acceptance and responsiveness of the selfobject during individual development that are related to grandiosity and the sense of failure, and thus reflect the danger in rejection and abandonment by the "significant object." However, it may not be the current interpersonal unresponsiveness of an external object that determines shame, but rather the repeated developmental experiences of empathic failure during development. A selfobject unresponsive to the self's needs for mirroring or idealized merger fosters instead the development of narcissistic shame-vulnerability. Thus, shame within the framework of Kohut's writings is neither social nor interpersonal, but a manifestation of deficits of the self.

Does this mean that shame can be experienced only in conditions of narcissistic vulnerability? Our clinical experience indicates that this is not necessarily the case. As suggested elsewhere (Levin, 1971; Morrison, 1983) for neurotic individuals, those with a firmly cohesive nuclear self, shame can also be external and secondary. Shame then can reflect microfailures in meeting the aspirations and goals of the cohesive ideal self, and thus it is only the *intensity* and *magnitude* of such failures that are at issue. I have suggested earlier that the neurotic experience of shame most frequently reflects a withdrawal from oedipal and interpersonal conflict into passivity, forming one part of the guilt-shame cycle of Piers (Piers & Singer, 1953). Thus, shame may represent the temporary, reactive retreat from competition of an otherwise healthy individual, that fortunate possessor of a firmly cohesive self, troubled "only" by intrapsychic conflict.

As the final element in this attempt to "reframe" our understanding of shame in terms of Kohut's contributions, I want to address the relationship of shame to depression and to rage. We have noted that shame may be experienced as "guiltless despair" from failure to realize ambitions and ideals, reflecting depletion of the nuclear self. Such self-depletion and shame may underly clinical *depression*, and closely approximates Bibring's statement: "depression sets in whenever the fear of being inferior or defective seems to come true, whenever and in whatever way the person comes to feel that all effort was in vain, that he is definitely doomed to be a 'failure' " (Bibring, 1953, p. 25). Again, "In depression, the ego is shocked into passivity not because there is a conflict regarding the goals, but because of its incapacity to live up to the narcissistic aspirations" (p. 30). Thus, Kohut and Bibring implicitly agree that shame and depression may be closely related, especially for those patients with narcissistic pathology for whom depression most frequently reflects failures in attaining the ambitions and ideals of the nuclear self. Too often, in the psychotherapy of such patients, only the depression itself is addressed, and not the shame which may underly it.

Similarly, I suggest that shame and *rage* bear a complementary relationship to one another. We have seen that Kohut viewed shame as a response of the self overwhelmed by unmirrored grandiosity; he considered rage to be the self's response to a lack of absolute control over an archaic environment (Kohut, 1972). Thus, outpourings of narcissistic rage reflect the experience of empathic failure by selfobjects or by the environment in meeting the self's needs for responsiveness or acceptance. I would suggest that shame and the related emotion of humiliation serve as stimuli to rage, a relationship which has been described in "shame cultures" (e.g., Singer, in Piers and Singer, 1953), and in the psychology of antisocial personalities (e.g., Gilligan, 1976). As with depression, the shame that underlies rage is frequently overlooked in psychotherapy, reflecting the tendency of shame to be hidden—in treatment, as in life.

I shall consider the psychotherapy of shame in greater detail in the next section, which will deal with issues raised in Nathanson's paper. However, at this point I want to emphasize several major therapeutic implications of the particular Kohutian perspective that I have been addressing. One major feeling that accompanies the core shame experience of narcissism is the conviction of *unacceptability*—to self, selfobject, or "significant other"—as a reflection of emptiness and of failure to achieve self-appointed, grandiose life tasks. This lack of acceptance (by self and other) relates to the deeply felt shame of the narcissistic patient, and should be a major focus in their treatment. Such feelings of unacceptability and shame are often difficult to detect because of the defenses which cover the grandiosity, defects, failures, and emptiness that generate them, but protracted "empathic immersion" in the treatment of these patients must inevitably lead to their unveiling. The discovery, examination, and working through of these painful feelings, and the ultimate realization that therapist and patient alike can accept them, constitute a major curative element in successful treatment. In achieving this goal, the therapist must be willing to face and acknowledge his or her own shame—his or her own failure to realize ambitions and ideals, his or her own grandiosity and defects. The therapist's avoidance of these feelings constitutes a major impediment to the treatment of shame, and explains in part the low profile of shame in the history of psychoanalytic writings.

## SHAMING SYSTEMS, AND THE CASE OF SAMANTHA

As I have indicated earlier, Nathanson's shame is essentially social, interpersonal. "Wherever there is shame, there is a shamer . . . we have in that moment relived the exposure of some hidden 'fact' before another person." Nathanson has emphasized the interactional, relational elements of shame, as exemplified by embarrassment and humiliation. Assisted by the system of self psychology elaborated by Kohut, I have tried to show that this is not necessarily the case—that shame may result solely from comparison of the self to the deficits and failures of one's "ideal self." I would emphasize that these perspectives are not contradictory, but are *complementary* in the broadest sense at that term. However, I think that our "self" perspective on shame invites a reexamination of some of Nathanson's observations and clinical material from a different point of view.

For example, in Chapter 8, Nathanson cites the exaggerations of a "fish story" to exemplify an attempt to deny embarrassment about a poor day's fishing, to hide lack of skill, to forestall ridicule by the listener. However, I suggest that the healthy person (s/he of a "firm nuclear self") would probably feel no need to concoct a fish story on returning with an empty catch, or work hard primarily to fulfill his or her own personal goals and ideals. Rather, it is the person riddled with narcissistic vulnerability who may feel the need to create a grandiose tale about the fishing expedition, in large part from a need to fill in the gaps in self-esteem resulting from the lack of adequate selfobject responsiveness during development. Such people, struggling against the emptiness and deficits, the shame and lack of self-acceptance that accompany their self-depletion, may work and study hard in an attempt to *compensate* for the resultant failures in their ideal self, in order to make themselves worthy of response from the mirroring or idealized selfobject. No external shamer need be present ridiculing our subject in order to account for his or her shame.

In the example of 12-year-old Johnny's sandlot homerun, Nathanson invokes embarrassment and ridicule from Johnny's social network to explain his shame at overvaluing his accomplishment. However, our understanding of self-vulnerability suggests another possibility. Supposing Johnny had grown up in a family in which his early, age-appropriate grandiosity and exhibitionism had been inadequately mirrored by an unresponsive, aloof maternal selfobject. He thus would not have been given the experience of transforming his grandiosity into appropriate and realizable ambitions. Instead, his grandiosity would have been disavowed and split off from awareness (Kohut's "vertical split") only to reappear in unmodulated form at the moment of this homerun. His resultant shame might then have occurred, not in a social context, but alone in his room as he contemplated his moment of triumph, and felt overwhelmed by the unrealistic outpouring of grandiosity which exceeded the merits of his accomplishment.

Nathanson usefully brings a "systems" perspective to bear on his view of the generation of shame in the family. However, I suggest again that his contribution is excessively "interpersonal" in its presentation of that perspective. For example, he notes that a family eager for the success of a child may treat that child as a narcissistic extension of itself. I agree with this suggestion, but I feel that it does not go far enough in elaborating the generation of narcissistic character structure in the offspring of such a family. For instance, Nathanson suggests that the resultant drop in self-esteem within the family system in response to a talented child may indeed lead to a "bitter shaming technique" used to devalue the child's actual accomplishments. However, alternative explanations are possible to account for the child's resultant narcissistic vulnerability.

Nathanson suggests that "an anxious parent makes an anxious family, as does an angry parent an angry family," emphasizing the role of affect transmission within family systems. While I agree with this observation, I would add with Kohut that a narcissistic, ashamed parent usually produces a narcissistically vulnerable child, but not exclusively through active shaming. As such a parent tends to view the child as a narcissistic extension of himself or herself, that parent will be insensitive, inattentive to the developmentally appropriate needs for affirmation of the child's exhibitionistic and merger needs. Such insensitivity to the needs of a developing self is experienced, to use Kohut's term, as "empathic failure," leading to the conviction that these needs are unacceptable, and, therefore, shameful. These narcissistic needs cannot then become modified or transformed into their more adaptive mature forms, but are, rather, walled off and disavowed, to return as self-disintegration and searing shame under conditions of provocation by internal or external triggers. The concept of empathic failure indicates that active shaming within the family system need not be invoked as the only explanation of such narcissistic vulnerability in the child, but that parental narcissistic needs themselves may prevent atunement to the selfobject functions that would have provided self-cohesion in the child. In this way, failure of the intrafamilial selfobject function to meet the needs of the developing child may account for later shame sensitivity, an explanation additional to the process of active, interpersonal shaming within the family.

Nathanson begins his chapter with an account of expressions of rage in another of his patients, described by her as a "mantle of hate." Elsewhere, he discusses rage in the context of a marital quarrel, suggesting that violence may result from the feeling that "our self-esteem has been reduced beyond our ability to tolerate this new view of ourselves," as from shaming phrases hurled in anger by the partner. I agree that rage most frequently occurs in an interpersonal context, as a result of embarrassment or humiliation. However, as I suggested in the previous section of this chapter, such active shaming must interact with the narcissistic vulnerability of a fragile and weakly established self. In other words, empathic failures of the infantile selfobjects have led to feelings of shame and unacceptability. These feelings have been walled off, only to reappear when triggered by an insult or insensitivity from the current interactive environment. The resultant embarrassment or humiliation is disavowed, and becomes transformed, rather, into intense expressions of rage and hate, aimed at recreating the shame experience in the person of the perpetrator.* Thus,

*I have detailed (Morrison, 1984a; 1986) my view that this "transformation" of shame into rage and hate reflects *projective identification* of the disavowed affect "into" the other person, just as the self begins to develop affiliation with the world of objects through projective identification of the ideal self into the idealized parental imago. I shall not divert the focus from this chapter through amplification of this (admittedly controversial) suggestion, except to point out that, with Ogden (1979), I share a view of projective identification shame and humiliation can be seen to underly most outbursts of narcissistic rage, as indicated in Nathanson's chapter.

I shall now turn to the complementary view of Samantha to exemplify the relationship of shame to the self. She was born into a family in which her mother ridiculed and demeaned her talent, and in which both parents were bitterly competitive. Her therapist (Dr. Nathanson) emphasizes that these parents actively shamed Samantha, which may indeed have been the case. However, in one incident described, it seems that the mother was insensitive to Samantha's need for mirroring affirmation, more than actually humiliating her. While engaged in sexual intimacy with Samantha, her boyfriend observed her mother's face "watching calmly." This example of inappropriate intrusiveness represents empathic failure of the grossest order as well as her mother's own shameless voyeurism, and no doubt reflects the absence of empathic attunement that must have occurred on numerous occasions during Samantha's early development. This mother seems to have taken no pleasure in her daughter's talents or strivings for autonomy, in addition to feeling them as threats to her own achievements. Thus, we can conjecture that her failures to affirm Samantha's attempts at self-expression and assertiveness represented repeated failures to provide the necessary mirroring selfobject functions required to enhance the self's development (the "glow of pride" in a child's accomplishments). In addition, this mother seems to have opposed such development through active shaming and humiliation. Apparently, Samantha's father failed too in offering the "second chance"—the opportunity for merger with calming power through idealization.

In emphasizing the family's "shaming propensity," Nathanson underscored the patient's quandry in knowing how to respond to such searing humiliation. In the language of childhood, to attack or return the shame may kill or drive away, thus increasing isolation of the self; alternatively, it may provoke further vicious retaliation. Thus, Samantha learned to suffer humiliation in silence, at least until her self-esteem was so affected that she retaliated with her "laser look" of rage. I have

---

as an *interactive process*, rather than solely as a formal (and confusing) mechanism of defense.

little to add to this description of Samantha's family dynamics, except to suggest that she must have experienced attacks on her assertiveness and talents as indications that her own needs and desires were unacceptable, and cause for shame. Thus, for her, defeat was not only humiliating, but also a source of self-depletion, the emptiness of a self devoid of hope, energy, and ideals. Her withdrawal from the real objects in her life represents not only a compromise in response to shame, but also a manifestation of the "guiltless despair" and depression which expresses emptiness and self-depletion, as well as shame.

So, Samantha's shame reflects withdrawal from objects with resultant isolation and feelings of abandonment, but also decreased self-esteem and self-depletion. I have discussed rage in regard to Samantha's stored-up shame, and would here like to add a comment on the related feeling of *contempt.* Nathanson mentions an ancient proverb which indicates that contempt is less bearable than anger or hate. In my view, contempt is closely related to shame and humiliation, but represents a good example of the process involved in the projective identification of shame. Contempt represents one way of handling the buildup of shame beyond a level tolerable to the maintenance of self-esteem. It is, I suggest, the process by which shame may be disavowed as a self-affect, projected into a willing external object (the scapegoat), who then *contains* the subject's shame while allowing him to maintain contact with it. How the object *processes* the contempt will determine, to a large extent, whether the subject is able to *reinternalize*, and acknowledge, his or her own shame. This is the language of our current conceptualizations of projective identification as process (Ogden, 1979; Morrison, 1986), but I think that it is also helpful in amplifying our understanding of one major manifestation of shame.

In Samantha's case, I suspect that the "laser look" and "vicious jabs of a verbal dissecting knife wielded with savage intensity and astonishing accuracy" reflected not only rage, but also the related feeling of contempt. In this way she transformed the buildup of shame (from experienced familial criticisms and "empathic failures" which triggered memories of her parents' insensitivities) into contempt, thus temporarily ridding herself of the painful self-doubts, emptiness, and failures which reflected her profound narcissistic vulnerability.

## DISCUSSION

In this chapter I have considered Nathanson's contributions and discussion of shame, and his clinical examples, from a somewhat different perspective. For Nathanson, shame, with his emphasis on embarrassment and humiliation, is embedded in a social matrix. Where there is shame, there seems always to be a "shamer." Shame, to him, is always the product of active shaming by another in the person's interpersonal environment. In contrast, I have offered a complementary view, in which the shame experience is, at times, a manifestation of the self's vulnerability, a response to internal feelings of failure, deficit, and weakness which reflect narcissistic character structure. I have suggested that Kohut's self psychology provides a useful framework from which to understand this perspective, with its emphasis on the narcissistic weaknesses of self development; the central place of shame in self-defects; and the role played by selfobjects in determining the strength and cohesion of the self. The lack of selfobject responsiveness during development determines to a great extent the vulnerability of the self to its unrealized needs (for mirroring affirmation and idealizing merger), and hence to its propensity for low self-esteem, lack of self-acceptance, and shame.

I agree with Nathanson that embarrassment and humiliation reflect the social edge of shame. I have suggested (Morrison, 1984b) that "humiliation represents the strong experience of shame reflecting severe external shaming or shame anxiety at the hands of a highly cathected object (a 'significant other')." Embarrassment represents the same phenomenon at a lower level of intensity. To this list of shame-related phenomena Nathanson (quoting Wurmser, 1981) has added ridicule, put-down, contempt, and mortification; I would add to his list disgrace, remorse, and apathy. One of these—mortification—is particularly powerful; its root indicates that shame "kills." I believe that this speaks eloquently to the importance of shame as a potentially overwhelming negative affect, the source, as suggested by Kohut in the passage cited above, of some suicides of later adulthood that reflects the "guiltless despair" of unrealized ambitions and goals.

I have used this discussion of shame to express what I

believe to be contradictions in Kohut's view of shame and the self, and in his theory of the bipolar self. As noted, he ascribes shame solely to the self's experience of overwhelming grandiosity, negating the role of failure with regard to goals and ideals. I have suggested that clinical evidence does not support this view, but that Kohut's position reflects his emphasis on the "self" side of the selfobject equation. Moreover, I have disagreed with his view of the bipolar self, in which its two poles (of ambitions and ideals) are seen as coequal anchors of the self's cohesion. Rather, I have suggested a developmental view of the self, in which it grows from the primary narcissism of archaic grandiosity to an early, object-seeking stage of idealization and a wish for merger with the perfection of the omnipotent selfobject.

It may seem to some that my argument is excessively detailed with respect to fine points of Kohutian theory, but it is Kohut's view of the selfobject that brings us to the heart of my understanding of shame, and to the distinction between my view and that of Nathanson. The selfobject construct may be seen as the "nutriment" that enables the development of a firm, cohesive self. Developmental failures in the availability of selfobject attunement—excessive empathic failures by the environment to meet the self's expressed, age-appropriate needs—lead to narcissistic vulnerability, and to accompanying shame sensitivity. Such self-deficit frequently accounts for the experience of searing shame that serves as the focus for this volume.

One controversy surrounding Kohut's writings is the importance of the role ascribed to reality (in this sense, the interpersonal environment) in human development. If narcissistic pathology is a reflection of selfobject failures in the person of mother and father, then what is the role of unconscious conflict in generating human misery? I will bypass this particular conundrum about the relevence of Kohutian theory to mainstream psychoanalytic thought except to acknowledge that Kohut *does* attribute more significance to actual parental behavior than that implied in conflict theory. But herein lies the paradox that brings us back to our consideration of shame. While the parental presence is crucial in the development of the self, that presence is significant principally in terms of providing the selfobject functions of empathic mirroring and idealized merger needed for self-development. In classical theory, parental presence may be less significant in determining the drive-related nature of unconscious/conflict, but the objects themselves have importance in libidinal/configurational terms, rather than as the representatives of functions.

So, again we come to the matter of the interpersonal, social nature of shame, and the paradox noted in the previous paragraph. Kohut finds the parents' role to be central in the formation of the self, through provision of the selfobject functions considered essential as nutriments for self-development. Once the self is formed, in its variable state of cohesion or deficit, it is this self-quality that will determine individual shame sensitivity.* On the other hand, from the classical perspective in which Nathanson is working, the individual's experience of shame reflects interpersonal manifestations of embarrassment and humiliation at the hand of a "significant other." Presumably, embarrassment can recall feelings about oedipal competition and failure with and desire for significant transference objects.

How, then, does shame relate to the significant objects in the life of the self? Nathanson (with Levin, 1971, and Wurmser, 1981) states that "shame has to do with separation anxiety," and thus creates the danger of "utter isolation . . . and fears of abandonment." In this context, shame primarily reflects relationships to objects. Thus, the withdrawal that accompanies shame would represent hiding, to protect the self from the potential object loss resulting from embarrassment and humiliation. Our "self" perspective on shame provides a complementary view, in which shame reflects decreased self-esteem—a manifestation of the self's sense of failure with respect to goals and ideals, its deficits with respect to the early insufficient functions of its selfobjects. Samantha's withdrawal is not only from her family, but also from self-awareness of the depth of her despair and lack of self-acceptance. She cannot tolerate facing her deep shame and diminished self-esteem, and therefore experiences intolerable emptiness. As indicated earlier, defeat causes not only humiliation, but also self-depletion.

*It should be noted that current work in self psychology is addressing the ongoing role of selfobject function on self-development throughout the life cycle.

Nathanson has made interesting suggestions relating shame to alcoholism, and to upper-class family systems. He also alludes to the therapist's potential participation in the shaming systems that influence our patients. I would add only that these forces operate as much through insensitivity to our patients' need for self-affirmation and to their deficits of self-acceptance, as to active shaming and provocation of embarrassment. With Nathanson, I suggest that the therapist attend to his or her participation in "the shaming systems of everyday life," but by being aware of his or her insensitivity to, and unawareness of shame as well as through active shaming. Each therapist must make a practice of facing and learning about his or her *own* shame experiences, his or her own lack of self-acceptance. Such awareness will inevitably foster attention to, and useful therapeutic work with the patient's shame, which constitutes one major treatment goal of every therapeutic encounter.

## REFERENCES

Alexander, F. (1938). Remarks about the relation of inferiority feelings to guilt feelings. *International Journal of Psychoanalysis, 19*:41–49.

Bibring, E. (1953). The mechanism of depression. In P. Greenacre (Ed.), *Affective disorders.* New York: International Universities Press.

Broucek, F. J. (1982). Shame and its relationship to early narcissistic developments. *International Journal of Psychoanalysis, 63*:369–378.

Gilligan, J. (1976). Beyond morality: Psychoanalytic reflections on shame, guilt, and love. In T. Lickona (Ed.), *Moral development and behavior* (pp 144–158). New York: Holt, Reinhart & Winston.

Grinker, R. (1955). Growth inertia and shame: Their therapeutic implications and dangers. *International Journal of Psychoanalysis, 36*:242–253.

Hazard, P. (1969). Freud's teaching on shame. *Laval Theologique et Philosophique, 25*:234–267.

Kaufman, G. (1974). The meaning of shame. Towards a self-affirming identity. *Journal of Counseling Psychology, 21*:568–574.

Kohut, H. (1971). *The analysis of the self.* New York: International Universities Press.

Kohut, H. (1972). Thoughts on narcissism and narcissistic rage. *Psychoanalytic Study of the Child, 27*:360–399.

Kohut, H. (1977). *The restoration of the self.* New York: International Universities Press.

Levin, S. (1967). Some metapsychological considerations on the differentiation between shame and guilt. *International Journal of Psychoanalysis, 48*:267–276.

Levin, S. (1971). The psychoanalysis of shame. *International Journal of Psychoanalysis, 52*:355–362.

Lewis, H. B. (1971). *Shame and guilt in neurosis.* New York: International Universities Press.

Lynd, H. M. (1958). *On shame and the search for identity.* New York: Harcourt, Brace and World.

Morrison, A. P. (1983). Shame, the ideal self, and narcissism. *Contemporary Psychoanalysis, 19*:295–318.

Morrison, A. P. (1984a). Shame and the psychology of the self. In P. E. Stepansky & A. Goldberg (Eds.) *Kohut's legacy: Contributions to self psychology* (70–91), Hillsdale, NJ: Analytic Press.

Morrison, A. P. (1984b). Working with shame in psychoanalytic treatment. *Journal of the American Psychoanalytic Association, 32*:479–505.

Morrison, A. P. (1986). On projective identification in couples' groups. *International Journal of Group Psychotherapy, 36*:55–73.

Ogden, T. H. (1979). On projective identification. *International Journal of Psychoanalysis, 60*:357–373.

Piers, G., & Singer, M. (1953). *Shame and guilt.* New York: Norton.

Thrane, G. (1979). Shame and the construction of the self. *Annual of Psychoanalysis, 7*:321–341.

Wurmser, L. (1981). *The mask of shame.* Baltimore: Johns Hopkins University Press.

10

# Pornography: Daydreams to Cure Humiliation

ROBERT J. STOLLER

*It would be difficult to describe succinctly the influence of Robert Stoller on contemporary psychoanalysis. It is through his meticulous psychoanalytic investigation of adult sexual fantasy that we began to learn about the early beginnings of gender identity and genitality. In* Sexual Excitement *(1979) he demonstrated that the script that functioned as a masturbation fantasy for a patient (code-named Belle) contained elements of early trauma, trauma that continued to affect her, but the pain of which could be decreased temporarily during the episode of excitement. Treatment involved the unraveling of a sadomasochistic character structure deeply intertwined with humiliation themes. The book reads like the best sort of detective novel (for Stoller is one of the best writers in all of psychiatry) and ranges from his recognition of the importance of gender identity in the formation of the self, to his suggestion that the content of all sexual excitement involves the reworking of early trauma.*

*I wondered whether "early trauma" might be a synonym for shame, and asked him to consider specifically the role of shame in sexual fantasy. In the exchange that followed I learned that he did indeed consider shame to be the proper term for the emotional meaning of this early trauma, and wrote that "at the center of my ideas on the dynamics of sexual excitement is humiliation, the effect of an attack acknowledged and accepted on one's self."*

Robert J. Stoller. Professor of Psychiatry, UCLA School of Medicine.

*Wurmser (1981) suggests that all shame words (embarrassment, humiliation, mortification, and so on) are best treated as cognates, simply because the shame experience is so personal that each of us has private definitions for these words. Agreeing with Morrison (1984) that humiliation implies shame in the presence of a highly cathected object, I offer the idea of a "humiliation index": If you assign, on a scale of 1 to 10, the intrinsic embarrassment value of the thing exposed (an unzippered fly means much more to an adolescent than revelation of his academic grades); and multiply that number by the value assigned (the degree of cathexis on a similar scale) to the person before whom one's secret is revealed, you will derive the humiliation index for the situation in question. Stoller gives his own personal understanding of humiliation in the body of this chapter.*

*The degree of humiliation encrypted in the pornographic scenes described herein suggests that the persons before whom the transvestite has been embarrassed, reduced, or ridiculed must be of the highest importance. What makes sexual daydreams so compelling for their authors is that constant repetition allows a temporary, fantasized reduction in the severity of the shame experience.*

## INTRODUCTION

In an episode of erotic excitement, I believe, is packed an individual's life history, the resultant character structure, and the more varied and movable defenses we call neurosis (Stoller, 1979). Therefore, analogous to decoding DNA in a cell, if we can decode a fragment of excitement, we could (someday; our knowledge so far is rudimentary) know the individual's past, his or her versions of what happened, and the import of that life to its author.

A fine way, then, to understand someone is by that person's typical erotic daydream. Before illustrating this idea, I can amplify the term "typical daydream." I am not using "daydream" as synonymous with "fantasy." (Fantasy, we know, is the shape we give desire. It can take the form of feelings, word-represented thoughts, unsought imagery, and nightdreams; these are mental states experienced as happening to us but not owned by us. So, though in us, they can, like hallucinations or a feeling of spirit-possession, be attributed to external agencies. On the other hand are daydreams.) By "daydream" I mean a consciously experienced, consciously controlled story for which its author acknowledges responsibility, knowing it was invented to satisfy him or her. One experiences it as one's own, a product of will, something to be shaped until it fits. By "typical" I mean that the daydreamer uses the same themes over the years, though the details may change. An erotic daydream can take several forms: a story worked out in one's mind, the usual experience labeled "daydream"; a story published by another, intended as pornography; or the preferred, perhaps necessary behavior that makes up one's erotic style.

Of these above forms, pornography is the most useful for my work. Like a laboratory specimen, it is available, can be repeatedly studied, can be shown to others, and represents the rest of its class. It makes a good biopsy. (Few other mental products have these qualities.)

I am surprised that erotic excitement (or even excitement in general) has not been studied much. It has concerned animal researchers, behaviorists, pornographers, and statisticians more than those, for example, psychoanalysts and philosophers, who should have been curious about its structure. Considering that this experience is among the most gratifying, the most compelling, and the most subject to restriction, frustration, falsification, and transformation, the lack of research interest has been downright peculiar. Daydreams—all, not just the erotic—are terribly revealing, as their owners know, and therefore demand greater care in handling. People almost never give the exact text to others,* even to their psychoanalysts, who are granted all sorts of other revelations. This truism should have indicated the importance of daydreams for those who wish to study human behavior, but instead, daydreams have been pretty much ignored. Certainly their study has not had the romantic appeal found in that of nightdreams. (I cannot account for the neglect but presume some of it has psychodynamic roots.)

*Exceptions, but still constructed with safety factors to prevent uninvited humiliation: using prostitutes to play parts (they are, one says, so degraded that, like slaves, children, and other incompetents, what they think does not count); acting our erotic scripts with a willing sexual partner (who, since willing, promises to be comparably undone by passion and therefore unlikely to humiliate). A tricky business, a tightrope walk that yields the highest excitement when we hide from ourselves that we have put up a safety net.

## DAYDREAMS AND HUMILIATION: PUBLISHED PORNOGRAPHY

My thesis is not startling: one function of daydreams—not just erotic ones—is to ward off and then undo the effect of humiliations that, striking from any direction, are defended against by each turn in the daydream's script. Daydreams are secrets pieced together from secrets. At their core is humiliation of two sorts. First; to reveal the exact details of the script would be humiliating, too revealing of one's needs. Second; those exact details are invented to hide from their author, and at the same instant reverse, knowledge of humiliations already suffered. Only when these problems are solved, that is, when safety factors have been put in place, can one move on to open pleasure.

In order to keep the argument lively, to get more participation from you as I trace the presence of humiliation as a goad to excitement, let me start with fragments from a pornographic story. Doing so should keep you from trivial (even when accurate) explanations such as saying that the excitement is simply the result of Mystery, or brain physiology, or psychobiology, or conditioned reflexes, or Culture, or some other nonintentional, nonmotivational, non-meaning-filled impulse. And, different from the usual psychodynamic explanation, I want you to experience in yourself the process of discovery, not get it second hand from a theory-loaded description and thereby be pressed to agree on faith.

Here is a drawing from a pornographic booklet (Figure 10-1). If, before I tell you what the picture is about, you remain unexcited, then you have entree into understanding the process

PANTY RAID

by Carlson Wade

As Bruce King made his way stealthily, under cloak of a velvet near-midnight darkness, toward the forbidden grounds of the sorority house, he began to feel apprehensive. Suppose he did not succeed in this panty raid? Suppose he failed to come back with the booty -- a pair of lacy-fringed bloomers or skin-tight peach panties, the silk-and-satin slip with red bows for straps,

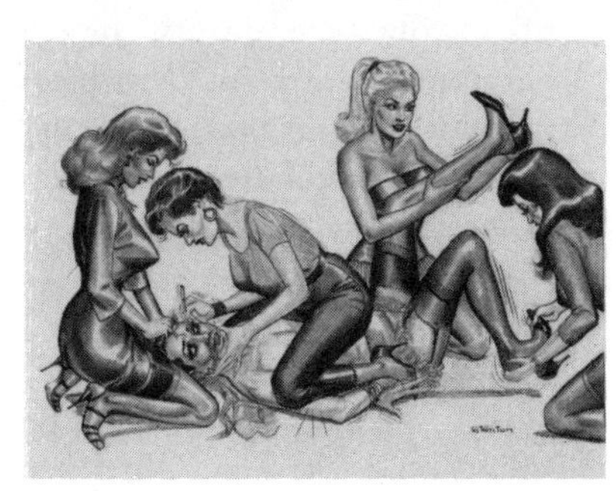

Figure 10-1.

of discovering what the picture brings to the person excited by it.

(As you read this next description, remember that, though the sentences may seem objective, they are nonetheless my interpretations. Keep that especially in mind if your version agrees with mine, for in that circumstance it is easy to think we are objective.) In this drawing, you see an anguished-faced, struggling young man held down by four young, pretty, feminine women, their faces gentle and benign, their clothes modest, their bodies clearly female, their movements graceful and easy. They are forcing him into intimate, unquestionably women's clothes and makeup. The power displayed by the women should not be sufficient to have trapped this man, for they show no evidence that they could so humiliate him, so arrest him.

If you are a transvestite, that is, a male, most likely overtly heterosexual, turned on by women's garments, you instantly know (your body tells you) the drawing is pornographic. If you are not, you will wonder how this fragment of a story could be exciting, for nothing manifestly erotic is going on. Quite the reverse. The man in the picture is being traumatized. What does the masturbating transvestite see that the rest of us cannot? Why should humiliation liven his biology?

The text underlines details present in the drawing but unnoticed by nontransvestites. The women, it is necessary for the transvestite to know, in being feminine and in not subduing the illustrated man by physical power, are thereby stating that their power comes from another source:

> Squeals and bubbling laughter suddenly enveloped him. . . . All were shrieking with joy. . . . They entwined his arms with silken robe belts. "Stop!" he tried to cry but suddenly found his mouth being filled with a silky-sheer stocking. . . . Lori . . . her heaving bosom thrust forth with a strange form of arrogance which demanded obedience and respect . . . Lori's waist was captivated (sic) by a hugh (sic: the spelling and prose style have their own unplanned aesthetic) patent leather belt of shining black; the contrasting silver buckle resembled a lock, with a tiny keyhole which defied entrance and exit. Her hips were forced into a figure-training position so that she walked with some difficulty, but with greater pride. . . . Lori stamped her dainty but powerfully strong foot.

The captured man, the text says, is masculine: his name is Bruce King, and he is given a clearly masculine history, physical attributes, and interests. He, a college fraternity pledge, has just been caught as he essayed a panty raid that "would really make him a hero." More; we are to understand that the women are fully female and the man fully male. With these emphases, the statement is subliminally made that the reader will not be threatened by intimations of bisexuality, homosexuality, gender conflicts. (The next illustration [Figure 10-2], an advertisement for a second pamphlet with the same sort of story, portrays these masculine qualities. We see another Bruce type, in the form appropriate for the era when these were published, the late '50s or early '60s.

With it established in these scripts that the men are men and the women women, the reader can know that the women humiliate the man *because they are women*. One is not to think that they did it because they were butch, with mannish bodies,

"PANTY RAIDERS"

by - Gilbert

* * *

. . . . has as its theme a 'sport' quite popular in most co-educational institutions. It deals with a group of under-graduated students who undertake a panty raid on a girl's dormitory. Unfortunately, for them, they are caught red-handed by three of the co-eds and their House Mother. By way of atonement, the boys are subjected to various forms of humiliation. They are even compelled to don the very panties they tried to steal as well as other bits of feminine apparel they never dreamed of wearing in public.

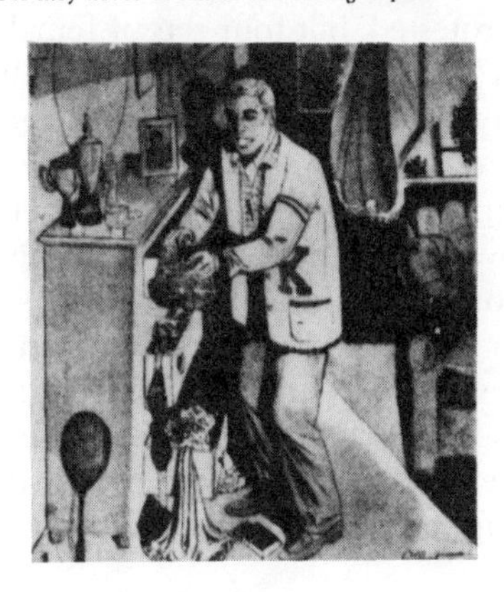

The tale is told in 48 exciting chapters. Each chapter is vividly illustrated and contains over four-hundred words. The chapters are reproduced on a heavy vellum stock (approx. 5½ x 8½ inches).

The first unit of 8 chapters is now ready . . . . . . . . . price $7.00

Figure 10-2.

with masculine personalities. The rule is: women (can, might, must, threaten to try to, enjoy the idea they could, have the skills to, are by nature equipped to, learn to, are amused they can, desire to, lust to, are gently moved to) ruin men because they are women. Such ruining is humiliation, with the attack aimed at males'—boys' and men's—masculinity:

> . . . much raucous laughter from the victorious vixens who thrilled at the helpless struggles of their male captives. . . . Before Bruce could protest, he found himself descended upon by the girls, who ripped off his simple white business shirt, cotton khaki trousers (he was grateful he wore protective boxer shorts), off went his moccasins, wool socks. "It's cold . . ." he shivered, feeling more embarrassed and humiliated than the elements of the weather in early Spring. To be stripped, bound and in the captivity of four domineering types of females was certainly an experienced (sic) that shattered his manhood. There was not telling what they could do to make good a threat that Lori not (sic) voiced: "We'll teach him that the female of the species are the *real* agressive (sic) members of the human race!". . . . "We're going to dress you, Bruce," purred Lori, her green eyes glittering with a strange fascination of the spectacle of a man being held in her captivity. "Now girls—get those boxer shorts of his and throw them out . . . good boys shouldn't wear such sloppy things. We'll teach our Brucie how to dress." "No! No!" he protested, but four sets of female hands yanked down his boxer shorts. With a sigh of relief, he remembered he wore his tiny athletic supporter which the girls ridiculed by giggling, "Look—he wears a G-string!" Lori then said, "Okay, girls, untie him. It'll be easier to get his clothes on. But Brucie-boy," she said in a falsetto tone, you won't get very far—in your G-string. So behave yourself, or we'll take that away from you, too." Bruce flushed and no sooner were his arms and legs freed then (sic) he tried to cover himself with his hands but his awkward knock-kneed position and round shouldered position of embarrassment only provoked more laughter. "Very funny! Very funny!" he gasped.

In the end Bruce is overcome and stops fighting, at which point he becomes happy, one of the girls, with the promise it will occur again. "These (women's) clothes were a perfect fit. He had gone through quite a lot to obtain them—nobody was going to take them away from him! No, sir! In fact, he already discovered that clothes can make the man! And these clothes made him feel just great! It was a start . . . THE END." And not one word or picture manifestly about sex—anatomy or actions. You can see now how transvestites wish for and in their erotic and nonerotic tales tell of being with an understanding woman, best of all a wife, who benignly and enthusiastically teaches them how to dress femininely. That theme is the happy ending for the chronicle that starts with humiliation.

The wish—the daydream–is that, for the moment, the power to humiliate is taken from the women. The story-line portrays that, and the erection and orgasm make it real. Beyond such success may be the thought that the women are a touch humiliated by having failed to destroy the man.

I also have in hand a drawing, which, so far as I know, is erotic to no one. (Certainly it was not drawn to be pornographic.)

Again we see four lovely, feminine, tranquil-faced young women, and again they are working-over a humiliated man. He, tiny, as unmanned as the transvestite, despite being a man—he is in a suit—is on his knees begging for mercy as the women (huge in comparison), looking, gently prepare either to dissect him or impale him on a hat pin. The drawing is entitled: "The Weaker Sex." I presume its audience is anyone in Western society in the last century or so. The artist understood us: all who are amused detect a truth in the exaggeration.

If you are familiar with Goya's painting, "The Straw Man," you recall that it shows, again, four lovely women, in the costume of the time, pitching a full-sized man of straw, dressed as a normal man, into the air with the aid of a blanket. He flies flaccidly upward. As with the first two drawings, this one can also touch on men's uncertainties about their gender and phallic competence and their fantasies regarding the deep, mysterious power immanent in women's femininity—and on women's wishes, reciprocating with men's fantasies, to reduce (with or without revenge) men's dangerousness.

What the men, transvestite or otherwise, cannot afford to recognize is that girls/women have been unendingly humiliated by boys/men. And there, as the cliche has it, is the battle of the sexes, the eternal misunderstandings. The effects of that battle energize the erotism of all the victims, not just those who are grossly perverse.

For some females, then, the punishment that best fits the males' crime is to rub out the accursed masculinity by putting into a boy the sign of what for these females is their deepest humiliation: femininity. The wonder, as we see in both this pornography's story and in the living transvestite's triumph by orgasm, is that the seemingly castrated male, on accepting the trauma, escapes it, retaining his manhood by disguising himself as a woman.

It is, however, a long way from one transvestite drawing to the belief that the function of perversion is to defeat humiliation, or even broader, that humiliation—ranging from trace element to massive component—is generally involved in erotic excitement. I ease my scientific conscience, as it wishes for better data, by realizing that when a pornographer publishes, s/he is a good enough businessman to know the piece will excite more than one person. We can guess, then, that the first drawing above suits at least some transvestites (though, within the category "transvestite," some will be more excited by the overtly sadomasochistic display and some less). If we move beyond transvestism to other pornographies and perversions, there are plenty—genres such as slave/master, S&M, excretory, dirty phone calls, rape, and infantilism—in which someone is manifestly humiliated. Our bag of specimens enlarges.

The thesis is better challenged when the perversion has, as in exhibitionism or voyeurism, no manifest humiliation. But even in these silent cases, talking with the performer reveals that, in his interpretation of his erotic act, he is, during the act, more or less conscious of invading, assaulting, degrading the objects of his attention (Stoller, 1975).

Finally, let us move on to "normal," that is, normative, by consensus, pornography. I suspect that men are stirred by the humiliation dynamic, for instance, when, on looking at pictures of nude women, they fantasize that, as in grosser voyeurism, they are invading the woman's privacy. And in women's pornography, which often (hundreds of millions of books published each year) takes form in romances, the story tells of threats of and triumphs over humiliation: yearning; unrequited love; tears and crinoline; strong, taut Bruce Kings—soldiers, sheiks, jewel thieves, and cowboys—resisting and finally succumbing to the soft, entreating woman.

For the men, the game is: "I humiliate in order to undo my humiliation." Women, more subtle in their pornography, think: I let myself be humiliated in order to humiliate" or, to use gentler phrasing, "in order to humble, disarm." (Men who manifestly look for humiliation are, of course, considered unmanly.)

The focus herein is on finding the humiliation dynamic, not (as done elsewhere [Stoller, 1975, 1979]), showing its origins in earlier trauma. I can, nonetheless, hint at how humiliation gets converted into a happier experience. When he was 2½ years old, the man who gave me the above transvestite pornography was separated from his mother, who had an illness from which she died a year and a half later. He was taken over by two women, one of whose first acts (memorialized in the family photo album) was to make him a suit that, in the community where he lived, marked him a sissy. Then on his fourth birthday, they dressed him as a girl and took a picture of him "as a joke." (This case is described elsewhere [e.g., Stoller, 1975]). Forced crossdressing is often reported by other transvestites, rarely by people with nontransvestic perversions.

## DAYDREAMS AND HUMILIATION: LIVE PORNOGRAPHY

To give the reader the sense that humiliation is a force in all pornography would require subjecting all pornography to examination. I cannot do this. Instead, by giving examples, I try to raise your interest to the point where you test the idea yourself. (This way of investigating, though not as well-honed as scientific method, can move us toward that method.) For this impressionistic technique to work, I must find examples that, though containing the challenge of being unusual, nonetheless are members of a universe.

Pornography is an extreme deadening—dehumanizing—of another person. I study it not to understand pornography but to have available, in the effort to find the dynamics of all erotic excitement, a specimen that stays still and lets itself be looked at and poked at without its running for cover. Pornography, then, is at the end of a continuum at the other side of which is erotic excitement caused by a real person accepted fully—intimately—in his or her selfhood, not fetishized. Between the two extremes are behaviors that more or less remove the other person. Let me now describe one, the jackoff call, that, though performed with another person, also has qualities found in the published pornographies: easy accessibility, protection against humiliation, custom-made fiction, sex object available but not encountered, stimulation restricted to only one system of perceiving (in this case, hearing). And, since pornography has a short halflife—boredom sets in quickly, the factor most proximate in making pornography lucrative—you will see another link between the jackoff call and more formal pornography: one can effortlessly get new samples.

The jackoff call is aural pornography with a heightened intensity. The system is ingenious, efficient, cheaper than negotiating with a person in-the-flesh, and quite private. The buyer, his* credit established, is connected by phone to the voice that is to service him. In the heterosexual case, it is a woman hired and trained to cater to callers' needs; she simulates excitement and is uncommitted. In homosexual servicing, however, the person at the other end is not hired but, rather, is another man also in need. They do not call each other directly, which could identify them, but make contact anonymously and randomly through the switchboard of the service. The callers may be anywhere in the country. They describe themselves to each other. Marvin, Herbert, or George become Brad, Rod, or Sean. "How big is your dick?" "9½" "How tall are you?" "6-2, slim, 175." "Hair?" "Blonde, curly." "How old are you?" "28." "What do you like?" And so forth.

They reduce each other to fetishes: though two live people are involved, each, as he would do with pornography, uses the other as if not a real person but simply as the emitter of suitable messages. Contact is one-dimensional, a voice on the telephone. One can have as many partners as desired. Truth—beer bellies, balding heads, tired faces, sad histories—never intrudes. Should it threaten, the episode—the voice, the person on the line—can be tossed aside. Fictions are invented as quickly as, in printed

*I suspect it is always a male.

pornography, one can turn the page. The action, with its so-minimal contact, is highly stylized, structured, ritualized, enclosed, protected, restricted, with the same attention to detail that is the pornographer's business. What seems an adventure in erotic aesthetics with a straightforward movement toward pleasure is actually, in every moment, a potentially dangerous mission. The danger is, of course, humiliation. "What if he knew my name, my age, the real size of my genitals, my business, my not-muscled body, my pain, my failure?"

## DISCUSSION

In this chapter I almost always use "humiliation," not "shame." Preferring shorter to longer words, I wondered why I chose the long one when, at first glance, they seemed synonyms. The dictionary, though using differently worded phrases, also makes them pretty much the same:

> humiliation: "fr. L. *humilis* low, humble . . . to reduce to a lower position in one's own eyes or the eyes of others: injure the self-respect of: HUMBLE, MORTIFY" *humus*, earth.

> shame: "fr. OE *scamu* . . . shame . . . la: a painful emotion caused by consciousness of guilt, shortcoming, or impropriety in one's own behavior or position . . . 2a (1): the condition of one that is in disgrace: IGNOMINY.

The dictionary (*Webster's New International Dictionary*, 1961) gives two connotations that might differentiate the words. First, it says, shame contains guilt. (Most of us, disagreeing, separate shame and guilt.) Second, in humiliation is injured self-respect. But the dictionary does not help us here, for we sense that humiliation, also, has (but is not the same as) guilt, and a part of shame is injured self-respect. (Let me note here that the words we use for affects—shame, humiliation, anxiety, anger, sadness, loneliness, joy, and so forth—are only approximations. After infancy, all affects, when in the body rather than as conjured up in a theory, are compound, made up of other affects, and are never experienced from one time to the next in the identical manner. And so, for instance, shame will never be experienced without intimations of, if not conscious awareness of envy, anger, anxiety, depression, guilt and lots more, besides. "In the adult, there cannot be, except manifestly and transiently, a contentless mental state" [Gediman, 1984, p. 191].)

Wurmser (1981) is extremely helpful in this regard, throughout his book but especially in his chapter on the phenomenology of shame. But as to "shame" and "humiliation," he says (1981, p. 51): "The sense of *humiliation* is just a strong form of . . . shame; humiliation itself is a shame-inducing situation. Disgrace, dishonor, degradation, and debasement are terms closely related to, if not largely synonymous with, humiliation." (See also Morrison, 1984.)

I, however, sometimes differentiate them. Shame connotes, to me, a more acute, fierce, flaming (as in a blush), face-manifested, exhibiting, and publicly broadcast set of qualities than does humiliation and its humbling. Shame is on the face, the front of the soul. It confesses itself, is harder to hide and therefore to transform. Humiliation is deeper, more hidden in muscle, bone, and mind; often more dangerous to others (as in paranoidness), more likely to provoke retaliation; and lower, in the body where *enteron* is becoming *humus*. (The way the words sound contributes to our feeling their differences.) Shame is more intense, more precise, more pointed, a faster burn, and, like guilt, a bit less likely to convert to anger and desire for revenge. With shame one cannot help but accept awareness of a personal flaw; with humiliation, the awareness is less complete, more involved with rationalizing that one's attacker is more responsible than are we for the awful feeling. But when anger and desire for revenge occur, then "shame" and "humiliation" are, for me, synonyms. (Words such as "sheepish" or "embarrassed" reflect how intimately "shame" and "humiliation" are entwined.)

Analytic theorists use "castration anxiety" as the dynamic that underlies the defenses of erotic life. Though it seems a most precise term, one that is evocative and full of drama, I find it lacks needed connotations. It points to anatomy when the issue is identity: who am I and is my "I" (selfhood) at risk? In muffling the identity meanings, "castration anxiety" fails to alert us to the shame/humiliation experiences that are the real essence of the sensed threats and the resulting reparative revenge fantasies. We do not fear amputation of our genitals but of our self. (Which does not deny that one can fear literal castration.)

Finding the dynamic of undoing shame/humiliation in erotic excitement only signals our awareness of its presence in energizing other behaviors, destructive and constructive, as this book indicates. Once alert to it, we see it at work unendingly in all of us*: the suffering and maliciousness ("masochism" and "sadism") in male–female relationships, highway accidents, warriorhood and impulses toward war, ambition and competitiveness, paranoidness, child–parent relationships, sibling rivalries, the defense mechanisms, in every case reported in the psychoanalytic literature (though often buried in grand obscurities such as "aggressive instinct"); in the construction of big cars; in table manners; in bowel habits; in words such as "vulnerability," "righteousness," "irritability," "sensitivity"; in such complex, uncertain gifts as art, science, humor, religious practice and theology, philosophy, politics, law. Even God is not exempt. Perhaps its most gracious form is humor, where we accept, willingly, even if wryly, insights that in shame/humiliation are forced on us.

Why are some shame/humiliation traumas transformed into erotism and others not? Until I get nonconfirming data, I shall believe that when the assault aims at gender/erotic parts of oneself, the trauma will be converted into gender/erotic character structure.

When we observe the wreckage associated with humiliation, including the ease with which people die for and kill for self-respect, we can accept that humiliation is a fundamental element of behavior.

It certainly is present in insight therapies. Yet discussions of treatment technique do not stress a common denominator that I think motivates resistances†: patients' fear they will be

*I have about reached the point where any clinical narrative is incomplete that does not either mention the humiliation at its core or that humiliation was looked for and not found.

†I am uneasy when colleagues say "resistance" or "the resistance" as if they believe in a special force with roots deep in mystery (e.g. "narcissism," "repetition compulsion"). Most resistance, to me, is simply a person's awareness—conscious, preconscious, and unconscious—of fearing feeling humiliated.

humiliated. That fear leads to a well-known problem in psychoanalysis, the lack of confrontation: patients can intellectualize forever, painlessly reporting fine associations and accurate interpretations, not noting that the most real, the most felt events, are often the start and end of each hour, when humiliation, in the form of nothing more dramatic than "hello" and "goodbye," threatens to strike. Wurmser, throughout his book on shame (1981), underlines the ubiquity of that state in life and in treatment, and the curious avoiding of its study. Much of my commentary herein could cite him.

How is one to avoid this awful affect, humiliation? The technique with the highest payoff is undoing, with which, as in mania to relieve depression, we not only anesthetize pain but replace it by pleasure (either directly, or, as in masochism and other symptom self-treating, indirectly). The trick is to take the power to humiliate away from someone who can spring it on us unexpectedly and therefore traumatically. We do this by becoming, ourself, the one who controls the mechanism, no longer helpless. In treatment, once they get the hang of it, patients can abnegate themselves unendingly—and it has no effect. Confession, the Church knows, is the ultimate defense against confession. It becomes an art form. Likewise, one humiliates oneself to avoid being humiliated and suffers guilt to avoid guilt.

Most psychoanalytic discussions go directly from a clinical report of overt, masked, or reversed hostility (e.g., anger, guilt, passivity) to an untestable theory of etiology: aggressive or destructive instincts. But we could, I think, move toward better understanding of much behavior if we would first search out that easy-to-find factor: humiliation "cured" by retaliation.

What a shame not to do so.

## REFERENCES

Gediman, H. K. (1984). Actual neurosis and psychoneurosis. *International Journal of Psychoanalysis, 65:* 191–202.

Morrison, A. P. (1984). Working with shame in psychoanalytic treatment. *Journal of the American Psychoanalytic Association, 32:* 479–505.

Stoller, R. J. (1975). *Perversion*. New York: Pantheon.
Stoller, R. J. (1979). *Sexual excitement*. New York: Pantheon.
*Webster's third new international dictionary* (1961) Springfield, IL: Merriam.
Wurmser, L. (1981). *The mask of shame*. Baltimore and London: Johns Hopkins University Press.

# 11

# The Sense of Shame in Psychosis: Random Comments on Shame in the Psychotic Experience

OTTO ALLEN WILL, JR.

*It has been said that European psychiatry derived from a philosophy of the individual, while the American temperament demanded a focus on the interactional. Freud's psychoanalytic stance draws us deep into the internal world of the patient, while Sullivan forces us to acknowledge that emotion frequently is triggered in the context of an interpersonal interaction. Although a later focus on object relations brought psychoanalysis out into the light of other people, it was mostly to ascertain the internal representations of those others rather than to determine a true understanding of the effects of one person on another. Only as a derivative of the recent work in infant observation has the psychoanalyst agreed to look at the ways infant and caregiver mold and form each other. Sullivan defined empathy as of critical importance in development more than a generation before any other significant figure in psychiatry.*

*Otto Will has been one of the great proponents of Sullivanian psychiatry, keeping us aware of our historical roots while himself advancing the treatment of seriously ill patients. Wurmser (1981) had suggested that shame conflict could produce such morbidity that, unrelieved, it might became a "shame psychosis." I asked Dr. Will if he*

Otto Allen Will, Jr. Private Practice, Richmond, California.

*would review his extraordinary experience in the treatment of psychosis in terms of our current interest in shame, something he had never before considered.*

*Using the language of interpersonal psychiatry, in which all negative affect is viewed as a subset of "anxiety," or "insecurity," he presents the interactional side of shame. Despite his assertion that "As a therapist, I have not found shame, in any simple form, to be a major topic of discussion." and that he has not seen shame as an important force in the lives of the schizophrenic patients in his practice, he proceeds to describe the phenomenology of shame conflict in minute detail. What he calls "A long-standing (often privately maintained) sense of estrangement from the world of others"; or "The absence of an intimate, enduring, trusting relationship with another person"; or "An increasing sense of isolation and social failure, emphasized by the many socializing demands of adolescence, threatening to a fragile self-esteem" would be viewed by many as psychopathology in the realm of shame.*

*Embedded in this contribution is the clear understanding that shame can be used as a device, or a weapon, in interpersonal affairs, especially through the powerful negative affects of contempt and disgust, which produce estrangement through a sense of inadequacy and shame. In Will's hands, treatment facilitates the return of the patient to normal interpersonal relatedness through interaction with a therapist who provides the acceptance and love necessary to overcome the estrangement produced by shame.*

## DEFINITION

Shame is a painful, unpleasant emotion experienced as an accompaniment of some awareness of wrong-doing, impropriety, shortcoming, or transgression of behavior and concepts of what is held to be "right," "good," or acceptable within a particular group. It is equated with feelings of disgrace, dishonor, infamy, humiliation, odium, or the like, and may be accompanied by physical sensations of apprehension, disgust, nausea, and dread. To be ashamed is to be faced with censure and the possible removal of the human support that is felt as necessary to exist with some semblance of comfort.

The sense of shame may be associated with the idea that one is deserving of punishment because s/he is, in some not clearly defined way, "evil" and "wicked." The punishment (pain or increased anxiety) is to be administered because the offender has not accepted, or acted in accordance with certain group standards which may, or may not be explicit or clearly comprehended by any of the participants. Many values and beliefs are presented—not only to the young—as beyond question; they exit "because that is the way things are." The most severe penalty for rule violation is the threat of being cast out or abandoned, that is, being exposed to a form of social, and sometimes physical death.

In the dictionary, shame is defined as a "painful emotion caused by consciousness of guilt, shortcoming, impropriety" (*Webster's New Collegiate Dictionary,* 1960). The dictionary definitions are, of course, given in words, and are adequate only if the person experiencing the emotion is aware of its significance in terms of current events. It should be noted, however, that the origins of shame, that is, the manifestations with which I am concerned, lie in early stages of human development in which self, object, and subject are not clearly defined, and gestures other than verbal are of primary significance. In brief, as here defined, no one would be expected to seek to be shamed, although there may be exceptions.

## ORIGINS

Shame, as I see it, is an expression of interpersonal phenomena, that is, it is an emotion (feeling, sentiment) that has its origins in a person's experiences with other people; it does not arise from the blue, and is not inherent in the human being. It is a reflection of human living.

Shame may have its most lasting origins in infancy, before the word itself has gained meaning. Certain behaviors of the infant may be met by forbidding gestures (facial expression, tone of voice, variants of the forms of physical contact, bodily withdrawal) which are not clearly understood but are nevertheless impressive as evidences of disapproval. The accompanying discomfort may contribute to the concept of "bad me" (in contrast to an acceptable or "good me"), and when more severe, may become part of a dissociated system of ideas not readily available to awareness—the "not me" as evidenced in some psychotic experiences.

There may be transmitted to the infant (child) in this fashion the mothering one's more personal feelings of distaste, disgust, and shame that may, or may not be in accordance with the mores of the family, society, and culture. In brief, at this early stage, there is no clear connection between the gesture of disapproval and the nature or consequences of a particular act or quality. Something "goes wrong" in a relationship, and the general feeling becomes one of being "bad," with the threat of the loss of a needed union with a caring person as the dreadful penalty.

In childhood, with the further acquisition of speech skills, the connection between act and shame may be seen more clearly. The child may learn that s/he should be ashamed to go naked in public, put a hand on the genitals, use "bad words," or whatever. Less clear are such prescriptions as "our kind of people don't do such things, as everyone knows."

In the juvenile period, with the need to be a member of a group of compeers, emphasis is placed on conforming to the standards and requirements of the group. Attention may then focus on personal characteristics that are valued, and one may be ashamed to be "weak," or "skinny," or "fat," or "a coward," and so on. The threat for being too different is ostracism. The needs and fears of the juvenile era are continued into later life, for many of us with little change.

In preadolescence, and later, the appearance of some form of love for another person carries with it the apprehension that something of which one is ashamed may disrupt the relationship. The specter of abandonment and loss that may have been experienced in infancy may then be painfully revived.

In all of these situations, shame is one of the expressions of anxiety defined as a threat to a person's sense of personal worth and self-esteem.

The following is a quotation from Sullivan (1950):

> What is it that the young are caused to learn? I must say that in spite of a very great deal of data about child psychology and educational psychology, we are not well equipped to answer that question. We know in a general way that . . . almost every home brings the child to the juvenile era ready

> to discover that the world is a much more complicated place than it had seemed so far, and a place in which various other people, compeers and nonfamily adults, will subject one to anxiety and pain. The experience of complex derivatives of anxiety, such as *guilt, shame, humiliation* by ridicule, etc., grows apace; and along with all this unpleasant experience, there goes the acquiring of more and more skill at various kinds of *security operations*—interpersonal activities for escaping from or minimizing anxiety. (p. 37; emphasis in original)

## USES

Shame has its uses, otherwise its continuance could not be explained. The arousal of anxiety, and one of its variants, shame, is a way of embracing cultural prescriptions of desired and undesired behavior. Such prescriptions, or customs, may in themselves not be simply rational and subject to ready explanation. Their teaching is, in the early years of life, irrational in itself, this is the result, in part, of the urgency to promote in the young such conformity to group standards that, at the very least, life itself can be preserved. The necessity for such learning through means other than verbal leads to an involvement of the "total person," that is, the disapproval is associated with general feelings of goodness and badness, and with the bodily sensations of nausea, repulsion, and smooth muscle activity leading to vomiting and loss of sphincter control.

Shame can, of course, be avoided or reduced by foregoing the acts that provoke it, and by accepting the prohibitions as correct. There are also a variety of magical verbal formulae for dealing with shame such as "I am ashamed," "I confess my shame," "I ought to be ashamed," or "I'm sorry."

Shame can be, and often is, used as a weapon. "You ought to be ashamed" at best raises doubt about one's deeds and thoughts, and "Shame on you!" can be a form of enduring curse. To "shame" is a way of putting onus on another person and can easily become a form of cruelty, accompanied as noted earlier, by the threat of abandonment, desertion, loss, ostracism, and death. The statement "I'd rather be dead than face such shame" is not uncommon, nor is its suggested act.

One of the unfortunate misuses, or unplanned results of shaming, is restriction of thought and imagination. It is very difficult to combine for all occasions freedom of thinking and security.

## APPEARANCE

In this context, shame is presented as one of the various expressions of anxiety. Although a sense of shame is common, it would not be useful to attribute to shame the many human emotional discomforts that may have other origins. Therefore, I will not attempt to equate shame with anxiety. The various manifestations of anxiety are often not easy to observe, identify, or understand in terms of origins and purposes. In the 1940s Sullivan (1953b) addressed this problem as follows:

> Anxiety appears not only as awareness of itself but also in the experience of some *complex* emotions into which it has been elaborated by specific early training. . . [such as] embarrassment, shame, humiliation, guilt, chagrin. The circumstances under which these unpleasant emotions occur are particularly hard to observe accurately and to subject to the retrospective analysis which is apt to be most rewarding.
>
> A group of security operations born of experience which has gone into the development of these complex emotions is equally hard for one to observe and analyze. These are the movements of thought and the actions by which we, as it were, impute to or seek to provoke in the other fellow feelings like embarrassment, shame, humiliation, guilt or chagrin. It is peculiarly difficult to observe retrospectively, and to subject to analysis, the exact circumstances under which we are moved to act as if the other person "should be ashamed of himself," is "stupid," or guilty of anything from a breach of good taste to a mortal sin.
>
> Disparaging or derogatory thought and action that make one feel "better" than the other person concerned, that expand one's self-esteem, as it were, at his cost, are always to be suspected of arising from anxiety. (p. 379)

As a therapist, I have not found shame to be, in any simple

form, a major topic of discussion. I do, of course, spend much time involved in accounts of how a person felt disadvantaged, humiliated, hurt, inferior, angry, contemptuous, and so on. My efforts are directed toward discovering something of the events associated with his or her experiencing a particular emotion, and the experiences in the life history that rendered the patient particularly vulnerable to a certain form of insult to self-esteem.

Some of the phenomena related to shame that are common in my therapeutic experience are summarized briefly as follows:

1. The therapist's personal experience with shame is of great importance. Depending on that experience, the concept of shame may be so painful and repugnant that its manifestations are avoided, minimized, or denied or, in contrast, the sentiment may be looked on as so commonplace as to be trivial and worthy of little notice. It is also possible to find shame everywhere, as it often seems possible to discover anger, anxiety, loss, sexuality, or other interests that may grab therapist's attention.

2. In reality a therapist may be ashamed of certain of his or her own behaviors, and thus become anxious when a patient reveals shame in a similar area. Here the therapist needs understanding and compassion for both the patient and himself or herself.

3. The person who has been shamed may well seek to shame others, including the therapist, and the therapist may discover that s/he will, on occasion, act to shame the patient. The hope in such situations lies in discovery, revelation, and discussion. This is no place for shame to go underground.

4. At times a patient may seem to seek shame, to acknowledge this emotion openly, and to ask forgiveness. This is an indirect way of seeking a form of relationship.

## PSYCHOSIS

My experience as a therapist with a wide range of psychotic manifestations is limited. I have not worked intensively, to any extent, with the aged, with children, or with people in the manic–depressive group. Most of the psychotic patients with whom

I have worked have been diagnosed as schizophrenic, range in age from 17 years into the fifties, and usually met with me after they had been obviously grossly disturbed for a year or more, and had been treated elsewhere with whatever methods were currently popular.

Shame, as such, has not been commonly revealed to me in this work. I think that this observation is, at least in part, a reflection of the idea that this sentiment in its articulated form is an expression of interpersonal experience in which the participants are recognized, as is the nature of the events of which one is to be ashamed.

In brief summary, the psychotic people with whom I have had much contact as a therapist have shown some variant of the following characteristics.

1. A long-standing (often privately maintained) sense of estrangement from the world of others.
2. The absence of an intimate, enduring, trusting relationship with another person.
3. An increasing sense of isolation and social failure, emphasized by the many socializing demands of adolescence, threatening to a fragile self-esteem.
4. A recurrent, and finally persistent, inability to limit the contents of awareness to ideas and emotions more or less clearly relevant to current activities.
5. The appearance, or eruption, of dissociated ideas into awareness, as in a waking nightmare.
6. The feeling of a loss of what has been familiar including a sense of self and others, accompanied by feelings of madness.
7. The transient state of panic, and the common accompaniments of delusions, hallucinations, ideas of reference, loss of ego boundaries, distortions of the body image, disturbances of speech, and terror.
8. Some form of resolution—hebephrenic collapse, paranoid restructuring of experience, "recovery" with possible expansion of personality, suicide, death by inadvertence, "chronic" psychosis, and so on.

In all of the above, the expression of shame in a direct way is, in my experience, generally absent. In the multiple and shifting events of developing psychosis, the person involved may feel overwhelmed by the threat of loss and the imminent dissolution of a personal universe—titanic events in which shame in its more sophisticated form is not apparent. As this intensity of feeling subsides, and increased security is found, as in the therapeutic relationship, there may then appear the concepts of being somehow evil and bad. These are more precise formulations of the earlier inchoate terror. Later, such ideas may be recognized as being related to earlier life situations in which shaming was used as a major means of controlling behavior and, perhaps inadvertently, of molding the personality.

The psychotic state is not a bed of roses (or a rose garden) but then, neither is reality. One young woman, long ensconced in a bleak, unchanging gray world of ice and silence, was frightened as movement, color, and sound came more into her awareness. "Don't make me wake up," she said. More recently, a patient said: "I hate you and your normal reality. People are more awful than what you call my imaginations."

Some aspects of the dreaded "reality" are commonplace and not to be denied:

1. To be, or to have been, psychotic is to be "different"; one has been labeled.
2. Having lost control of one's very self in the exposure of terrors previously, at least partly, hidden and dissociated—having "gone crazy"—it is difficult not to feel less than human.
3. There comes a recognition of being a member of a group of people that as a whole is feared and unwanted, and in some instances has been done away with in the practice of triage.*
4. With the loss of fictive characterizations of psychotic experience, loneliness in the human society must be faced.
5. In the process of "recovery" come sorrow and grieving about lost opportunities.

With all of these phenomena come feelings of anger, hurt, despair, and often shame. It is easy to become lost in such emotions, and even to "make a career" of their experience which may function as an attempt to deny one's humanity.

Sullivan (1953a) spoke of this when he said: "In most general terms, we are all more simply human than otherwise, be

*Triage refers to the selection of people who are to be—or can be—saved, as in military casualties. Psychotic people have been killed in some societies, as in Nazi Germany. In many cultures such people are given only the minimum of care—not being "worthy"—or considered to be "hopeless."

we happy and successful, contented and detached, miserable and mentally disordered, or whatever" (p. 16).

That is, there is no escape from the human condition by resort to such concepts as being bestial, inhuman, or saintly. Our survival as human beings may depend on our taking ourselves seriously and moving beyond the many subterfuges that may prevent us from facing the essential question: How much do we value life itself—including its human variant?

## References

Sullivan, H. S. (1950). Tensions interpersonal and international: A psychiatrist's view. In H. Cantril (Ed.) *Tensions that cause wars*, (pp. 79–138). Urbana: Univerisity of Illinois Press.

Sullivan, H. S. (1953). *Conceptions of modern psychiatry*. New York: Norton.

Sullivan, H. S. (1953). Towards a psychiatry of peoples. In H. S. Perry & M. L. Gawel (Eds.), *The interpersonal theory of psychiatry*. New York: Norton.

*Webster's new collegiate dictionary*. (1960). Springfield, MA: Merriam.

Wurmser, L. (1981). *The mask of shame*. Baltimore: Johns Hopkins University Press.

# 12

# Shame and Envy*

JOSEPH H. BERKE

*In a supervision session some years ago, a young therapist asked me to help her refer away to another therapist a patient who made her unacceptably uncomfortable. The large diamond engagement ring recently acquired by this patient proved such a distraction that the therapist could not concentrate on the case. "I will never have a ring like that, and I want one more than anything in the world."*

*Jealously, envy, greed (in the therapist) are usually dismissed as transient emotions, beneath dignity for serious discussion and not likely to interfere with therapy. Generally considered derivative of perceived inadequacy or deprivation, which release shame, they are frequently denied by the therapist and ignored in supervision. Yet somehow such issues must be addressed, and this chapter (in its casual recognition of them) allows the therapist new focus on these unpopular emotions.*

*Berke takes an unusual approach in this poetic and lyrical chapter, stating that envy and greed are* primary *emotions related to shame but not derivative of it. Many of the authors in this book would disagree with him, yet his case is well stated and well documented. I find most useful his concept of "envious tension," the noxious state of mind which can only be resolved by destructive action. For some time I had been puzzled by a shift in the format of horror movies—where previously*

*This chapter includes material from Dr. Berke's forthcoming book *Envy, Greed and Jealousy*, which will be published by Summit Books in 1988.

Joseph H. Berke. Director, Arbours Association, London, England.

*one could discern some motive for the grotesque actions around which the plots were loosely draped (jealously, unrequited love, and so on) now it seems that people are destroyed merely because they are attractive or likeable. Reading Berke one sees immediately that envy is the unifying theme, and envious tension the unbearable (and uncontrolable) force that impels horrible action.*

*Here too the therapist will find another word usually avoided in contemporary therapy: sin. How unpopular are considerations of morality in psychotherapy today! It has been said that until the work of Freud most psychological counseling was based on the model of confession perfected by the Roman Catholic Church. Since Freud it has become impossible to ignore the omnipresence of libido, to treat sexuality as something that "should" merely be repressed or controlled. During the first half-century of the psychoanalytic movement the Church steadfastly refused to accept the teaching of Freud, and the populace shifted its allegiance to counselors who would deal with sexuality differently. During this period it became fashionable for psychotherapists to eschew all involvement with moral ("superego") issues.*

*Now, of course, pastoral counselors are free to talk about matters sexual and secular, as well as religious. Perhaps the rest of us therapists had better pay attention to the avalanche of interest in evangelical Christianity, to great masses of people once again focused on sin. Where for two or three generations one might seek excuse for misbehavior by claiming that "My unconscious made me do it!", now people adduce diabolic influence. It seems likely that the "me generation" has swung the pendulum too far in the direction of "freedom," for narcissism and exhibitionism are more the rule than exception today. To be a fundamentalist or a "born-again" Christian one must adopt a strict set of external rules that define the ideal self (acting as a reference standard for shame) as well as ideal behavior (failing which one experiences guilt). By Berke's inclusion of sin, of the patient's understanding of an action as sinful, and of the existence of a state of sin, he returns these complex affective and cognitive states to psychotherapeutic consideration.*

Shame is a tormenting sense of inferiority and sinfulness. It signals a loss of face and a state of disgrace. It reveals social inadequacy and moral degeneracy. It revels in worthlessness whether in light of oneself, or of others. Shame appears when goodness disappears.

In describing shame I have deliberately used the word *sin*, because it is in the nature of shame to expose sin, or to be exposed as a sinner. Sin means a fundamental wickedness, a transgression against God, against man, against self. Nowadays it is not fashionable to think in these terms. When it is applied, sin is generally mentioned in relation to guilt. However, the concept is useful and relevant in understanding shame, both from the perspective of the shamed person, and the shamer.

Shame is not a mild emotion. It denotes a state of self-damnation brought about by the sudden annihilation of personal integrity. To be ashamed is to feel devoid of goodness, full of sin, and utterly reprehensible. Therefore I shall begin my analysis of shame by focusing on sin.

Throughout recorded history, many people have commented on sin, or evil, or wickedness, and there have been many attempts to systematize the essential qualities and quantities of the sinister side of human life. Christian theologians carried out some of the most formidable investigations, describing seven deadly sins. For hundreds of years these seven sins "explained" evil and contributed to a basic model of reality which permeated popular consciousness.

In *The Canterbury Tales* Chaucer (1982) detailed *pride, envy, anger, accidie, avarice, gluttony,* and *lechery*. He considered envy to be the worst because "all other sins oppose one virtue, but envy is against all virtue and all goodness."

On closer examination the seven sins reduce to three: envy, greed, and jealousy. Of these, envy is the most prominent. It includes pride, anger, and accidie. Greed comprises avarice, gluttony, and lechery. And jealousy touches on lechery and anger.

The sin of "anger" was not simply a state of justified displeasure, rather it was "a wicked will to vengeance" that encompassed "malice aforethought" and conjured forth an essential malevolence towards love and life. "Accidie" is usually translated as "sloth," but this sin did not depict only laziness. It meant a vengeful passivity, something we might see in a malicious passive–aggressive character who seeks revenge on life by deliberate inaction. Finally "pride" did not mean a pleasure in self. On the contrary it implied hubris, a hateful self-inflation, an arrogant overstepping of bounds designed to put down and hurt others, a maneuver typical of pathologic narcissism. Together with "envy," these evils comprise an entity which Chaucer linked with the Devil, who always rejoices in human suffering.

The other three sins are but variations of greed, that is, an excessive and insatiable desire for goods, possessions, riches, sex, and so forth. Jealousy is less obvious because it is less bad. It is concerned with love, love lost and love denied. Lechery means an excessive desire for another's body, really for love. Should the desire be frustrated or threatened, then great rage and humiliation will occur, consistent with the idea of sinful anger, revenge against an allegedly unloving person.

Therefore the seven deadly sins can really be viewed as three primary pernicious impulses, and comprise what I consider to be the three fundamental negative constituents of character and culture. In the next few paragraphs I will discuss these destructive impelling forces in greater detail.

Envy is an inborn, destructive motivating force, opposed to love and antagonistic to life. Writing in *The Metaphysic of Morals* in 1797 Kant (1797/1922) had no qualms abut describing envy as "the vice of human hate," a moral incongruity that delights in misfortune (*schadenfreude*) and ingratitude. He called envy a "hate that is the complete opposite of human love" and concluded:

> The impulse of envy is thus inherent in the nature of man, and only its manifestation makes it an abominable vice, a passion not only distressing and tormenting to the subject, but intent on the destruction of the happiness of others, and one that is opposed to man's duty towards himself as towards other people (p. 316).

Still, many theorists believe that envy is too sophisticated a state of mind and pattern of behavior to exist at birth, and that the cognitive faculties and sensitivity to relationships, such as in malicious comparison, only develop in the second or third year of life. From this point of view envy would have to be a "later derivative" because the infant does not have sufficient "ego strength" to be envious. Recent studies of neonates demonstrates that this is not the case. They are enormously sensitive not just to physical stimuli, but to human relationships, and can respond according to what they see and feel. Obviously these capabilities expand as the infant grows older, but sufficient evidences does exist to confirm a potentiality for envious attack from birth (Restak, 1982).

Over a hundred years after Kant, Freud also commented on envy as a hatred that opposes love. This is hatred directed against "any source of unpleasurable feeling" including, for example, the absence of something needed, the presence of noxious sensations, and overexcitement. Common to these experiences is an intolerable inner tension associated with the very things a person wants (Freud, 1924).

Mere relief from the distress does not assuage such a degree of unpleasure. On the contrary, it remains as a passionate hostility toward any stimulation, even rooted in desire that has become too painful to bear. The description fits a rudimentary envy that averts love and transforms intense interest and excited desire into malevolence.

At first Freud believed that these angry attacks on the world were secondary to what he called Eros, or the life instinct. Later he concluded that destructive forces were equal in importance and power to life-enhancing ones, and that the life instinct, Eros, was opposed by a death instinct, Thanatos. This view was strongly supported by Melanie Klein (1957/1975) who argued that envy is the earliest direct externalization of the death instinct.

The concept of a "death instinct" is not easy to accept, not the least on ethical grounds. To many, "death instinct" has seemed ominously close to "original sin." I think the duality, life–death, can best be understood as a struggle between forces aiming at growth, order, integration, and structure (an upward energy flow) and forces leading to contraction, disorder, fragmentation, and chaos (a downward spiral). Conception is a psychobiological impetus to structure which draws upon all the possibilities of the genetic code and the energies that flow from the mother's body to combat a return to randomness (entropy). "Life instinct" implies the former, "death instinct" the latter. In fact, "impulse" is a much better term than "instinct" because it denotes an impelling force rather than an unalterable one.

Greed is also a primary emotional impulse. It is an insatiable desire to take for oneself what another possesses. It is damaging because of its ruthless acquisitiveness. However, a greedy person sees what he wants as good and valuable, while in contrast, an envious person is not concerned with possessing, just with preventing others from possessing.

Two different kinds of housebreaking illustrate the difference. In one the person is concerned to steal as much as he can, money, jewels, furniture, "valuables." He wants to get in and get out with as few difficulties as possible, then sell his loot. He tries to avoid making a mess except as may be necessary to break into the house or make off with a particular item. In the second instance the person aims to create havoc. He is not concerned with stealing things—often valuable items are left in place. But the house will be wrecked, with paint sprayed on the walls, the water left on, and even shit smeared all over. The former has to do with greed, the latter with envy.

Envious anger is different from that aroused by frustration, revenge, rivalry, or indignation. The latter presuppose actual hurt, deprivation, or injury and are assuaged when the cause of the hostility is overcome or removed. Envy lingers on even after a frustration has been overcome, a specific hurt repaid, a rival removed, or an injustice made right. Envy may be associated with real events, but it is more than a reaction to them. Envy is both the tension and the hostile reaction to this tension in the envier, a tension that is not dependent on, or necessarily related to anything actually happening. Quite the contrary, this preverbal state of unpleasure is highly sensitive to mental activity, especially perception, and the power of the imagination. Aeschylus (1925) conveyed the envious state of mind through the voice of Agamemnon after he returned from Troy:

> For not many men, the proverb saith,
> Can love a friend who fortune prospereth
> Unenvying; and about the envious brain
> Cold poison clings and doubles all the pain
> Life brings him. His own woundings he must nurse,
> And feels another's gladness like a curse. (p. 35)

Envious tension is aroused by the awareness of vitality and prosperity, indeed, by life itself. The envier aims to eliminate the torment in himself or herself by forceful, attacking, annihilatory behavior. This discharge, directed against the alleged source of the envy, constitutes a means of self-protection as well as other-destruction. *Therefore, envy can be seen as a mechanism of defense at the service of the death impulse.* It is opposed, mitigated, but never entirely vanquished by the opposite impulse associated with love. This view is consistent with Freud's theories of the life and death impulses, and the pleasure principle. Life energies, or libido, promote pleasure when a person achieves growth, integration, and structure. Pain is the result of the inability to achieve libidinal needs, that is, reduce libidinal pressures. It also results from breakdown, chaos, and disorder.

The energies of the death impulse, akin to envious tension, continually resist libidinal fulfillment. This is the action of entropy on the organism whereby *pleasure* consists of a return to randomness. Conversely, *pain* lies in structure, order, and growth. The two sets of tensions and tendencies are inborn. They can never be resolved, but both contribute to the richness, variety, and complexity of existence (Berke, 1985).

The envious person feels inferior, rather than empty. He can't stand to see others full of life and goodness, because he is preoccupied with his own limitations and defects. So he aims to debunk, debase, and defile what others have.

Envy is a graspingness for self. Greed is a graspingness for life. Both are never satisfied because the envious person can always imagine someone else has more, or is worth more than he, while the greedy person can never imagine that he can get, or will have, enough.

But greed recognizes life. The greedy person can acknowledge and value care, tenderness, nourishment, beauty, and love. That is why greed is not as shameful as envy, which denies all these things.

Developmentally, jealousy is a later emotion concerned with possessive love and bitter hatred. It has to do with rivalry with a second person for the affection of a third. Jealousy always involves a triangular relationship even when one member of the triangle is an internal figure, that is, a part of oneself. In contrast, envy is dyadic. It only comprises an envier (the subject) and the envied (the object). Envy is pure malice. Jealousy is wicked inasmuch as frustrated love leads to murderous attacks on the rival and on the original loved person.

Shame essentially puts us in touch with these three basic

sins or destructive forces. Envy is the most devastating of them all because it is the most destructive to integrity and propriety. Therefore, envy is the most shameful experience and the one most defended against.

The anthropologist George Foster believes that it is almost impossible for the inhabitants of competitive, contemporary Western societies like the United States to concede the fundamental importance of envy because of the comparative elements involved which, when acknowledged, threaten the envier with a massive loss of self-esteem. In recognizing envy in oneself, Foster (1952) comments: "a person is acknowledging inferiority *with respect to another*; He measures himself against something else, and finds himself wanting. It is, I think, this implied admission of inferiority, rather than the admission of envy, that is so difficult for us to accept" (p. 184).

Foster's conclusions are drawn from the work of Harry Stack Sullivan who was one of the first psychiatrists to study envy thoroughly. Sullivan (1956) wrote: "we find that the people who are much at the mercy of envy have learned to appraise themselves as unsatisfactory—that is, as inadequate human beings" (p. 129).

I think the issue is not simply one of inferiority, but rather the hatred aroused by people's perceived or imagined sense of inferiority in relation to each other, and the extent to which this reaction transgresses established values. Unlike ancient Greece or Renaissance Italy, we live in a world where envy is continually unleashed and collusively denied. In this respect envy is to this century what sex was to the Victorians, an obsession best avoided and forgotten.

Shame arises from a sudden insight, often a forced insight into what we want to keep hidden. This especially applies to envy, a feeling which confirms inferiority and imposes an awareness of dependency, fragility and impotency. Interestingly, there is a significant connection between the experience of shame and the experience of those intolerable states of mind which I call envious tension.

Envious tension is a deep, gnawing, tormenting, excruciating awareness of disparity between oneself and something else, inevitably something desirable, beyond one's reach, like the bright vitality of the girl in a Coca-Cola ad. An immediate wish for discharge follows the tension. The envier aims to eliminate the torment in himself by forceful, attacking, annihilatory behavior. So envy has to be seen as both the tension and the hostile reaction to the tension in the envier. The latter, the discharge, is what most people recognize as envy.

Shame is also a powerful inner tension experienced as an exquisitely painful sense of inferiority at variance with one's wished-for image of personal goodness, like the wholesomeness of the girl in the Coca-Cola ad. The quality and degree of emotional pain is comparable to that of envious tension, so much so that it is likely that shameful tension is a variation of, as well as a contributor to, envy. If this is correct, we would expect that shame will be followed by rage. This is generally the case. The shamed person either wants to hide further away (as the envier at times), but also wants to destroy the alleged source of the shame. So the model is the same, for with shame as with envy, a tormenting tension leads to an angry discharge. But with shame, it is the former, the tension, that most people recognize as shame. They tend to overlook the subsequent response.

In order to appreciate why someone should suffer shame, we have to look at the relationship between the shamed and the shamer. Like envy, shame is an interpersonal event. Again like envy, shame has to do with comparison, malicious comparison. The envier is always looking around with a jaundiced eye. The shamer functions in a similar way, always drawing attention to disparities between how he is and how he should be. He arouses shame by self-inflation and other-deflation. This transaction can occur in the outside world, or inwardly, between a shaming internal figure and a representation of oneself.

But who does this, who puts others to shame? The shamer is a person who may act inadvertently, but usually acts aggressively, to put down another. He is like a parent who disciplines a child maliciously. The issue becomes more than moral convenience or control, but the systematic demoralization of one human being by another who gains considerable sadistic pleasure by so doing. I can think of many examples of mothers and fathers who have accosted their youngsters in this way: "Sam, will you please stop picking your nose, pleeese, *stop* picking your nose."

Sam was a 4-year-old who was invariably reprimanded in public by his mother. She seemed to delight in making him appear bad and in destroying the pleasure he took in his body. The nose picking seems innocuous enough, hardly a sin, but the tone of her voice, the persistence of the rebukes, the context in which these occurred, all led the child to believe he had committed a major crime and to feel ashamed in the face of his friends and relatives. He responded with temper tantrums which then evoked further rebukes: "Oh you *naughty* boy, wait till your father hears about this."

Other incidents often concern eating (greed) or sibling rivalry (envy and jealousy): "*Must* you eat so sloppily!" "Why *must* you take two apples when you *know* one will do?" "*Are* you fighting with your sister again?"

Whether these are shaming comments or not depends on the tone of voice, the gestures, the context, and indeed, the sensitivity of the child. Unnecessary, excessive shaming exchanges are inevitably malicious and force an awareness of badness onto an immature or fragile ego before a child or adult is capable of coping with his or her own feelings, and those of the shamer. The sequence reinforces envious torment, for the shamer is usually trying to discharge his or her own envious/shameful tensions. Thus the mother who deflates or puts down her child in an irritated, vengeful voice is likely to feel ashamed herself. She identifies with the antics of her son and immediately seeks to get rid of the tension her parents evoked. Simultaneously she might feel envious of the boy for enjoying pleasures which she feels have been denied to her. The same holds true for the mom who attacks her child's eating habits. Maybe he *is* biting off more than he can chew, maybe his eyes *are* bigger than his stomach. That is for him to find out. Her intervention may have less to do with morals, and more to do with her own envy of her child's vitality. It is in the nature of envy to attribute greed, so shaming comments about greed usually have envious antecedents.

Dr. Nathanson provides excellent examples of aggressive putdowns which evoke shame in his chapter on "Shaming systems in Couples, Families, and Institutions" (Chapter 8 of the present volume). In particular, he discusses Samantha, a woman born to bitterly competitive parents, and her mother, "a cruel, jealous, angry woman" who used to demean her daughter's talents as a painter. Ostensibly this was because the daughter did not carry on in the family tradition. Really it occurred because the mother could not stand Samantha's creativity. The ridiculed creativity represented demeaned and devalued sexuality, vitality, and happiness, all that the mother had lost, or never had, and couldn't stand to see in another.

This mother was not totally destructive. Samantha did grow up and create a family of her own. Her mother's put-downs were selective. But her annihilatory comments did make an obstacle that Samantha could never surmount. As an adult, Samantha still contained and was attacked by a malicious mother who had become a part of her internal world, an "inner object" that continued to shame and abuse her.

Dr. Hanna Segal (1979) has pointed out that the envious internal figures contribute to the construction of and are comparable to what Freud called the "over-severe superego":

> The projection of envy into the (internal) object gives rise to an envious superego. The over-severe superego which Freud describes as the basis of psychical disturbance, often turns out on analysis to be an envious superego. That is, its attacks are directed not only against the individual's aggression, but also, and even predominantly, against the individual's progressive and creative capacities. (p. 143)

Internal shamers are comparable to and close cousins of internal enviers. They perpetuate highly charged shaming put-downs as well as the damaging relationships that initiated them. Hence shame can be activated by an actual person or an internal figure. The latter are probably the most devastating.

Internal figures also contribute to a second kind of transaction that evokes shame. I refer to the shamer's self-inflation. This represents an indirect, but nonetheless extremely effective form of attack. Relative to the shamer's hubris, the shamed feels as deflated as if he has been personally demeaned. Self-inflating shamers are usually severely narcissistic people whose grandiose overestimation of their own capacities and virtues serves as a basic defense against underlying inferiority and self-hatred. In fact pathological narcissism and envy are variations of the same problem—excessive mental pain consciously perceived as overweening inferiority and inadequacy. To begin, the envious and the narcissistic persons attack this problem differently, the envier by deflating others, the narcissist by inflating himself or herself, but their thinking, feeling, and actions run along convergent tracks.

Aggressive narcissism is identical to envious self-assertion, as Samantha's mother illustrates so well. Her child's creativity was a narcissistic wound that she could not tolerate, because it shattered the fragile balance between her inadequate self-esteem and intense self-deprecation. This aroused the most murderous rage, self-murder, and soul murder. She shamelessly set out to annihilate her daughter's creative soul while concurrently murdering her self as located in and reflected by her child. For the narcissist the act of shaming is an emotional attack that can feel as satisfyingly destructive as if she had taken a knife and actually injured another's body.

It is well known that shame and narcissism are closely associated. I have emphasized the action of the narcissist as shamer. But narcissism is an important feature of the easily shamed individual. S/he may be a fragile adult or child who feels vulnerable to the actions of relatives, friends, associates, and so on. They may not behave in a derogatory, hurtful, shaming way, but they tend to be perceived as if they had done, or might do so. The anticipation of shame brings to the forefront root difficulties in psychotherapy. Increasingly we see a host of narcissistically vulnerable individuals, often diagnosed or diagnosable as "borderline personality disorder," who put up tremendous resistance to therapy. A major reason for the resistance is because they view the therapist as a dangerous aggressor who, in the guise of conveying beneficent insight, is out to destroy their self-integrity and drive them mad. These patients projectively identity the therapist with their own envious and shaming selves. So they will do anything to defend themselves against the shame of therapy.

Protective measures to avoid shame parallel defenses deployed against envy. They include concealment, denial, magical self-defense, appeasement, and aggressive counterattack. Concealment includes the wish to hide the act, the thought, the wish—anything that might attract shame, as well as to hide from the shamer. Sam, for example, went to great lengths to pick his nose in private rather than expose his activity to his mother. Samantha would periodically withdraw in therapy. Presumably she did this in order to hide her feelings and avoid comments and interpretations that she found as shameful as those of her mother.

In Chapter 8, Dr. Nathanson also points out: "Shame is about eye contact. We lower our eyes, avert our gaze when embarrassed. This certainly interrupts whatever had been going on between the participants."

Lowering the eyes is a widely recognized gesture indicating shame and the wish to avoid the shaming gaze or eye of the shamer. In exactly the same way the envied person tries to avoid the malevolent look and eye of the envier which has been known since antiquity as "the evil eye." The evil eye is the envious "I"—penetrating, provocative, controlling, and poisonous. It inserts slander just as the shaming eye inserts disgrace. When patients expect to receive criticism, shame and blame, they will do anything to avoid insight, that is, taking the sight from inside their therapist's eye/"I." Far from being helpful, they see these insights as mind and soul destroying. No wonder so many therapies go on interminably, but without change. All the patients want to do is keep shame and blame at bay. Their continued presence is a form of appeasement. They will attend sessions and pay fees as a sop to the therapist so long as s/he doesn't focus on anything shameful.

Denial is a further defense against shame. Denial includes self-effacement and self-inflation, which are protective facades designed to avoid shameful realizations about thoughts, wishes, feelings—all the essential components of personal identity. Quite often denial is an important "meta-defense." People deny the denial so they can honestly say that they are who they aren't.

"Sue-Ann" was a patient of mine who came from a wealthy Southern family. She had spent 7 years in various private and public mental hospitals and had received diagnoses ranging from psychopathic personality to chronic schizophrenia. Over the years she had received medication, electroshock, insulin shock, group therapy, milieu therapy, individual therapy, and had been offered a lobotomy. Needless to say, she was considered to be incorrigible. As a last resort her family brought her to see me in London, after hearing about the Arbours Association Crisis Centre, a mental health facility that provides intensive, personal, psychotherapeutic care, of which I am a founder and the director (Berke, 1982).

Initially I met with Sue-Ann and her parents in various combinations, alone and together. I soon concluded that she was a relatively "normal" young woman who had taken up a career as a mental patient in response to various incidents that had occurred at the onset of puberty. I thought she wanted to protect her family from their disappointments in her, and to protect herself from her disappointments in herself, all by a self-punishing facade. I suggested this to her, and, after some hesitation, she confirmed that my comments were essentially correct. With lowered eyes, she said she had felt terribly shamed by what had happened. Afterward she had discovered that hospitalization and treatment were useful ways in which to hide. Now she didn't know how to change things. She wanted to help embark on a new career as a "normal person" and to shed her previous life-course.

I think that many patients, like Sue-Ann, use their diagnoses, and identify with them, in order to conceal and deny the shame involved in their original family disputes. In many instances their new stigma as a mental patient is far less shameful than the original issues. That is why they hold on to it so tenaciously. Moreover, the medications, electroshock, and social therapies all serve as magical talismans that keep shameful feelings and a shaming family at bay. These treatments work, like Roman fascini, to avoid the shaming eye/"I."*

Aggressive counterattacks are also part of the shame reaction and a protection against shameful tension. The angry actions involve acting-out and acting-in, that is, vengeful, shaming attacks on external and internal figures. In therapy, noncooperation, seduction, or suicide is a literal rubbing of the doctor's nose in the same shameful morass that s/he has been asked to clean up. Moreover, many individuals try to turn the tables on shame by flaunting their condition. Sue-Ann, for example, enjoyed being dismissed as an "hysteric" or a "schizophrenic." The outrageous behaviour enabled her to shame her parents and doctors and become more of a persecutor to them

*The fascinum was a little statuette of a phallus which the Romans used to wear around their necks to protect themselves from the evil eye.

than they were to her. During the withdrawn, silent periods she tried to accomplish the same thing by destroying her own feelings and thoughts. Her morbid self-annihilation represented a further shaming attack on hurtful inner images of herself and her parents.

Of course, aggressive flaunting measures are not limited to patients. Many people display their shameful feelings or thoughts or possessions for the same reasons, to discharge intolerable inner tensions and stick them somewhere else. When he wasn't hiding away, Sam used to pick his nose in public. He loved to watch others' discomfort. I have noticed that the daughter of a neighbor flaunts her messiness and greed whenever her mother deploys shame to control her. Adults do likewise when they ostentatiously flaunt established values in public. Instead of feeling ashamed by vulgarity or adultery, they splash it about, like neon advertisements. The whole point is to avoid shame by becoming the shamer and making others look bad. In this way, shame and envy act in tandem. *Shame rubs one's nose in the dirt, while envy rubs the dirt in one's nose.*

The practices I have outlined are concerned with protecting honor and pride from shameful attack. My discussion assumes that a person identifies with the wish to be good and feels vulnerable to activities and relationships, or insights and dreams, anything from the outer or inner worlds that might question his or her standards. Essentially the shamed or potentially shamed individual finds the awareness of destructive wishes and impulses to be unacceptably painful. I think that all shame, no matter how innocuous the provocation or issue, is unconsciously connected to a threatened exposure of the sinister side of the self, a side that hates life and revels in death. But there is an important variation of shame that delights in destruction and finds goodness disgraceful. This occurs in people who have dealt with an intolerable split between good and bad, and have turned around shame and envy, by dismissing goodness and identifying with the omnipotent, hateful side of their personality. Dr. Herbert Rosenfeld (1971) calls this phenomenon "destructive narcissism." He comments:

> The destructive narcissism of these patients appears often highly organized, as if one were dealing with a powerful gang dominated by a leader, who controls all the members

> of the gang to see that they support one another in making the criminal destructive work more effective and powerful. However, the narcissistic organization not only increases the strength of the destructive narcissism, but it has a defensive purpose to keep itself in power and so maintain *the status quo*. The main aim seems to be to prevent the weakening of the organization and to control the members of the gang so that they will not desert the destructive organization and join the positive parts of the self or betray the secrets of the gang to the police, the protecting super-ego, standing for the helpful analyst, who might be able to save the patient.

These people find shameful any indication that they are not bad. They experience the therapist as a persecutor whenever he threatens to unmask kernels of goodness. This is akin to a situation where a Hell's Angel would fear exposure for not being cruel enough, or a Nazi for not killing enough Jews. Patients who have identified with their criminal selves are notoriously difficult to treat, because they take any sign of therapeutic progress, any weakening of their criminality as extremely shameful, aside from being an insufferable affront to their sense of superiority.

In these circumstances the therapist has to be exceptionally sensitive to flurries of shame, to interpret them, and to try to nourish areas where the good side is beginning to flourish. He also has to tolerate the envious hatred that the patient feels toward him as the embodiment of the patient's own denied goodness. At best there may be periods without progress. But it is possible to sustain, if not create conditions where seemingly incorrigible people can flip over and reverse their destructive impulses. I think Sue-Ann did this of her own accord. She had begun to change even before she knew me. But by being attuned to her shame-filled past, and by articulating her present struggles, I enhanced the possibility of change and enabled her to cleanse old wounds.

Certainly an awareness of shame, of shameful tension and shaming attacks presages progress, not only in the chronically destructive narcissistic individual, but in all patients who, at some point, revert to this facade as a means of self-protection. Then we have to wait, and hope, and allow that a detailed exposure of the whole shaming system will enable goodness to reappear as the shame disappears.

## REFERENCES:


Aeschylus (1925). *Agamemnon* (G. Murray, Trans.; 1–35). London: Allen & Unwin.

Berke, J. (1982). An alternative sanctuary: The Arbours Crisis Centre. In U. Rueveni, R. Speck, & J. Speck (Eds.), *Therapeutic intervention: healing strategies for human systems* (pp. 33–57), New York: Human Sciences Press.

Berke, J. (1985). *Envy Loveth Not: A study of the original, influence and confluence of envy and narcissism. British Journal of Pyschotherapy, 1* (3): 171–186.

Chaucer, G. (1982). *The Canterbury Tales* (N. Coghill, Trans.) New York: Penguin.

Foster, G. (1952). The anatomy of envy. *Current Anthropology, 13* (2): 184.

Freud, S. (1957). Instincts and their vicissitudes. In J. Strachey (Ed. and Trans.), The *standard edition of the complete psychological works of Sigmund Freud* (Vol. 14, p. 138). London: Hogarth Press. (Original work published 1924)

Kant, I. (1922). Metaphysik der Sitten [The metaphysics of morals]. In K. Vorlander (Ed.), *Samtliche Werke* (Vol. 3, 4th ed.). Leipzig: (Original work published 1797).

Klein, M. (1975). Envy and gratitude. In *Envy and gratitude and other works 1946–1963*. (pp. 176–235). London: Hogarth Press. (Original work published 1957)

Restak, R. (1982). Newborn knowledge. *Science 82, 3* (1): 59–60.

Rosenfeld, H. (1971). A clinical approach to the psychoanalytic theory of the life and death instincts: An investigation into the aggressive aspects of narcissism. *International Journal of Psychoanalysis, 52*, (2): 174.

Segal, H. (1979). *Klein*. London: Fontana.

Sullivan, H. S. (1956). *Clinical studies in psychiatry*. New York: Norton.

13

# Shame and Domestic Violence

MELVIN R. LANSKY

*Shame makes some people withdraw and others attack. Lewis (1971) suggests that the difference lies in the degree to which one is willing or able to experience shame as an emotion—expressed shame acts as a social signal, allowing the one before whom we are embarrassed to recognize and accept our awareness; while unexpressed, blocked, or bypassed shame initiates a sequence which results in humiliated fury. It is this humiliated fury that powers shame–guilt cycles (Alexander, 1938; Piers and Singer, 1953) characterized by inhibition of an action (usually hostile but occasionally affectionate action); followed by a period of passivity and inaction (unexpressed shame); next by humiliated fury which seeks to reduce the accompanying feelings of incompetence; and finally by guilt—as punishment for this untoward action—with consequent inhibition of further action until the bypassed shame accompanying this passivity initiates the next cycle. Shame anger may be as benign as a door slammed after an argument or as malignant as murder.*

*I have found some correlation between parental attitudes toward shame and the later development of the many contrasting adult responses to shame; in general, people tend to respond pretty much in a way colored by their family of origin. Patients who flare up when embar-*

Melvin R. Lansky. Adjunct Professor of Psychiatry, UCLA Medical School; Staff Psychiatrist and Chief, Family Treatment Program, Brentwood V.A. Medical Center; Faculty, Los Angeles Psychoanalytic Institute.

*rassed frequently describe one parent as "like a tinder box," while those who are comfortable expressing their embarrassment grew up in a family system more characterized by banter than by destructive shaming attack. Given adequate provocation, however, most people can be goaded to anger.*

*Stable organizational systems, including successful marriages and families, generally involve what is best termed a "good fit" of personalities—constellations of attributes that (although not necessarily mature and optimally healthy) reinforce the strength of the union. Terms like "folie à deux," or "sadomasochistic relationship," or "an affirming marriage" convey this mutuality of defensive structure. And unstable relationships are just as likely to involve defensive systems that amplify the forces leading to destabilization.*

*Rarely do we get an opportunity to study marital chaos in such detail as offered herein by Lansky. A marriage about to splinter was frozen in time just long enough for Lansky to record and study the interaction at his Family Treatment Program. Lansky makes it clear that despite the intuitive stance that leads us to protect attachment and assist in the preservation of marriage, some unions are ill-fated simply because the defensive styles of the partners are irremediably mutually destructive. In this case, the wife felt more centered and at ease when attacking her husband's self-esteem; this inherently shaming attack ("I can sit there for 3 hours and listen. But I can't speak for about 1 minute before she steps on me, stomps, and I have to start all over.") duplicated the behavioral control techniques utilized by his Marine drill sargeant father. Further, she allowed him no opportunity to recover from the frequent episodes of humiliation to which he was prone, thus leaving no outlet for shame but humiliated fury ("It's almost like I have to hit her to get her attention") which functioned as a stimulus to further rage from the wife.*

*The abuse of power within the family, whether in the form of rape, incest, or battery is the legitimate concern of psychoanalytic investigation. Wherever there are levels of power, wherever there is distance in perceived power between participants in a system, there is the opportunity for shaming interaction. Lansky notes that when innate disparity in levels of power is compounded by the presence, in one or more members of the family system, of impairment in the degree of integration of the self, there is urgent need for therapeutic strategies that can reduce the propensity for violence.*

## INTRODUCTION

In this chapter, I will consider domestic violence in the light of the extreme vulnerability of the individuals involved, and in light of how vulnerability to narcissistic injury is handled within the attachment behaviors of such persons, that is, within the family. This is a point of view that encompasses both individual dynamics and a family systems perspective. The problem of domestic violence will be looked at in terms of tendencies of the personalities involved to disorganize and of the collusive defensive operations that are those persons' attempts to minimize the chaotic effects of those vulnerabilities.

I am assuming, then, that in a marriage characterized by overt violence where violent episodes are repeated, *both* spouses usually have a high vulnerability to personality disorganization and, as a result, have to deal with a great deal of shame that floods them not only when they become aware of this lack of cohesion, but also when they become aware of the maneuvers in close relationship that they use to hide it. Persons with such vulnerability have sought out spouses with similar personality organization who are available for collusive relationships that keep the marital system from being flooded with shame. Within such relationships, complex regulatory maneuvers that I have previously called pathologic distance regulation (Lansky, 1985) keep persons within the family from getting too close or too far away, and thus risking personality disorganization and the attendant amplification of shame.

## NARCISSISTIC VULNERABILITY IN THE FAMILY

In previous writings on narcissistic vulnerability in family systems, I have attempted to delineate the clinical phenomenology of pathologic distance regulation within collusive relations (Lansky, 1981, 1984). Seemingly chaotic behaviors or emotional absences are invariably found to have complex regulatory effects on the family. Personality disorganization and attendant shame is often minimized, or at least made tolerable, by adjusting distance among intimates to a reasonably comfortable level, one that is neither too close nor too far away, and by restoring control over the situation to the participants in these defensive operations. I will comment briefly on defensive maneuvers typified by blaming (Lansky, 1980), by pathological preoccupation (Lansky, 1985), and by impulsive action (Lansky, unpublished).

In marriages dominated by blaming transactions, verbal conflict is characteristically at the forefront of the couple's activities. Often some transgression by a spouse serves both as a precipitant to disorganization in the blamer and a provocation to blame. Such blaming attacks may be precipitated by major transgressions or by events so small as exclusion from a conversation, or other types of seemingly mild narcissistic injury. Underneath the apparent chaos seen in blaming transactions is a tightly bound, cohesive dyad, guarded by the blaming transactions themselves from too much intimacy, on the one hand, and from too much distance on the other.

The blaming transaction conveys to the blamed person that they have hurt, let down, deserted, or abandoned the blamer. Such transactions carry with them the implication that the blamed person could, if s/he only would, be a perfectly satisfactory person. In that sense, despite tumult and hostility, both the blamer and the blamed person may feel a greatly enhanced sense of power during the act of blame; the blamer by the discharge of the self-righteous accusatory attack, and the blamed person by the attribution of near-omnipotent power in the attributions of the blamer. This sense of enhanced power is in striking contrast to the overt shaming that takes place in relationships that involve domestic violence.

Overt shaming, as opposed to blaming, has a deviation-amplifying effect on the family system. Defects, instead of being hidden in the marital system are exposed by it; and the dyad, instead of being a refuge from humiliation, is the source of it.

Relationships characterized by pathologic preoccupation involve some person or persons whose activities are felt by the family system to confer great prestige or promise on the family. These persons are emotionally absent even when physically present, the absence usually rationalized as preoccupation with the prestigious activity. This kind of emotional absence is often found to precipitate a great deal of depression, blaming, and impulsive action in other members of the family. Families so organized often have several members with high vocational attainment and a great deal of responsibility in their relationships outside of the family.

Collusive systems organized around impulsive action in one of its members are often found to have a specific regulatory structure. Often, the impulsive actor, that is, an overdoser, binge drinker, slasher, or sexually uncontrolled person, is found to act impulsively following some sort of change in a relationship. That change is usually some sort of a narcissistic wound, that is to say, an experience of disorganization when intimates either become too close or too far away.

What follows this precipitating experience is some type of personality disorganization which may be consciously experienced as an uneasy or paranoid prodromal phase, or may not be consciously noticed at all. The prodrome is followed by the impulsive act itself, which often has an organizing effect on people, for example, by spreading fear of suicide or violence or desertion, or loss of control. Often this sort of control over distance is exercised without actual harm being done. Such impulsive acts are often followed by waves of guilt that serve, among other things, to take attention away from disorganization in the disorganized or prodromal period. Impulsive action often has a regulatory effect on intimates, reorganizing them, sometimes by intimidation, sometimes for other reasons in a protective array around the impulsive actor, so that again they are neither too close nor too far away.

I hope to extend this line of investigation to the family system characterized by domestic violence. I will consider the problem both in terms of extreme narcissistic vulnerability in the spouses themselves, and in terms of the failure of collusive defensive operations in which that narcissistic vulnerability lodges. Domestic violence is here viewed as a type of impulsive action, but unlike the type of impulsive action that merely intimidates and so reorganizes intimates, domestic violence fails both to restore a feeling of control to those in the system and to keep those persons relatively safe. My attempt will be to get a view of the problem that will be of use no matter what treatment strategies are actually decided on.

In marital systems characterized by habitual domestic violence, shame dynamics are of central importance. Unlike the collusive operations typified by blame, pathologic preoccupation, and intimidating (as opposed to actually violent) impulsive action, transactions in marriages characterized by domestic violence are typified by maneuvers that sharply increase shame in the system, that is, by *overt humiliation* as a typical transactional mode. Such deliberate humiliation shows up prominently in the family history of at least one spouse, and disposes that person to a sensitivity to humiliation; in the transactions of the spouses as they deal with each other; and often in the experience both spouses have of the therapist's comments. The volatility of the system can better be understood in light of the shame dynamics, that is, in light of the erosion of a marital defensive system organized around minimizing shame by transactions within the marriage that actually amplify shame.

## A CASE IN DETAIL

In this discussion I will deal entirely with material drawn from one case. In so doing, I am fully aware of the dangers of overgeneralizing. I do not presume that every case of domestic violence is like the present one. Nonetheless, I think enough of the pertinent dynamic material is in evidence to make the detailed case material valuable. Any attempts to generalize the results are of course at risk, unless further studies or extensive clinical experience give independent testimony to the accuracy of such generalizations.

I have presented a very detailed case for several reasons; first, because many aspects of the case that portray both individual and systems dynamics have to be appreciated to gain a clear view of the way in which interlocking character pathology is the problem, and not something simpler such as troublesome behavior or uncontrolled impulse. Second, because treatment of these volatile emergency situations is difficult to conceptualize and involves more than one modality. Containment by hospitalization, medication, protective custody, or shelter usually are short-term measures and may have to accompany more long-term strategic therapy aimed at the shame-amplifying transactions that are usually woven into the fabric of the relationship. Any treatment approach, then, will be drawn from a complex array of possibilities. Only a detailed, perspicacious grasp of the interlocking of individual and systems dynamics together with an appreciation of how shame dynamics pervade the relationship will be suitable for the formation of overall strategies to address the problem.

## CASE ILLUSTRATION

The case material consists of four interviews with a husband and wife. The man, Mario, is 32. His wife, Anna, is 46. They were referred on an emergency basis to the Family Treatment Program, an inpatient psychiatric unit, after they appeared for consultation. Mario had struck Anna three times in the last week. This was the first violent episode, the first time in their marriage of 6 months and relationship of a year and a half. Both were horrified; both came to the hospital wanting emergency intervention, and both wanted him hospitalized. The initial interview was to decide on the advisability of hospitalization, and took place in an open staff interview.

### *SESSION 1*

The couple came in, and both commented on the presence of other staff together with the interviewer. The therapist inquired what the difficulties were. Anna spoke first. She mentioned in a tearful way that she was frightened, and spoke of Mario's being out of control. Mario had humiliated her. Driving to church, she had seen him driving the other way with another woman in a car that she had bought for him. He had not been home the previous evening. As she described this beginning of the week that culminated in the violent episodes, she noted flippantly, "He does not work." She went on to speak of some of the marital difficulties, and then a little bit about her own background. She had had several previous marriages. She went on to describe one with an older man, by whom she had two children. He could not satisfy her sexually, but despite the long time since the divorce he still supports her. Then she married a younger man, an alcoholic. "Mario doesn't drink," but she hastened to add, "He doesn't work either. At least Paul worked." Her commentaries on Mario and the other two husbands were peppered with disparaging remarks, either about sexual inadequacy, drinking, or lack of working. She described briefly the family in which she was born. Her mother, she said, had yelled a lot. There were seven children. Anna was the sixth. Father avoided facing problems in the marriage constantly. He drank. He let her down all the time. He couldn't face things at all. She, Anna, had almost always sided with her mother in the marital disputes. She was unhappy at home and ran away from home.

The therapist then turned to Mario for his thoughts.

*Excerpt 1*

THERAPIST: "What's your view of the marriage?"

MARIO: "Of our present marriage. We don't share, either one of us or the other. I can come out with an idea which is probably a good one, but she looks at it and says it's a pipe dream."

THERAPIST: "As you say it, the wind gets knocked out of your sails."

MARIO: "Yeah. Anna says I don't follow through on things, but she's going to knock it right from the beginning. If she's going to do that, what chance does it have to begin with. It has no chance of succeeding, if she's not going to back me with it. She's got to be able to sit down there and talk to me and say, 'It looks like a good idea, but maybe this won't work out of it, or maybe that won't work out of it.' We've never had those kinds of discussions over any ideas I've had."

ANNA: "Can I interject?"

The therapist stops her from interjecting, but assures her that she will have her turn later. Mario goes on to speak of his broken line of thinking, and of Anna's disorganizing effect on him.

*Excerpt 2*

MARIO: "We don't communicate as well as we could. It's funny. We've had three physical confrontations, break-down, knock-down, drag-out fights."

THERAPIST: "Why with this marriage?"

MARIO: "Because Anna seems to have a talent for pushing buttons that make me go. . . . Nobody's been able to get to those buttons before because I always protected them very well. With Anna I'm much more open in that area. I'm much more emotional with her than I ever would get with anybody else . . . I know what can set me off. Unfortunately, she does too."

ANNA: "I don't realize it."

THERAPIST: "Well, if you can tell me, then she'll have a chance to listen. Perhaps we'll have something to work on."

MARIO: "Okay. Anna and I, you know, had an affair before my marriage was ended."

ANNA: "You were separated and divorcing." (*Mario becomes flushed.*)

THERAPIST: "What happened just now?"

MARIO: "She aggravated me because she stepped in."

THERAPIST: "You look furious at her. Do you feel that way?"

MARIO: "Yes I do. She stepped in. She stepped all over what I was trying to say. She's broken a train of thought."

THERAPIST: "Is that at all typical of what goes on between the two of you?"

MARIO: "Yes. Very much so."

THERAPIST: "Let's stick to that for a moment . . . If Anna doesn't know what she's doing, or you can't put it exactly in words, this way she'll have a chance to hear. When you started to talk, and said you had an affair before the divorce, she spoke up and said that actually you were separated, and you looked furious."

MARIO: "I looked furious because I was angry about it. She does this constantly. I mean it's a matter of I can sit there for 3 hours and listen. But I can't speak for about 1 minute before she steps on me, stomps, and I have to start all over. And she can go, like in the car on the way here today, she kept saying this and saying this and saying this and . . ."

ANNA: "Mario, I'm at my end, honey, I've broken down, I've had it."

MARIO: "That's what I mean, she can't keep her mouth shut. I say, 'Anna please stop! You've made your point, don't repeat it.' From the end of that sentence to the time she repeated it you couldn't measure with a stop watch . . . That's exactly how I feel. I can't make a point with her, but it seems that after every time we have a physical confrontation she's willing to shut up, back off, let me talk and let me say what I've got to say. It's almost like I have to hit her to get her attention . . . I feel like it's every time that something has to be done it has to be done when Anna wants it done. I'd like to see where I go with my own talents and abilities and thoughts."

When the therapist inquired whether this was a lifelong difficulty, Mario went on straightaway to talk abut his own upbringing. Mario's father was a Marine drill sergeant, a career soldier who had deliberately put him in humiliating situations.

*Excerpt 3*

MARIO: "He'd come in in the middle of the afternoon and say, 'Well we're going down to the post. I'd say well, let me change clothes. He'd say, no, no, that's what you're wearing, wear it, go on. He made me feel like an idiot. . . . He didn't know how to handle a kid this high when he was used to handling 18-year-olds on the drill field and using that kind of thing on them. They understood it, why couldn't I? But I wasn't old enough to understand it. Now I'm at the age I'm at, I can look at what he did and say,"He really didn't do that badly, he just picked the wrong age to do it to me.' "

THERAPIST: "What effect do you think it had on you? Has it spilled into your marital problems?"

MARIO: "I got so that in school I'd take a piece of paper out of a notebook, and if it had a speck of dirt on it I'd throw it away because it wasn't neat enough, and that's ridiculous. Then as I got older I went to just the opposite. I don't really give a damn. Anna will tell me, 'You need a haircut.' I don't need a haircut. In my estimation, I won't need a haircut for at least 3 weeks. Maybe 4."

THERAPIST: "You don't need a drill sergeant to tell you you need a haircut."

The therapist, feeling that the situation was by no means resolved, during the interview inquired about hospitalization. Both Anna and Mario wanted Mario to be hospitalized.

## *SESSION 2*

(*A week later, in private in the therapist's office.*) The couple both tell the therapist how unsettling it has been to open things up and at the same time leave them unfinished. Anna resents Mario's getting therapy on the ward, and wants some herself. Mario brings up how confusing it is and how difficult it is to have things opened up and so little time to finish with them. Anna then mentions that she hadn't told him about two other marriages prior to the one with the older man. The first was when she was 15. Mario, then, is her fifth husband.

They began arguing about whether or not he should have friends that were just his and not both of theirs. Anna then brought up the fact that he had had six jobs in the preceding year.

*Excerpt 4*

ANNA: "He's had six jobs this year and six jobs last year. There's no reason for it. There are one or two reasons, and it's not all home problems. Either he is not experienced enough, or he's—or his emotional problems have affected his ability to work. He hasn't been easy to get along with. I can't carry everything if he's not working somewhere. I can carry if he's working somewhere and getting, you know, maybe a small salary, but if he's not getting anywhere, or if he's not being educated, he's not getting anywhere either, it would be very nice if he could get into some kind of training where he could draw something or get benefits while he's being trained. I don't think he can hold a job. We've talked about it, we've gone through it. He gets jobs easily and loses them all the time. This has gone til it hurts him, it hurts me, and hurts the marriage."

THERAPIST: "I guess you feel that if he doesn't work you're doing all the work, or that he lets you down all the time. You, on the other hand, Mario, might be very upset by all this criticism and feeling very picked on, feeling there is no way out. How can you do something that matters right now? Where are you both now?"

MARIO: "You pretty well explained where I'm at."

ANNA: "You pretty well explained where I was. Mario came

to me practically from his other wife and moved into my house and I kept carrying things, and by the time we got married—before we got married—I co-signed a loan because my credit was good and his wasn't. And I'm stuck with that loan. And I'm making payments on cars because Mario's here and not working, and it's getting to be a little more than even I can handle. You know, the house and everything. At least with Mario here, while it doesn't help a heck of a lot economically speaking, it helps. . . ."

MARIO: "I'd like to be able to contribute. I'd also like to be able to work at something. I worked at retail for 6 years. I'm good at it. But I don't like it. You get the position where you're in between somebody above wanting something done one way and a customer wanting to do it another way. You get caught in that all the time, and if you're not extremely stable in all other aspects of your life, you're really in a stress pattern, and I'm not very fond of that."

THERAPIST: "I'm getting a feeling, Mario, that it's a little more complicated than that you don't like it. You feel really trapped, as I'm hearing it, and you feel you need to produce an income, but then are forced to put up with so many indignities that you won't be able to do anything that matters. That's what I thought I heard."

MARIO: "Yeah, you heard it pretty good. You see, as a mechanic everything you do has a purpose. Nobody bothers you, and you do it. They come and say this needs to be done, and you do it. Take the car out, and that's it. Nobody comes and looks over your shoulder, and the customer isn't allowed there. You do it, get it done, and get rid of it."

THERAPIST: "So that line of work, rather than a people-centered kind of thing, is much more suited to your personality, because where you deal with the public and deal with a supervisor and everything gangs up on you, I take it, it's just the wrong fit for you."

MARIO: "If I feel like telling the brake lining to go to hell, I do that. There's nobody around to worry about whether I said it in front of the wrong person."

In the midst of Mario beginning to talk about how humiliated he is in the job situation, Anna interrupts to correct him. The therapist intervenes, but she continues.

*Excerpt 5*

ANNA: "What you have heard from Mario and what I have lived with Mario for over a year are two different things. He wants to start at the top. Everybody would like to, but unfortunately everybody doesn't get to. Mario, you know, last week he was talking about his ideas. Every time he has an idea he brings it up, and I squash it. Unfortunately, he doesn't carry these ideas out and so he comes and puts them on me because I've got the credit and I can go on and say hey, I'd like to borrow some more money to put him in business. We'd only been married a very short time and he wanted me to start a business with him but he wouldn't carry through with it. He would just be, you know, because Mario doesn't carry through. He's got a lot to learn. He's got to go out and work and he's got to make a minimum pay for a while, and then go slowly. You just can't reach for it and it's going to be there. It's just not going to be there that fast. Mario has a wonderful mind, he has ideas, great ideas. But he doesn't know how to put them through without me, and I can't help him. I can't handle that part of the marriage."

MARIO: "Okay, let me make a comment on that. First of all, you don't know what the hell I've done for the last 20 years of my life. You don't know what kind of training I have, whether I can handle a job or not. You don't have any idea." (*Shouting.*)

THERAPIST: "Mario, that really hurt you, when she said that."

MARIO: "Yeah, it knocked the shit out of me, as a matter of fact, because she has no idea what kind of training I've got, how I've dealt with people, what business experience I've developed. Hell, I've handled six or seven thousand dollars and come out only a few cents off in the cash register."

ANNA: "That's an accountant's job."

MARIO: "No it isn't, it's a manager's job to do that. What the hell do you mean, it's an accountant's job. (*Shouting*) I've made schedules for people that covered a goddamn month at a time, 7 days a week, 24 hours a day, with nine people, and had everybody happy."

THERAPIST: "You sound so angry and put down. Do you feel that way?"

MARIO: "Yes, I feel that way. She still doesn't know what the hell I'm capable of doing. She has no idea what my experience levels are, and she'll sit there and say that I'd better crawl before I can walk, and I've heard my father say that all my goddamn life."

THERAPIST: "The drill sergeant again."

MARIO: "Yeah."

ANNA: "All right, let's go back to the mechanics, okay?"

THERAPIST: "Is this typical of what you get into in the marriage? You know, he's so hurt that no matter how much truth there is in what you're saying, nothing's going to get done right here unless we understand how you both feel, and work with that for a while. Because I think you're so hurt, Mario, by what she's saying, that the content's going to get lost. (*To Anna*) Do you follow what I'm saying? He's going to hear it like his father telling him he's not good enough."

ANNA: "All right. Why should I have to work, wash dirty, greasy clothes because he won't take the time to do them, and put up with this when he's going to think he's too good for the job anyway, and quit it or walk out or fool around and get fired over something silly. I don't really think he's all that incapable. I think a lot of it is his attitude. He walked out on a couple of bosses and didn't even give notice. You don't do that on a job—you can't. People can't live with themselves and build up anything out of life doing things like that and then running."

Anna fulminates about Mario's irresponsibility. The therapist interrupts, and attempts to get the focus onto their anxieties and their method of communicating them. He inquires of Mario what he would like from Anna to help him, even when she disagrees and even when she is very firm in feeling that he's wrong. Toward the end of the session both Anna and Mario turn to the therapist for the solution to their difficulties, expressing resentment that their problems were just thrown back on them. Anna again stated that she wanted her own therapist. Both were upset and angry with the therapist for opening up hostilities and leaving them vulnerable when the session ended. The therapist empathized with this plight and agreed to make inquiries concerning an individual therapist for Anna.

just an off-day for me, or maybe I just—Why are you so sensitive to my criticism anyway?"

At this point the therapist interrupted, noting Mario's anger, and asked if this sort of interaction were typical—Anna vehemently pointing to Mario's irresponsibility, and Mario feeling totally disorganized by her so doing. They both agreed. The therapist went on to explore with Mario what ways might be that Anna could make him feel supported and still have her own opinions, even differing with him. Mario implored to be allowed to make his own mistakes. Anna started to interrupt, but the therapist instructed her to listen, to get an understanding of him, and to rest assured that her point of view would also be discussed. He again talks of his sensitivity and of his humiliation-proneness.

*Excerpt 7*

MARIO: "It's sometimes difficult for a person to learn from another person's mistakes. Now, she's assuming that I've been through all these things before and I've made these mistakes and I know how it's going to go and there's no sense in doing it that way because I've done it that way before. . . . What I'm saying, what I would like her to do is shut up and let me make my own mistakes . . ."

ANNA: "But you haven't. . . ."

MARIO: " . . . A lot of movement within my framework, the one I'm living in, to have the opportunity either to become what I want, or falling down the tubes, one or the other. . . . I'm not a real easy person to give criticism to."

ANNA: "You can say that again."

MARIO: "I don't particularly care for it. Number one, because I have succeeded in a number of things that other people have not succeeded in trying the same damn thing. It may not have been a job. It may have been way of doing something that they didn't learn. You know, like everybody all through school told me that if you didn't study, you'll never pass. And I didn't, but I carried a B-plus average all through school, with a 90% comprehension rate. And I have a 95% retention rate of anything I read or hear."

ANNA: "So you should be in college, then."

MARIO: (*Yelling*) "Probably I should, but that's beside the point."

The therapist tries to calm Mario and to link the current turmoil in the discussion to Mario's history of debunkings from his father.

THERAPIST: "I understand what you don't like about what she does. Tell me what you would like her to do."

MARIO: "No, no. What I'm saying, what I would like her to do is shut up and let me make my own mistakes."

THERAPIST: "Well, specifically, if you decide you want to go to real estate school. . . ."

MARIO: (*Interrupting*) ". . . and if it turns out to be a mistake, at least I made the decision and it wasn't a compromise on my part."

ANNA: "But you haven't."

MARIO: "Between what I wanted and what she wanted."

THERAPIST: "Let me interrupt. Let Mario and I talk, and then you and I will talk, and that way the two of you will both have a chance to listen without preparing your argument, and you'll each be assured that you'll get a chance to talk, too. I get a sense it's very difficult to resolve things. You both keep ending up in the same stalemate. So, (*to Mario*) she should appreciate that you need to have your space, so to speak, and to make your own mistakes, or at least to have enough. . . ."

MARIO: "A lot of movement within my framework, the one I'm living in, to have the opportunity either to become a success or what I want, what my idea is, or falling down the tubes, one or the other."

THERAPIST: "And I guess we know from our previous talks, I'm sure she knows better than I, that you are very sensitized to debunking comments from your father and that you are very vulnerable to that. . . ."

MARIO: (*Interrupting*) "You know what the greatest pleasure in my whole life was? My father was a crack shot with a pistol and a rifle, and the greatest pleasure in my whole life was he was firing his pistol and I took the pistol and left-handedly beat him. It was the greatest—that shining hour . . . because everytime I had picked up a weapon he said, 'You're handling it wrong, you don't know what you're doing.' The man's an expert no doubt about it. He can take any one of the military makes, take it apart and put it back together, and fire it. But the shining hour of my life was when I beat him left-handedly." (*Calms*)

THERAPIST: "But you talk very much as though being told what's good for you isn't really advice, it's a method of undermining you and knocking the wind out of your sails, and putting you in your place."

MARIO: "Yeah. That can't be done that way or this way, or I don't think anybody's done it. I don't think you can do that, a lot of that."

THERAPIST: "Would you agree that you're quite sensitive to every sort of advice given that way."

MARIO: "Yeah, I'm very sensitive to it."

THERAPIST: "And your wife gets a fair amount of that sensitivity."

The therapist had a chance to draw their attention to the process between them by labeling their mutual reactivity as one major problem between them. They began to talk about their communicating, and in particular about Mario's need to feel heard, and finish his line of thinking, especially if this would not endanger Anna's right to disagree with him. Mario was calmed greatly by the process, but Anna, far from drawing her attention to the process in the marriage and calming her anxieties about losing her point of view, seeming fired to even more criticism about Mario's half-baked ideas. She seemed oblivious to his escalating shame and anger, and continued talking about his inability to follow through with anything. The therapist again tried to mediate. Anna talked about her own needs and how much he had let her down. Mario talked more about the process and how it disorganized him.

Near the end of the session the therapist noted that both seemed to be a long way from feeling safe with the other's point of view. Mario talked angrily of her excluding him from a big part of her life. She said that he meant the way she invested and spent her money given to her by her third husband to provide for the children. She had kept the money separately and followed that man's advice to keep Mario out of the arrangements. It wasn't community property. Mario began shouting. The therapist closed with a vain attempt to get them to look at the process and understand what their anxieties were.

## *SESSION 4*

(*Three weeks later*) In this session the therapist, recently returned, hears for the first time that Mario's demands for more and more passes from the ward are presenting a management problem. Anna began the session angrily, again saying that she had nobody to talk to, that she called in angrily and was written up as an angry person. Mario said jeeringly that she was written up as a drunken person. She talked angrily about the hospital pass on which he played bridge with the other woman. Another argument about his refusal to join her at a dance class ensued. Mario said that the level of the class was too advanced for him, and the mutual anger mounted.

The therapist commented that Mario seemed to be setting himself up to leave angrily, both in the session and with his behavior on the ward. Mario then petulantly challenged the need to be in the hospital. He wasn't getting any medications, he wasn't being helped. The therapist commented on the fact that there was less and less structure, more and more passes, more and more anger, more confusion and provocation. Mario asked again why he had to be in the hospital. The therapist noted that the original reasons were first for protection, and also for therapy, and then inquired about Mario's anger, wondering if it wasn't what he had felt in other situations, on jobs and in the marriage. Mario talked about being very offended and insulted and humiliated by these limits.

When he started to feel calmer talking about this, Anna interrupted, saying that it was her feeling that he should stay in the hospital and get no passes whatsoever. He screamed that she should be locked up in a place for alcoholics. A furor developed between them. Mario turned to the therapist and asked about a form applying for disability benefits that he had given to the therapist shortly before. The therapist asked whether or not he thought he was disabled. Mario proceeded to blame Anna for his difficulties, and an argument ensued between them. Mario turned back to the therapist and asked what the therapist thought was wrong with him. The therapist said that he saw Mario's personality as such that he became chaotic without structure, and that he became very resentful if structure was applied, and that that difficulty caused him difficulties in many areas: jobs, marriages, and now even the hospital.

The therapist continued that the vulnerabilities and lability might suggest a kind of depression. Mario was furious at this, and asked the therapist to justify the diagnosis, saying that he was upset at the idea of medication. The therapist clarified that any medication would be optional, but might help with his vulnerability and disorganization. Mario vented fury at Anna, saying that he couldn't have a normal life because of her.

*Excerpt 8*

MARIO: "You know why I'm angry?" Because she's using the hospital as a way of keeping me out of a normal life structure right now."

ANNA: "That's not true. You life should be here. You should be here. You're a patient."

MARIO: "She's telling me I should be in the hospital when I don't really feel I should be, and she's using it as a wedge between us, and I'm not going to allow that. Either we're going to have a marriage or we're not going to have a marriage, but we're not going to have a half-marriage."

ANNA: "Well, we had a half-marriage before because you laid all the responsibility on me. You said that you needed structure to get up and go to work. Well, honey, I had to get you up. The responsibility was on me every morning to get you up. That alarm went off for an hour before you'd get out of bed, and with me yelling at you. I was the one at you every morning, yelling, 'Mario, get out of bed.' That was the way every day started. Let's talk about your job."

MARIO: "Okay, let's talk about it."

ANNA: "Okay, you're going into an unstructured job, you're going to be your own boss. I've seen you in a job. The day we married I started you. Monday, you went into an unstructured salesmanship job and you blew it, babe, because you went down and gambled. You weren't taking care of business, and so instead of quitting you just left. You know, I mean you left on really bad terms. Okay, this is the type of person you are now. All right, we laid out the money which we couldn't afford to give you another chance at another job because you're not making with the mechanics. I'm going to sit by, and I'm going to watch, and see how you do with that, and hope to God you don't blow it."

Anna went on to talk about how poorly he did at unstructured jobs. Mario got back to the disability. The therapist pointed out that there seemed to be two ideas in his head that didn't go with each other. One, that he was disorganized and upset and very needy of help and disability and relief from responsibility, but also that he was very patronized, manipulated, and humiliated by people telling him that he could not come and go as he pleased when he was perfectly capable of it. The therapist thought that Mario had great difficulty in figuring out in his own mind what to do with those notions of himself. Mario became defiant on the matter of continued hospitalization. Anna said that she refused to have him home if he signed out. Mario became more and more furious and asked why he had to be here, and a furor ensued between Anna and Mario. The therapist hoped that Mario wouldn't feel he had to leave just because Anna said that he must stay. An appointment time was set for the following week, and the session ended. Mario left the hospital on the next day, and did not return.

## *THE STRUCTURE OF DOMESTIC VIOLENCE*

Domestic violence, as I have noted above, is a kind of impulsive action. But the kind of domestic violence here considered is a type of impulsive action where impulsivity does not take place in the context of a system that can absorb and minimize the disorganization, impulsivity, and reorganization that follow narcissistic wounding. With intensely humiliation-prone individuals so constituted that they provoke shame, habitually shame others, and react strongly to being shamed, the collusive marital system amplifies each spouse's vulnerabilities rather than minimizing them. Distance regulation, that is, the reorganization of the system around a *safe* distance among intimates, fails, leaving both spouses ashamed, powerless, and aware at some level of their basic destructiveness within relationships. The collusive relationship has basically failed to bind and absorb narcissistic vulnerability within the system in such a way as to minimize the sense of shame.

I will attempt to get perspective on the case material from the point of view of the structure of impulsive action within a collusive relationship. These features include vulnerability to personality disorganization; a precipitating event; the prodrome or experience of disorganization; the act itself; emotional reactions to the act; and a distance-regulating effect. Mario, the "violent" person, will receive somewhat more emphasis than will Anna; nevertheless, her role in the destructive relationship is evident. I will make some comparisons between the type of violent impulsive action here illustrated and more cohesive types of collusive relationships, that is, blaming transactions.

1. *The tendency to personality disorganization:* Beneath his bluster and his considerable verbal dexterity, Mario's extreme narcissistic vulnerability, that is, his tendency to disorganize, is evident in a number of areas. The consequences of this tendency are convincing in his history of job losses and marital failures. Another dimension emerges from his vividly recollected history of humiliation at the hands of his father. He defends against this humiliation with a kind of characterologic swagger and provocativeness that is evident in Excerpt 6. The neediness and disorganization are evident throughout the case material, but especially at the beginning and at the end of Session 2 which show in both spouses, a neediness and a shame over it that is not relieved in any useful way by the marital system. Anna's vulnerability is also evidenced by a history of five marriages, all of them devalued in some way. Her method of handling her own shame is to disorganize, debunk, and shame the other person. Her neediness is also apparent throughout.

2. *Precipitant:* The circumstances that cause events to escalate to the point of violence are prominent in both spouses. Mario's provocativeness is first talked about in the episode described in the first session, his being seen by his wife with another woman in the car that Anna had bought for him; later it

shows up by his provoking limits on the ward and by his presenting a constant and inconsistent array of plans to his wife. Noteworthy throughout the transcript is Anna's style of expressing her anxieties and criticism (however well founded) in a manner that disorganizes, humiliates, and publicly shames. Mario is able to talk about this time after time in many of the excerpts. When Mario is wounded by some remark, talk about the process and clarification calms him down rather easily, and when he is able to feel understood talking about the process, he is able to calm down and admit his responsibility in the difficulties, and proceed to talk constructively. When he talks to Anna, however, his disorganization is compounded, and his line of thinking and sense of an organized self scarcely lasts more than a few sentences.

3. *The prodrome* is the disrupted state of disorganization that precedes an impulsive act. Such a state may be experienced as confusing, eerie, or persecutory, or may not be in conscious awareness at all. Mario's ability to talk about his experience of disorganization, and the amplification of this in the process between Anna and himself gives a good view of the broken line of thought resulting from the overt shaming transaction. This is evident in Excerpts 2, 4, 5, and 6. The degree of overt disorganization is much more than is usually seen, for example, with couples who blame. Blaming couples often give the implication in their accusatory outbursts that the blamed person *could* do almost anything if s/he only *would*. However unpleasant they may be, blaming transactions are usually not overtly shaming.

4. *The act* itself is most strongly characterized by the fact that actual harm was done. Both spouses feel frightened, out of control, and weak. This is in sharp contrast to blaming transactions in which the blamer feels self-righteous and powerful, and the transgressor who is blamed is also accused in a certain way of being very powerful. The blamed person feels wronged, perhaps, but not frightened, humiliated, and disintegrated in public. The result of the act of actual violence (as opposed to intimidation transactions with the threat of violence) is that both Mario and Anna feel weak, out of control, frightened, and more ashamed.

5. *Reaction to the act:* Very often with an impulsive actor,

for example, a binge drinker or a pathological gambler, there is some guilt expressed over what has been done—some genuine concern for the other. This guilt may be of such intensity that it overshadows the disorganization and accompanying shame. But Mario's reaction to the act is much more aimed at buttressing his shameful sense of self. He says in a passage shortly after Excerpt 3:

*Excerpt 9*

MARIO: "Well, it's like I never really had a temper that manifested itself in violence. I had a temper where I yelled a lot, but I never am aware of my size. I'm six feet three—I can take a pipe and bend it into a pretzel with my wrist. I can take a can that's closed—a soda can that's closed—I'm right-handed, and with my left hand pop it open. So I know what kind of power I generate with my physique and size and weight, and I hesitate to use this."

Mario's reaction to his loss of control is a certain amount of fright and wish to exert control, but no real concern, not even temporarily, for Anna. His guilt is voiced in a kind of amazement of his own power, not as a sense of pain on having harmed a love object. He covers over weakness with even more provocativeness. Neither spouse seem to have moments when they are protective of each other and concerned about the other.

6. *Pathologic distance regulation:* The totality of these factors add up to a failure of effective defensive operations in the collusive relationship. That is to say, the act itself, far from reorganizing the marital system in the way that blame and intimidating impulsive action do, tears the system apart, and gives the spouses' lack of confidence in the protectiveness offered by the marriage itself. This security is a common feature of the other types of defensive operations that I have described: in blaming transactions, the blamer and the blamed are locked in a self-righteous transaction which may have a tremendous emotional cost, but actually binds the system securely together. The preoccupied person who is physically present but emotionally absent may bind the system together by supplying enormous reliability and prestige to the system even if family members'

emotional needs are not met. The impulsive actor may organize rescuers or those intimidated by the impulsive act so that the system persists or even reorganizes. Not so with the present case of actual violence. The sense of shame and the vulnerabilities are too intense to be bound by the defensive activities that can be handled by the maneuvers of blame, preoccupation, and impulsive action. The defenses simply are not powerful enough to deal with the overwhelming amount of vulnerability. There is a failure of effective regulation of a safe distance to intimates and a basic failure of restitution, that is, of the way back to objects after the process of detachment that follows personality disorganization.

## IMPLICATIONS FOR TREATMENT

In this case, the act of overt violence within the marriage can be seen as a failure of restitution, a failure of people to bind together in a protective collusive system. There is too much vulnerability, too much shame generation, too much reactivity, too much humiliation-proneness, too much overt shaming, and too much shameful disorganization and provocation for the system to absorb. Too many shame-producing features are present that must be bound in the system, so the narcissistic vulnerability spills over as provocation on the part of Mario and overt shaming on the part on Anna. They are underscored in the history of her marital failures and his job failures. The couple as a unit is too busy with internal turmoil to maintain any sort of directed purposive activity, within the marriage or outside of it. This chaos goes far beyond what can be contained even with the high-cost defensive operations that are seen in blaming and preoccupied families, and even those with habitual intimidating impulsive action. Shame in the therapeutic process, that is in relation to the therapist, is seen in the beginning and end of Session 2, and mounting in Mario's whole relationship to the ward, evidenced at the end of Session 4.

The presence of so much shame in the system has vast implications for treatment. Drawing attention to shame does not minimize it: this is not true of guilt, which is often based on an exaggerated phantasy of the effects of one's actions or hostilities. The shame when one appears disorganized, defective, and out of control in the presence of the other is not based simply on fantasied aggressions or attack or hurt. Humiliation tends to be about genuine deficits and to feed on itself. Mario is provocative. He has incompatible views of himself, one as perfectly competent and merely misunderstood, and the other as genuinely damaged and in need of help. His provocativeness and swagger in relationships where he is dependent put his employers and those in helping relations to him in a position where they must set limits. Such limits humiliate him even further. When Mario's difficulties combine with his wife's pathologic propensity to disorganize and inflict shame, the tension in the system escalates to the point where the system flies apart, fails to offer security or a sense of specialness or power, and eventuates in violence.

This case, with its vulnerable spouses exerting an undermining effect on each other's integrity, demonstrates a type of marital bonding that is both incohesive and dangerous. The spouses have a more ominous prognostic status than do those who can bond to form stable protective family systems, even if those systems come at a high emotional cost. Persons who can become part of families with blame, pathologic preoccupation, or intimidating impulsive action as organizing transactions have a better prognosis than those described here. These patients prognostically are closer to those who later in their careers as psychiatric patients present as solitary "borderline" patients with families that refuse to be involved with them (Lansky, 1986; Lansky, Bley, Simenstad, West, & McVey, 1983).

This point of view has enormous significance for an approach to treatment. Such patients have chaotic character pathology that does not in any real sense remit or become dormant. They attract equally chaotic mates to form unions that are both incohesive and dangerous. Interventions must usually be on many levels in this type of domestic violence. Protection of the victim and restraint of the violent spouse are obviously of first priority in the short run, but measures such as confinement in hospital or shelter fall short of addressing the long-term propensity each spouse has for reestablishing or recreating the same situation. These spouses have neither the cohesion of personality nor the ability to control themselves that are the prerequisites for learning from experience.

It is not possible to talk of definitive treatment strategies for these vulnerable and volatile persons. Maneuvers designed to restrain the violent person or protect the victim must be combined with long-term nurturant therapeutic experiences that allow such vulnerabilities slowly to heal. Conjoint psychotherapy sessions should focus empathetically on disorganizing effects of the couple's reactivity to each other. An intergenerational approach is decidedly useful in pointing to patients' reactivity to each other without shaming them (see Excerpt 3). Antidepressant medication is frequently of help. Nonetheless, with the degree of vulnerability and chaos present in cases such as these, a clear view of the difficulties and of the central role of shame is necessary for effective treatment strategies of any type.

## REFERENCES

Alexander, F. (1938). Remarks about the relations of inferiority feelings to guilt feelings. *International Journal of Psychoanalysis, 19:* 41–48.

Lansky, M. R. (1980). On blame. *International Journal of Psychoanalytic Psychotherapy, 8:* 429–456.

Lansky, M. R. (1981). Treatment of the narcissistically vulnerable couple. In M. R. Lansky (Ed.), *Family therapy and major psychopathology* (pp. 163–182). New York: Grune & Stratton.

Lansky, M. R. (1984). Violence, shame and the family. *International Journal of Family Psychiatry, 5:* 21–40.

Lansky, M. R. (1985). Preoccupation and pathologic distance regulation. *International Journal of Psychoanalytic Psychotherapy, 11:* 409–425.

Lansky, M. R. (1986). Shame in the family relations of borderline patients. In J. S. Grotstein, M. Solomon, & J. Lang (Eds.), *The borderline patient: Emerging concepts in diagnosis, psychodynamics, and treatment.* Hillsdale, NJ: Analytic Press.

Lansky, M. R. (unpublished). The explanation of impulsive action.

Lansky, M. R., Bley, C., Simenstad, E., West, K. R. & McVey, G. G. (1983). The "absent" family of the hospitalized "borderline" patient. *International Journal of Family Psychiatry, 4:* 155–171.

Lewis, H. B. (1971). *Shame and guilt in neurosis.* New York: International Universities Press.

Piers, G., & Singer, M. (1953). Shame and guilt. Springfield, IL: Thomas.

# Index